Molecular Biology of Cancer

Molecular Biology of Cancer

Mechanisms, Targets, and Therapeutics

SECOND EDITION

Lauren Pecorino

University of Greenwich
Fellow of the Royal Society of Medicine

OXFORD

UNIVERSITY PRESS

Great Clarendon Street, Oxford OX2 6DP

Oxford University Press is a department of the University of Oxford.
It furthers the University's objective of excellence in research, scholarship,
and education by publishing worldwide in

Oxford New York

Auckland Cape Town Dar es Salaam Hong Kong Karachi
Kuala Lumpur Madrid Melbourne Mexico City Nairobi
New Delhi Shanghai Taipei Toronto

With offices in

Argentina Austria Brazil Chile Czech Republic France Greece
Guatemala Hungary Italy Japan Poland Portugal Singapore
South Korea Switzerland Thailand Turkey Ukraine Vietnam

Oxford is a registered trade mark of Oxford University Press
in the UK and in certain other countries

Published in the United States
by Oxford University Press Inc., New York

First published 2005
Second edition published 2008

British Library Cataloguing in Publication Data
Data available

Library of Congress Cataloging in Publication Data
Data available

Typeset by Graphicraft Limited, Hong Kong
Printed in Great Britain
on acid-free paper by
Ashford Colour Press Ltd., Gosport, Hampshire

ISBN 978–0–19–921148–7

3 5 7 9 10 8 6 4

This book is dedicated to my mentors:

Raffaela and Joseph Pecorino

Professor Frank Erk

Professor Sidney Strickland

Professor Jeremy Brockes

In memory of:

Marie Favia

Mildred Maiello

Kerry O'Neill

■ PREFACE

The Molecular Biology of Cancer: Mechanisms, Targets, and Therapeutics is intended for both undergraduate and graduate-level students (including medical students) and employees in the pharmaceutical industry interested in learning about how a normal cell becomes transformed into a cancer cell. Signaling pathways of a cell detect and respond to changes in the environment and regulate normal cellular activities. Cells contain many receptors on their membrane that allow a signal from outside the cell (e.g. growth factors) to be transmitted to the inside of the cell. Signaling pathways are composed of molecules that interact with other molecules, whereby one triggers the next in a sequence, in a way similar to the actions of team members in a relay race. The relay of information may cause a change in cell behavior or in gene expression, and results in a cellular response (e.g. cell growth). Interference in these signal transduction pathways has grave consequences (e.g. unregulated cell growth) and may lead to the transformation of a normal cell into a cancer cell. The identification of the malfunctions of specific pathways involved in carcinogenesis provides scientists with molecular targets that can be used to generate new cancer therapeutics. I have chosen to present the biology of cancer together with a promise for its application towards designing new cancer drugs. Therefore, for most chapters in the text, the first half discusses the cell and molecular biology of a specific hallmark of cancer and the last half of the chapter discusses *therapeutic strategies*. To help form a link between particular molecular targets discussed in the first half of the chapter and the therapeutic strategies discussed in the last half of the chapter, a target symbol (◎) is shown in the margin. I hope that this presentation stimulates interest and motivates learning of the subject matter.

Several new chapters have been added to this second edition. Deservedly, the cell cycle now has a chapter of its own. The new chapter 'Infections and inflammation', celebrates the approval of the first preventative cancer vaccine that targets a cancer-causing infective agent. Another new chapter 'The cancer industry: drug development and clinical trial design', may be valuable for special career interests and supplementary for some cancer courses.

Personally, I believe that the use of diagrams and illustrations is an extremely powerful tool of learning. A picture paints a thousand words . . . and more. I strongly suggest that the reader studies and enjoys the figures, artistically created by Joseph Pecorino. Major points and new cancer therapeutics are illustrated in red, and the target symbol (◎) is used to identify molecular targets. Detailed descriptions of the figures are found in the body of the text. New to this edition is the inclusion of color plates of experimental data.

Several additional features that are used throughout the text to facilitate learning and interest are described below:

Pause and think

These features are often presented in the margins of the text and are designed to engage the reader in thought and to present additional perspectives of core concepts. Many times questions are posed; sometimes they are answered and other times they encourage the rereading of particular sections of text.

How do we know that?

This is a new feature for this second edition. These features examine experimental evidence from the scientific literature and ask the reader to analyze raw data or understand the details of an experimental protocol.

Special interest boxes

Shaded boxes are used to highlight special topics of interest such as the box entitled 'Skin cancer' in Chapter 2. They are also used to provide additional explanation of more complex subjects such as 'A little lesson about ROS . . .' in Chapter 2, 'A little lesson about the MAP kinase family . . .' in Chapter 4, and 'A little review of immunology basics . . .' in Chapter 13.

Lifestyle tips

These are suggestions about lifestyle choices and habits to minimize cancer risk, based on our current knowledge.

Leaders in the field of . . .

Scientists around the world have made contributions to the concepts presented in this text. Short biographies of several leading scientists, including their major contributions to a particular field of cancer biology, are presented. This feature is meant to give a human touch to the text. It may also be used as a tool for professional use and for following a continuing interest in the research literature. It may be of interest to listen to leading scientists in a particular subject area, by attending scientific conferences.

Analysis of . . .

Specific molecular techniques used to analyze particular biological and cellular events are described. It is important that science and medical professionals ask themselves 'How do we know that?'. Each of the major concepts underlying our current state of knowledge is the result of numerous experiments that generate data, suggesting possible explanations and mechanisms of cellular events. The information retrieved is governed by the techniques that are used for analysis.

Chapter highlights: refresh your memory

Summary points are listed in order to consolidate major concepts and provide a brief overview of the chapter. These may be particularly useful for revising for examinations.

Self tests and activities

Several features are included to strengthen your understanding of particular concepts presented in the chapter: *Self tests* presented within the text ask you to immediately reinforce material just presented and often refer to a figure. This causes a break from reading and engages you, the student, in 'active' learning. *Activities* that are aimed at strengthening your understanding of particular concepts and encouraging additional self-centered learning are presented towards the end of a chapter. Some require web-based research while others are more reflective. Multiple choice questions can be found on the companion website.

Further reading is a list of general references found at the end of each chapter. These references consist mostly of reviews and support the contents of the chapter. They are not referenced in the main body of the text.

Selected special topics mainly lists specific primary research papers that *are* referenced in the main body of the text and may be pursued for further interest. Several relevant **web sites** are also included.

Appendix 1 is a summary diagram that links key molecular pathways to the cell cycle.

Appendix 2 lists centers of cancer research as a starting point for searching for research posts and employment in the field. Entries are separated by location (USA and UK).

Glossary

Over 140 entries are defined in a clear and concise manner in order to provide students with a handy reference point for finding explanations of unfamiliar words.

It is my hope that the readers of this text will learn something new, become interested in something molecular, and ultimately, somehow, contribute to the field of cancer biology. This field is evolving at a tremendous rate, and so by the time of printing the information contained within these pages will need to be updated! This does not concern me because my aim is to present a *process* of how the pieces of science are put together and how we may attempt to apply our knowledge to cancer therapies. Many new drugs will fail but a select few will not. These select few will make marked improvements in the quality of life for many.

■ ACKNOWLEDGMENTS

First, I would like to express my deepest gratitude to Jonathan Crowe, Commissioning Editor, at Oxford University Press (OUP). I am indebted to him for his faith that I could turn a one-page proposal into a complete textbook for the first edition and for his continued support during the writing of the second edition. He nurtured the synthesis of the book with special care, and provided a wealth of helpful suggestions and advice. With love, I thank my father, Joseph Pecorino, for his never-ending encouragement and I acknowledge his artistic talent used to translate dozens of my stick drawings into precise illustrations for the book during our visits across the Atlantic Ocean, over the years. Stephen Crumly kindly reproduced the illustrations using his fine skills in computer graphics under tight deadlines. Thanks also to Anna Reeves, Production Editor, and her production staff, especially Bridget Johnson and Rose James, and Ross Bowmaker, Alla Vaynshteyn and Sarah Broadly, for additional assistance, at Oxford University Press.

Kind appreciation is expressed for the precise and critical comments given by my official reviewers for the first edition: Tony Bradshaw, Oxford Brookes University, UK; Moira Galway, St Francis Xavier University, Canada; Maria Jackson, University of Glasgow, UK; Helen James, University of East Anglia (UEA), UK; and Ian Judson, Cancer Research UK, London, UK. The value added to the text by these scientists cannot be underestimated. Their comments have had tremendous impact and provided a foundation for the second edition. Kind appreciation is expressed for the critical comments given by my official reviewers for new chapters of the second edition—Michael Carty, NUI Galway, Irish Republic; from the UK: Joanna Wilson, Glasgow, Jonathan Bard, Edinburgh, Phillipa Darbre, Reading, Stephanie McKeown, Ulster, Penka Nikolova, KCL, Elana Klenova, Essex; from the USA: Annemarie Bettica, Manhattanville College, Nancy Bachman, Oneonta, and James Olesen, Ball State University.

Many improvements in the second edition are due to casual feedback from many people from different places—so many thanks to all of you and apologies to those I have not named. I thank Ken Douglas, Dario Tuccinardi, Ricky Rickles, and Anne Schuind for providing unofficial scientific critical comments. I thank my colleagues Alistair Bishop, Babs Chowdhry, John Spencer, Laurence Harbige, and Mike Leach and students, Sarah Thurston and Azzaya Kingham, at the University of Greenwich for feedback and communicating cancer news. Thanks also to the Head of School, John Newbery, for support of this project. Dylan Edwards, UEA,

Nicole Bournias-Vardiabasis, University of Californa at San Bernadino, and Young-Joon Surh, Seoul National University, have contributed greatly by suggesting new topics to add to this second edition.

I acknowledge the support of The Biochemical Society which provided me with a travel grant to attend the American Association of Cancer Research (AACR) Annual Meeting in 2006 and the School of Science, University of Greenwich who provided me with support to attend the AACR Annual Meeting 2007. The information gained and contacts made were important resources for this edition. Appreciation for their kind gestures of support of the first edition is given to Michael Caligiuri, Ohio State University, Jules Harris, University of Arizona, and Candace Ritchie, Merck, who I met at these conferences.

Many fellow scientists have made suggestions or other contributions to the book, including: Jeremy Griggs, several members of the Kuriyan Laboratory, Gerd Pfeifer, Mariann Rand-Weaver, and Jerry Shay. Special thanks are expressed to Andrea Cossarizza, Sarah Cowan, Xiuhuai Liu, M.-A. Shibata, Emma Weir, and Kelly Dobben-Annis for helping me to obtain electronic figures. The Wellcome Library, London, provided an ideal scientific sanctuary.

I admire and acknowledge the work of all those scientists whose research efforts have contributed to the field of cancer research.

I am especially grateful to the support that came from my family, especially Raffaela Pecorino and Teresa Rapillo, and from friends, especially Rita Canipari. I am grateful for the tremendous support given by Marcus Gibson.

OUTLINE CONTENTS

■ DETAILED CONTENTS

Chapter 1

Introduction

Introduction

The aim of this text is to provide a foundation in the molecular biology of cancer and to demonstrate the conceptual process that is being pursued in order to design more specific cancer drugs. Common threads are woven throughout the different chapters so that the terminology becomes familiar and the logic of cellular mechanisms becomes clear. The text also provides guidance for everyday decisions that may lead to a decrease in cancer risk. The translation of the knowledge of molecular pathways into clinically important therapies (linked throughout the text by the target symbol, '◎') will be communicated and will breathe excitement into learning. Academically, you will gain a foundation in the cell and molecular biology of cancer. More importantly, you will develop an intellectual framework upon which you can add new discoveries that will interest you throughout your lifetime. My goal in writing this book is to inspire. It would be most gratifying for me if, by reading this book, you the reader will be compelled to contribute to the cancer research field directly. Knowledge is powerful.

Cancer statistics are shocking. Cancer affects one in three people. Jemal *et al.* (2007) estimated that 559,650 Americans would die from cancer in 2007, and the mortality rate (number of cancer deaths per year per 100,000 people) was over 200 for the UK in the 1990s. The worldwide **incidence** (number of new cases) is about 10 million cases per year, a figure that is due to double in 20 years. These numbers are cold, stark, and impersonal. Hidden behind them are tears, fears, pain, and loss. No one is excluded from the risk. There is a need to understand the disease and to translate our knowledge into effective therapies. In order to understand the process of **carcinogenesis**, whereby a normal cell is transformed into a cancer cell, we must know the intricacies of cell function and the molecular pathways that underlie it. We must consider the cell in the context of the entire body. We have a lot to learn! However, knowledge of the molecular details in important cellular and biochemical pathways can be applied to a new wave of cancer therapies. What better reward for these efforts?

1.1 What is cancer?

Cancer is a group of diseases characterized by unregulated cell growth and the invasion and spread of cells from the site of origin, or primary site, to other sites in the body. Several points within this definition need to be emphasized. First, cancer is considered to be group of diseases. Over 100 types of cancer have been classified. The tissue of origin gives the distinguishing characteristics of the cancer. Approximately 85% of cancers occur in epithelial cells and are classified as **carcinomas**. Cancers derived from mesoderm cells (e.g. bone, muscle) are called **sarcomas**, and cancers of glandular tissue (e.g. breast) are called **adenocarcinomas**. Cancers of different origins have distinct features. For example, skin cancer has many characteristics that differ from lung cancer. The major factor that causes cancer in each target tissue is different: ultraviolet (UV) radiation from the sun can easily target the skin while inhalation of cigarette smoke can target the lungs. In addition, as will be examined in detail later, there are differences in the molecular mechanisms involved in carcinogenesis within

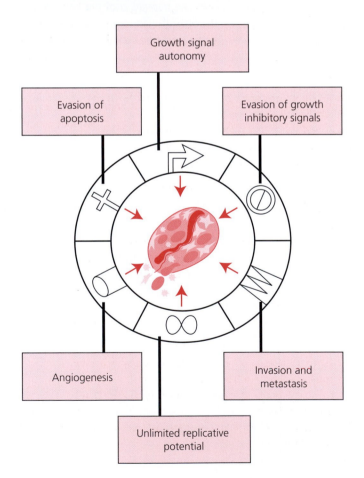

Figure 1.1 The six hallmarks of cancer. Reprinted from Hanahan, D. and Weinberg, R.A. (2000) The hallmarks of cancer. *Cell* **100**, p. 57, copyright (2000), with permission from Elsevier Science.

each cell type and the pattern of spread of cells from the primary site. Treatment must be applied differently. Surgical removal of a cancerous growth is more amenable for the skin than the lungs. This initial view presents layers of complexity which may seem insurmountable to dissect in order to improve the conventional therapeutic approaches. However, even though the underlying cellular and molecular routes are different, the end result is the same. Upon fine analysis, Hanahan and Weinberg (2000) have defined six hallmarks of most, if not all, cancers (Figure 1.1). They propose that acquiring the capability for autonomous growth signals, evasion of growth inhibitory signals, evasion of apoptotic cell death, unlimited replicative potential, angiogenesis (the formation of new blood vessels), and invasion and metastasis are essential for carcinogenesis. Each will be examined in detail in this text and each is a potential target pathway for the design of new therapeutics.

The six hallmarks of cancer (see Figure 1.1)

- Growth signal autonomy:
  - Normal cells need external signals from growth factors to divide
  - Cancer cells are not dependent on normal growth factor signaling
  - Acquired **mutations** short-circuit growth factor pathways leading to unregulated growth

- Evasion of growth inhibitory signals:
  - Normal cells respond to inhibitory signals to maintain homeostasis (most cells of the body are not actively dividing)
  - Cancer cells do not respond to growth inhibitory signals
  - Acquired mutations interfere with the inhibitory pathways

- Evasion of **apoptosis** (programmed cell death)
  - Normal cells are removed by apoptosis, often in response to DNA damage
  - Cancer cells evade apoptotic signals

- Unlimited replicative potential
  - Normal cells have an autonomous counting device to define a finite number of cell doublings after which they become senescent. This cellular counting device is the shortening of chromosomal ends, **telomeres**, that occurs during every round of DNA replication
  - Cancer cells maintain the length of their telomeres
  - Altered regulation of telomere maintenance results in unlimited replicative potential

- Angiogenesis (formation of new blood vessels)
  - Normal cells depend on blood vessels to supply oxygen and nutrients but the vascular architecture is more or less constant in the adult
  - Cancer cells induce angiogenesis, the growth of new blood vessels, needed for tumor survival and expansion
  - Altering the balance between angiogenic inducers and inhibitors can activate the angiogenic switch ➜

> → ● Invasion and metastasis
> - Normal cells maintain their location in the body and generally do not migrate
> - The movement of cancer cells to other parts of the body is a major cause of cancer deaths
> - Mutations alter the activity of enzymes involved in invasion and alter molecules involved in cell–cell and cellular–extracellular adhesion

Cancer is characterized by unregulated cell growth and the invasion and spread of cells from their site of origin. This leads to the distinction between a **benign** tumor and a **malignant** tumor. A benign tumor is not evidence of cancer. Benign tumors do not metastasize, although some can be life-threatening because of their location (e.g. a benign brain tumor that may be difficult to remove). Malignant tumors, on the other hand, do not remain encapsulated, show features of **invasion**, and metastasize.

PAUSE AND THINK

Why are malignant tumors life-threatening? They are physical obstructions and as they invade other organs they compromise function. They also compete fiercely with healthy tissues for nutrients and oxygen.

Cancer cells can be distinguished from normal cells in cell culture conditions

Normally, cells grow as a single layer, or monolayer, in a Petri dish due to a property called contact inhibition; contact with neighboring cells inhibits growth.
   Transformed cells acquire the following **phenotypes**:

● they fail to exhibit contact inhibition and instead grow as piles of cells or 'foci' against a monolayer of normal cells

● they can grow in conditions of low serum

● they adopt a round **morphology** rather than a flat and extended one

● they are able to grow without attaching to a substrate (e.g. the surface of a Petri dish), exhibiting 'anchorage independence'

1.2 Evidence suggests that cancer is a genetic disease at the cellular level

Interestingly, most agents that cause cancer (**carcinogens**) are agents that cause alterations to the DNA sequence or mutations (**mutagens**). Thus, similarly to all genetic diseases, cancer results from alterations in DNA. A large amount of evidence indicates that the DNA of tumor cells contains many alterations ranging from subtle point mutations (changes in a single base pair) to large chromosomal aberrations such as deletions and chromosomal **translocations**. The accumulation of mutations in cells over time represents a multi-step process that underlies carcinogenesis. The requirement for an accumulation of mutations explains why there is an increased risk of cancer with age and why cancer has become more pre-valent over the centuries as human lifespan has increased. There have been more cases of cancer in recent years because we are living longer. The longer we live the more time there is to expose our DNA to accumulating mutations which may lead to cancer. Interestingly, only 5–10% of the mutations observed are thought to be directly involved in causing cancer based upon mathematical modeling. This estimate provides the basis for the current optimism in the field of molecular therapies. Almost all of the mutations identified in tumor cells are somatic mutations whereby the DNA of a somatic (body) cell has been damaged. These mutations are not passed on to the next generation of offspring, and therefore cannot be inherited, but they are passed to daughter cells after cell division. Thus, cancer is considered to be a genetic disease at the cellular level. Only alterations in the DNA of sperm or egg cells, called germline mutations, will be passed on to offspring. Some germline mutations can cause an increased risk of developing cancer but are rarely involved in causing cancer immediately. Cancer cells continue to change their behavior as they progress. The progressive changes of a cell resulting from an accumulation of genetic mutations that confer a growth advantage over its neighbors proceeds in a fashion analogous to Darwinian evolution: chance events give rise to mutations that confer changes in phenotype and allow adaptation to the environment, resulting in the selection and survival of the fittest. This classifies the mechanism of cancer as obeying 'natural order' and being statistically inevitable and is discussed at length by Mel Greaves, in his book *Cancer, the evolutionary legacy*. The accumulation of mutations occurs only after the cell's defense mechanisms (e.g. DNA repair) have been evaded. Any alterations of DNA that are not repaired before the next cell division are passed on to the daughter cells and are perpetuated. The cell relies on several processes to repair damaged DNA. In cases of severe DNA damage, cell suicide is induced in order to protect the whole body from cell transformation. The molecular details of these processes and the mutations that compromise them will be described in Chapters 2 and 7. Thus, many mechanisms exist for blocking carcinogenic events, but over-burdening the system increases the probability that a cell carry-ing a deleterious mutation will escape surveillance.

Growth, apoptosis, and differentiation regulate cell numbers

There are three important processes that contribute to the overall net cell number in an individual. Cell proliferation (cell division, cell growth) is the most obvious. Cell division results in two daughter cells. Secondly, the elimination of cells by programmed cell death also affects the net cell number. Lastly, during the process of differentiation cells can enter an inactive phase of cell growth and thus differentiation can affect net cell

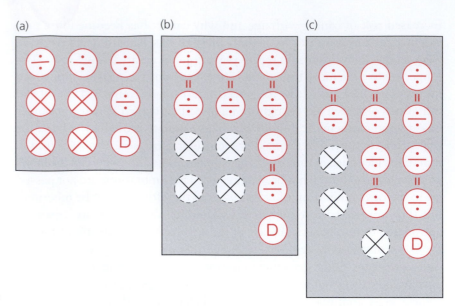

(a) (b) (c)

Figure 1.2 Growth, apoptosis, and differentiation affect cell number (see text for explanation).

numbers. DNA mutations that alter the function of normal genes involved in growth, apoptosis, or differentiation can affect the balance of cell numbers in the body and lead to unregulated growth. Examine the simplistic model shown in Figure 1.2. If four of the nine cells shown in Figure 1.2(a) divide ⊝, and four are programmed to die by apoptosis ⊗, and one differentiates ⊚ (so the cell neither dies nor divides) the cell number will remain the same (Figure 1.2b; remaining cells shown in red). However, if apoptosis is blocked in one cell and that cell divides instead, the total number of cells will increase to 11 (Figure 1.2c). Similarly, if differentiation in a cell is blocked and that cell divides, as is the case of some leukemias, the number of cells will also increase. Thus an alteration in the processes of growth, apoptosis, or differentiation can alter cell numbers. Normal genes that can be activated by mutation to be oncogenic are called proto-oncogenes. Proto-oncogenes play functional roles in normal cells. The term reminds us that all normal cells have genes that have the potential to become oncogenic.

PAUSE AND THINK

So, is a mutation in the hemoglobin gene likely to cause cancer? No, because the function of hemoglobin does not affect cell growth, differentiation, or death and does not lead to unregulated growth of blood cells. The hemoglobin gene is not a proto-oncogene.

Oncogenes and tumor suppressor genes

Growth is regulated by both positive and negative molecular factors. Thus, to increase growth, enhancement of positive factors or depletion of negative factors is required. There are two major types of mutated genes that contribute to carcinogenesis: oncogenes and tumor suppressor genes (Figure 1.3). A general description of an oncogene is a gene mutated such that its protein product is produced in higher quantities, or has increased

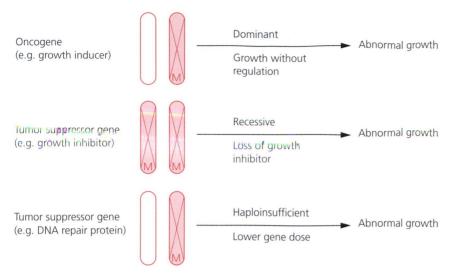

Figure 1.3 Oncogenes and tumor suppressor genes.

activity and therefore acts in a dominant manner to initiate tumor forma-tion. For example, one oncogene produces increased quantities of a specific growth factor (e.g. platelet-derived growth factor) which stimulates growth inappropriately. Another example is an oncogene that produces a growth factor receptor with increased activity because it has been altered so that it is always in the 'on' state and does not require growth factor to transduce a signal into the cell. 'Dominant' refers to the characteristic that a mutation in only one allele is sufficient for an effect.

Analysis of oncogene function by cell transformation assays

The prototypical experiment used to demonstrate the presence of an oncogene is to test for cell transformation in culture. The DNA of interest is isolated and introduced into a standard cell line called NIH/3T3 (mouse fibroblast cells) by calcium phosphate precipita-tion or electroporation. If the test DNA contains an oncogene, foci (mentioned above) will form and will be easily identifiable against a monolayer of untransformed NIH/3T3 cells.

   Tumor suppressor genes code for proteins that play a role in inhibit-ing both growth and tumor formation. Loss of growth inhibition occurs when mutations cause a loss of function of these genes. Consequently, growth is permitted. Tumor suppressor mutations are mainly recessive in nature because one intact allele is usually sufficient to inhibit growth; thus both alleles of the gene must be mutated before the loss of function is actually seen phenotypically. Recessive mutations support Knudson's two-hit hypothesis, the classical model used to explain the mechanism behind tumor suppressor action (see Chapter 6 and Figure 6.2). It states that both alleles need to be mutated (recessive) to trigger carcinogenesis. This model has been used to explain the mechanism behind conditions that predispose individuals to an increased risk of cancer. Patients inherit one mutated tumor suppressor allele and may acquire a second somatic mutation over time. Therefore, these patients have a 'head start' towards a cancer phenotype in the race for accumulation of mutations. Recent evidence suggests there is an alternative mechanism for particular tumor suppressor genes, called haploinsufficiency, whereby only one mutated allele can lead to the cancer phenotype. As the term suggests, one normal allele produces half ('haplo-') of the quantity of protein product produced by normal cells and this is not enough to suppress tumor formation in these cases. This has been demonstrated for genes that regulate DNA repair and the DNA-damage response, such that reduced activity leads to genetic instability. Gene dosage may also affect the spectrum of tumors observed; haploinsufficiency may cause cancer in some cell types and recessive mutations may cause cancer in other cell types (Fodde and Smits, 2002).

All of the cancer cells in a patient arise from a single cell that contains an accumulation of initiating mutations; in other words, the development of cancer is clonal. It is generally assumed that only one of the 10^{14} cells in the body needs to be transformed in order to create a tumor. However, studies of adult stem cells have made recent contributions to our understanding of carcinogenesis. Stem cells are undifferentiated cells that have

HOW DO WE KNOW THAT?

Types of evidence

Like all science, cancer biology depends on evidence. Gilbert's textbook, *Developmental Biology*, classifies evidence into three types: *correlative evidence*, *loss-of-function evidence*, and *gain-of-function evidence*.

Correlative evidence ('show it' evidence) documents observations between two events and weakly intimates that one may cause the other. For example, a gene from a tumor sample has a mutation compared with the same gene isolated from healthy tissue. This type of evidence provides a good starting point but is not particularly strong evidence and may even be coincidental.

Loss-of-function evidence ('block it' evidence), uses different techniques to inhibit the function of a gene, gene product, or other factor of interest. Antibodies that block protein function and knock-out mice are common experimental techniques used to investigate loss-of-function. Appropriate controls must be in place to ensure that only the target is affected.

Gain-of-function evidence ('move it' evidence) is the strongest type of evidence and is obtained when your factor of interest is moved to a new location and triggers a causative event at a time or place where it normally does not occur. This is strong evidence. Recombinant DNA plasmids may be constructed whereby the coding region of a gene of interest is placed under the control of a promoter that directs expression of the gene in a different tissue or at a different time. DNA transfection of cells in culture and the production of transgenic animals, with such recombinant plasmids, are important experimental techniques used to demonstrate gain-of-function.

As you read the scientific literature, try to classify the evidence presented into 'show it', 'block it' or 'move it' types in order to develop your ability to critically analyze the data (Adams, 2003). Overall, the field of cancer biology relies on the sum of many types of experimental techniques that must be critically evaluated.

the ability to self-renew and produce differentiated progeny. Normal stem cells may be a main starting point for carcinogenesis in some cancers since both cancer cells and stem cells utilize and rely on **self-renewal** molecular programs. Also, cancer is more likely to develop in cells that are actively proliferating since there is a greater chance for mutations to accumulate; normal stem cells continue to proliferate over long periods of time. These concepts will be discussed further in Chapter 8.

The concepts described above suggest that cancer is a genetic disease at the cellular level.

1.3 Influential factors in human carcinogenesis

Environment, reproductive life, diet, and smoking are four factors that play an important role in carcinogenesis. These lifestyle factors can, in principle, be altered to prevent most cancers. Exposure to carcinogens, hormonal modifications influenced by childbirth and birth control, and exposure to viruses, underlie these lifestyle factors. Epidemiology, the study of disease in the population, has been instrumental in elucidating the contributions of these factors towards different cancers. Although molecular details will be discussed in later chapters, a brief introduction of each factor is given below.

Environment

Observations by a British surgeon in 1775 resulted in the first correlation between an environmental agent and specific cancers. Percival Pott concluded that the high incidence of nasal and scrotal cancer in chimney sweeps was due to chronic exposure to soot. Not only where you work, but also the choice of where you relax can contribute to your risk of cancer. Unprotected exposure to the sun exposes your skin to UVB radiation which can directly alter your DNA by forming **pyrimidine** dimers and cause mutations. Sun blocks that have UV-absorbing ingredients have been developed to protect your skin from UV radiation and are a good defense if you do decide to relax in the sun.

Reproductive life

Another early observation was that nuns are more likely to develop breast cancer than other women. We now know that having children reduces breast cancer risk for women compared with not having children. The age of a woman at the time of giving birth for the first time and the age of a woman at the initiation and termination of her menstrual cycles also

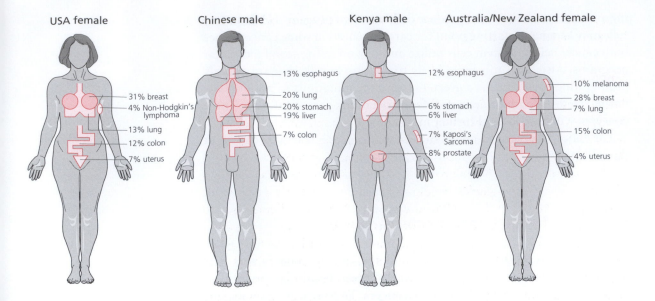

USA female   Chinese male   Kenya male   Australia/New Zealand female

USA female:
- 31% breast
- 4% Non-Hodgkin's lymphoma
- 13% lung
- 12% colon
- 7% uterus

Chinese male:
- 13% esophagus
- 20% lung
- 20% stomach
- 19% liver
- 7% colon

Kenya male:
- 12% esophagus
- 6% stomach
- 6% liver
- 7% Kaposi's Sarcoma
- 8% prostate

Australia/New Zealand female:
- 10% melanoma
- 28% breast
- 7% lung
- 15% colon
- 4% uterus

Figure 1.4 Leading new cases of cancers differ among different populations. Data from Globocan 2002, IARC (Ferlay *et al*., 2004).The percentage of new cases of a specific cancer is reflected in the degree of red shading.

influences cancer risk. Hormonal contraception and fertility treatments also affect cancer risk because they alter a women's ovulation schedule (active ingredients prevent and promote ovulation, respectively). Sexual promiscuity can also contribute to increased risk of cancer. Sexually transmitted human papillomaviruses can be found in all cervical cancers worldwide. It is not surprising therefore that nuns have a low incidence of cervical cancer. Barrier methods of contraception can protect against this infectious pathogen. One can see in Figure 1.4 that Kaposi's sarcoma is a predominant cancer in Kenyan males which correlates with the AIDS epidemic in Africa.

Diet

The incidence of a specific cancer varies greatly between different populations in different geographical locations. Observation of immigration patterns has revealed that local cancer rates strongly influence cancer risk, with diet being one of the most influential factors. Figure 1.4 shows a comparison of cancer prevalence between US females and Chinese males (Ferlay *et al*. 2004). Stomach cancer is a predominant cancer in the Chinese population and a minor cancer in the population of the USA. Interestingly, the risk of stomach cancer in Chinese people who have migrated to the USA decreases only if they adopt the American diet, but not if they retain an Eastern diet. The Mediterranean diet, which is rich in fresh fruit, vegetables, and red wine has been promoted to be beneficial in reducing cancer risks. Recently, studies of the molecular interactions of individual dietary constituents (e.g. polyphenols, carotenoids, and allium compounds) with cellular signaling pathways have begun and some will be examined in Chapter 11.

Smoking

The clearest example of lifestyle factors underlying a specific cancer is the discovery that smoking causes lung cancer (it is also implicated in pancreatic, bladder, kidney, mouth, stomach, and liver cancer). Since 1985, lung cancer has remained as the main cancer worldwide. Smoking accounts for 40% of all cancer deaths: 1.18 million deaths. At least 81 carcinogens have been identified in cigarette smoke. Smoking became particularly fashionable in Europe and the USA during World War I and World War II and resulted in an epidemic of lung carcinoma. After vast public education campaigns and a subsequent reduction of smoking, lung cancer death rates have fallen dramatically in the USA (Figure 1.5). Unfortunately, lung cancer rates are still rising in other parts of the world. These countries should consider implementing restrictions on smoking in public places and imposing tobacco taxes. A significant increase in the incidence of lung cancer in China can be noted between data collected for the first edition (6%) and second edition (20%; see Figure 1.4) of this book (though this may be due in part to improved data reporting and collection).

It is clear that some future cancer deaths can be avoided by changes in lifestyle factors.

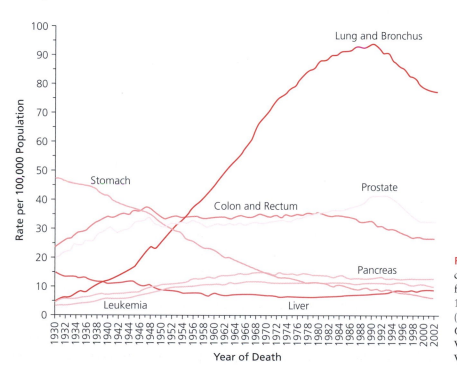

Figure 1.5 Annual age-adjusted cancer death rates among males for selected cancers, USA, 1930–2002. From Jemal, A. *et al.* (2006). Cancer Statistics, 2006. *CA Cancer J. Clin.* **56**: 106–130. With permission from Lippincott, Williams, and Wilkins.

Additional influences

In addition to lifestyle factors, there are risk factors inherent in our own physiology. By-products of our metabolism and errors that occur during DNA replication contribute to carcinogenesis. Aerobic metabolism produces by-products of oxygen radicals that are mutagenic. Several inherited metabolic diseases also produce mutagenic by-products. For example, tyrosinemia type I patients have a defect in the enzyme fumarylacetoacetate hydrolase which is involved in tyrosine breakdown. As a result of this block, the by-products fumarylacetoacetate and maleylacetate accumulate and increase the risk of cancer due to their ability to covalently modify DNA and cause mutations. During DNA replication and repair, polymerases can introduce mutations directly in DNA because of their associated error rates. There is a perpetual inherent risk of mutation during the lifespan of a cell by the nature of cell processes.

1.4 Principles of conventional cancer therapies

The earliest therapeutic strategy used against cancer was surgically to remove as much of the cancer as possible. Obviously this is relatively easy in some types of cancer and impossible in other types. It is not a precise procedure at the cellular level and does not address the question of cells that have spread from the primary site (metastasized cells). Therefore chemotherapy and radiotherapy have been used to inhibit or eradicate metastasized cells. The objectives of cancer therapies are to prevent proliferation (**cytostatic** effect) and to kill the cancer cells (**cytotoxic** effect). The aim with all drugs is to achieve an effective result with the minimum side-effects. This is indicated by the **therapeutic index**. This is the value of the difference between the minimum effective dose and the maximum tolerated dose (MTD) (Figure 1.6). The larger the value, the better the drug. Many conventional cancer treatments are administered at maximum tolerated doses (MTDs).

Chemotherapy

Conventional chemotherapy uses chemicals that target DNA, RNA, and protein to disrupt the cell cycle in rapidly dividing cancer cells and thus has broad specificity. The ultimate goal of cytotoxic chemotherapy is to cause severe DNA damage and to trigger apoptosis in the rapidly dividing cancer cells. The side-effects of chemotherapy, which we are all too aware of, such as alopecia (loss of hair), ulcers, and anemia, are due to the fact that hair follicles, stomach epithelia, and hemopoietic cells are also rapidly dividing and therefore they too are greatly affected by these

PAUSE AND THINK

Let us 'create' an example purely to illustrate the concept of the MTD. Two aspirins may be the minimum for an effective dose against a headache and 30 may be the dose that can be tolerated before harmful side-effects are observed. However, if harmful side-effects were seen after three aspirins the therapeutic index would decrease and the drug would be much less favorable.

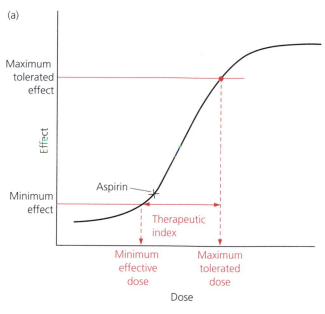

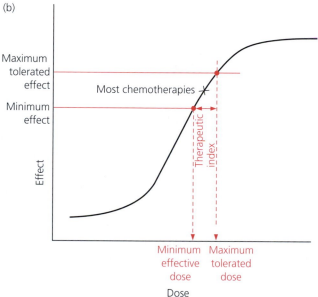

Figure 1.6 The therapeutic index is the value of the difference between the minimum effective dose and the maximum tolerated dose (MTD). (a) The value for the therapeutic index of aspirin is higher than that of (b) the therapeutic index of most chemotherapies.

drugs. Often, prescribed MTDs induce toxicity in sensitive tissues and require a pause in drug administration so that normal cells can recover. We must appreciate that conventional chemotherapies (e.g. cisplatin and methotrexate, discussed in Chapter 2) have had results in treating cancers and continue to extend lives but at the same time we must desire drugs with better efficiencies and less severe and debilitating side-effects. We must strive to develop drugs that rise to these expectations.

Table 1.1 Clinical trials

	Purpose	Number of patients
Phase I	Safety	20–100
Phase II	Efficacy	Up to several hundred
Phase III	Efficacy often tested against conventional treatments	Several hundred to several thousand

1.5 Clinical trials

Testing of new drugs in humans must progress through staged clinical trials (Table 1.1). Phase I trials examine dose responses for assessing drug safety, using a small number (20–80) of healthy volunteers or patients. Many parameters of the metabolism of the drug in humans (e.g. How long does the drug remain in the body?) are obtained at this time. About 70% of drugs tested in Phase I will progress to Phase II studies. Phase II trials are designed to examine efficacy in a larger group of people (100–300). Phase III trials should not be initiated prior to knowing the effective drug dosage. Phase III trials are large-scale studies (1000–3000 people) to confirm drug effectiveness, monitor side-effects, and also to compare the efficacy of the new drug with conventional treatments. Only terminally ill patients may be recruited for clinical trials, by law, in many countries. This has implications for the outcome of testing particular drugs and will be discussed later in the text. About 30% of drugs tested successfully complete Phase III studies. Drugs are also tested against control populations. These people either receive no treatment or receive a placebo, or inactive substance. In order to reduce the risk of bias, trials can be randomized. That is, patients are randomly assigned to either a treatment group or a control group, guaranteeing that the two groups are similar. In addition, the trial may be conducted as a single-blind study, whereby patients do not know which group they are in, or as a double-blind study, whereby neither patients nor investigators know who has received the treatment or placebo until after a code is broken that identifies the people in the two groups. Unlike conventional chemotherapies, targeted therapy may not require MTDs. Experience is teaching us that the design of trials for molecularly targeted drugs needs to be well thought out. It is important to consider the stage and type of cancer to be treated, patient populations with the correct molecular profiles (that is, does the patient carry mutations in genes of interest), assessment of the compound in inhibiting its molecular target, and assessment of the relationship between molecular inhibition and clinical response.

PAUSE AND THINK

Is tumor shrinkage a suitable assessment criterion for cytostatic drugs? No, because direct cell death is not anticipated with this class of drugs. Cytotoxic drugs are expected to kill tumor cells.

1.6 The role of molecular targets in cancer therapies

The major flaw in the rationale of most conventional therapies is the lack of selectivity against tumor cells versus normal cells. As a result the side-effects of most therapies are very harsh, as mentioned above. There is a need to learn about the differences between normal and transformed cells at the molecular level in order to identify cancer-specific molecular targets. In this way, we can design drugs that will be specific for the cancer cells, have increased efficacy, and cause fewer side-effects.

Molecules of fame

As we examine the molecular pathways that underlie carcinogenesis we must keep in mind that the pathways do not act in isolation but are interconnected (see Appendix 1). Despite the many hundreds of molecules involved in carcinogenesis, there are several families of 'star players' in the story of carcinogenesis. Many of these 'star players' act as nodes that receive signals from many pathways and can exert several effects in response to a specific signal.

The family of protein kinases, one of the largest families of genes in eukaryotes, must be included in any introduction to cancer biology. Protein kinases phosphorylate (add a phosphate group to) a hydroxyl group on specific amino acids in proteins. Tyrosine kinases phosphorylate tyrosine residues while serine/threonine kinases phosphorylate serine and threonine residues. Phosphorylation results in a conformational change and is an important mechanism for regulating the activity of a protein. Kinases can be found at the cell surface as transmembrane receptors, inside the cell as intracellular transducers, or inside the nucleus. Kinases play a critical role in major cell functions including cell cycle progression, signal transduction, and transcription, and are important molecular targets for the design of cancer drugs. Phosphorylation is also regulated by phosphatases, enzymes that remove phosphate groups. Mutational analysis of all known human protein tyrosine phosphatases suggests that several of these act as tumor suppressors in some types of cancer (see Chapter 6).

The Ras family is another 'star' set of genes which are found mutated in over 50% of certain cancers (e.g. colon cancer). Ras is an intracellular transducer protein that acts subsequently to binding of a growth factor to its receptor and is involved in transmitting the signal from the receptor through the cell. As G proteins, they reside on the intracellular side of the plasma membrane and are activated by the exchange of GDP for GTP.

Tumor protein p53 (TP53; p53) and its related family members hold pivotal positions in guarding the integrity of the genome by coordinating responses of the cell (e.g. cell cycle arrest, DNA repair, apoptosis) to different types of stress (e.g. DNA damage, hypoxia). The *p53* gene is a tumor suppressor gene that has a key role in inhibiting carcinogenesis. It is mutated in more than half of all cancers and over a thousand different mutations have been identified. It acts as a transcription factor and induces the expression of genes required to carry out its functions.

The retinoblastoma gene (*Rb*) is also a tumor suppressor gene that plays a central role in regulating the cell cycle. It is commonly mutated in several cancers. The retinoblastoma protein normally functions as an inhibitor of cell proliferation by binding to and suppressing an essential transcription factor of cell cycle progression. Its activity is regulated by phosphorylation by cyclin D and the cyclin-dependent kinases (4/6).

The introduction of cancer genomics

The completion of the Human Genome Project, whereby every nucleotide of a human genome has been sequenced and mapped, has paved the way for cancer genomics. Learning about the details of the genome of a cancer cell and how it differs from a normal cell will provide us with the fine distinctions needed to design more powerful and specific drugs. Several projects are under way. The Cancer Genome Anatomy Project (CGAP) is aimed at developing cancer-specific gene data sets for public access (Strausberg *et al.*, 2001). Both academia and biopharmaceutical industries can mine the databases and utilize the online informatics tools. It is envisaged that *in silico* (computer) analysis of these data sets will help define specific molecular signatures for specific cancers and promote the development of new methods of diagnosis and treatment. New human genes and tumor-specific gene deregulation have been discovered through use of the CGAP database. The human genome has recently been subdivided into the 'kinome' by the mapping of the complete set of 518 protein kinase genes in the genome (Manning *et al.*, 2002). Since aberrant regulation and mutation of these genes are involved in carcinogenesis, this will be an important tool for the design of new molecular therapies. The International SNP Map Working Group is analyzing single nucleotide polymorphisms (SNPs) to identify mutations within the genome that may be linked with cancer. A recent demonstration of a genome-wide analysis of SNPs in one type of leukemia revealed frequent targets of somatic mutations (e.g. *PAX5* altered in 32% of cases), many of which code for regulators of differentiation (Mullighan *et al.*, 2007). Discoveries about the functional role of small RNAs have led to new tools (e.g. RNA interference) to help elucidate the function of genes in an organism. The findings from studies of functional genomics promise to provide insights into cancer biology.

Analysis of gene function by small interfering RNAs (siRNAs)

Gene function is often determined by abolishing the expression of a gene product and observing the resulting phenotype. RNA interference is a cellular mechanism for regulating **gene expression** in most eukaryotes. Short RNA duplexes (approximately 21 nucleotides long with two nucleotide 3′ overhangs) called small interfering RNAs (si RNAs) mediate the expression of genes by causing the degradation of homologous single-stranded target RNAs. Experimentally, we can use siRNAs to target endogenous genes in mammalian cells. Using the known sequence of a segment of target mRNA, sense and antisense RNAs are designed, synthesized, and annealed to produce siRNA duplexes. The siRNAs are delivered to cells by classical gene transfer methods (e.g. electroporation). Specific antibodies against the targeted protein are often used to ensure that target protein levels have been diminished. (See Kamath *et al.* (2003) as an example of the use of this approach.)

Good news

The nature of the 'now' generation of drugs is small molecules and antibodies targeted against selective gene products. Soon it is likely that methods to prevent expression of specific target genes (e.g. antisense RNA, siRNAs) will also enter the clinic. Several therapies based on these designs that can treat specific cancers will be described later in the text. The good news is that in the USA the absolute number of cancer deaths decreased for two consecutive years (Jemal *et al.*, 2007). Progress is beginning to show.

■ **CHAPTER HIGHLIGHTS—REFRESH YOUR MEMORY**

- Cancer is a common disease that will affect one out of three people worldwide.
- Cancer is a group of diseases that results in the spreading of mutated cells throughout the body.
- There are six hallmarks of cancer. They are:

    Growth signal autonomy
    Evasion of growth inhibitory signals
    Evasion of apoptosis
    Unlimited replicative potential
    Angiogenesis
    Invasion and metastasis.

- Most carcinogens are mutagens.
- Carcinogenesis is a multi-step process that requires the accumulation of several mutations.

- Cancer is a genetic disease at the cellular level.
- Genes that are involved in growth, differentiation, or cell death when deregulated can give rise to the cancer phenotype.
- A gene containing a dominant mutation that results in inappropriate activation of growth is an oncogene.
- Tumor suppressor genes are usually inactivated by mutations in both alleles (recessive) and this results in inactivation of growth inhibition.
- Haploinsufficiency, whereby only one allele of a tumor suppressor gene is inactivated, also contributes to carcinogenesis.
- Changes in lifestyle factors can affect cancer risk.

- Many conventional therapies are broad-acting drugs administered at MTDs resulting in severe side-effects.

- Protein kinases, enzymes that phosphorylate proteins, are important molecules in carcinogenesis.

- Cancer genomics is being used to define molecular targets for tumor-specific effects.

- Some cancers can already be treated by specific molecular approaches.

■ ACTIVITY

1. Become familiar with the Cancer Genome Anatomy Project web site (http://cgap.nci.nih.gov).
   On which **chromosome** is the *p53* gene located?
   Is it expressed in bone and mammary gland tissues? Name three genes regulated by this transcription factor.

2. Become familiar with the Globocan 2002 web site and see how epidemiological data can be formatted in different ways (go to http://www-dep.iarc.fr/).
   Select Globocan on the right side of the top tool bar. On the left-hand side, select **Tables, By population**. Enter different countries and look at pie charts etc. How do the cancer profiles differ between continents? Select to run a cancer map for lung cancer. What are your conclusions?

■ FURTHER READING

Alison, M.R. (2002) *The Cancer Handbook*, Nature Publishing Group, Macmillan, London.

Ferlay, J. *et al.* (2004) *Globocan 2002. Cancer Incidence, Mortality and Prevalence Worldwide*. IARC CancerBase No.5, Version 2.0. IARC Press, Lyon.

Gilbert, S.F. (2000) *Developmental Biology*, 6th edn. Sinauer Associates, Inc., Sunderland, MA.

Greaves, M. (2001) *Cancer, the Evolutionary Legacy*. Oxford University Press, Oxford.

Hanahan, D. and Weinberg, R.A. (2000) The hallmarks of cancer. *Cell* **100**: 57–70.

Jemal, A., Siegel, R., Ward, E., Murray, T., Xu, J., Smigal, C., and Thun, M.J. (2006) Cancer Statistics, 2006. *CA Cancer J. Clin.* **56**: 106–130.

Jemal, A., Siegel, R., Ward, E., Murray, T., Xu, J., and Thun, M.J. (2007) Cancer Statistics, 2007. *CA Cancer J. Clin.* **57**: 43–66.

King, R.J.B. and Robins, M.W. (2006) *Cancer Biology*, 3rd edn. Pearson Education Ltd, London.

Parkin, D.M., Bray, F., Ferlay, J., and Pisani, P. (2005) Global Cancer Statistics, 2002. *CA Cancer J. Clin.* **55**: 74–108.

Peto, J. (2001) Cancer epidemiology in the last century and the next decade. *Nature* **411**: 390–395.

Reddy, A. and Kaelin W.G., Jr (2002) Using cancer genetics to guide the selection of anticancer drug targets. *Curr. Opin. Pharm.* **2**: 366–373.

■ **WEB SITES**

American Cancer Society. Cancer Statistics 2007
http://www.cancer.org/docroot/stt/stt_0.asp

The Cancer Genome Anatomy Project homepage http://cgap.nci.nih.gov

The Food and Drug Administration. Educational materials about good clinical practice and clinical trials http://www.fda.gov/oc/gcp/education.html

Globocan 2002 http://www-dep.iarc.fr/

■ **SELECTED SPECIAL TOPICS**

Adams, D.S. (2003) Teaching critical thinking in a developmental biology course at an American liberal arts college. *Int. J. Dev. Biol.* **47**: 145–151.

Kamath, R., Fraser, A., Dong, Y., Poulin, G., Durbin, R., Gotta, M., Kanapin, A., LeBot, N., Moreno, S., Sohrmann, M., Welchman, D., Zipperlen, P., and Ahringer, J. (2003) Systematic functional analysis of the *Caenorhabditis elegans* genome using RNAi. *Nature* **421**: 231–237.

Fodde, R. and Smits, R. (2002) A matter of dosage. *Science* **298**: 761–763.

Manning, G., Whyte, D., Martinez, R., Hunter, T. and Sudarsanam, S. (2002) The protein kinase complement of the human genome. *Science* **298**: 1912–1934.

Mullighan, C.G., Goorha, S., Radtke, I., Miller, C.B., Coustan-Smith, E., Dalton, J.D., Girtman, K., Mathew, S., Ma, J., Pounds, S.B., Su, X., Pui, C.-H., Relling, M.V. Evans, W.E., Shurtleff, S.A., and Downing, J.R. (2007) Genome-wide anlaysis of genetic alterations in acute lymphoblastic leukemia. *Nature* **446**: 758–764.

Strausberg, R., Greenhut, S., Grouse, L., Schaefer, C., and Buetow, K. (2001) *In silico* analysis of cancer through the Cancer Genome Anatomy Project. *Trends Cell Biol.* **11**: S66–S71.

Chapter 2

DNA structure and stability: mutations versus repair

Introduction

Genetic information, coded within DNA, requires stability. DNA directs the production of proteins needed for the structure and function of cells over a lifetime, through an adaptor molecule, RNA. Unlike RNA and protein, which have a limited existence before they are degraded and/or recycled, DNA must maintain its integrity over that lifetime. However, our genes are subject to a myriad of attacks by both environmental agents and endogenous processes that result in mutation and scission. Changes to the DNA sequence may have severe consequences for the cell and its progeny. Cancer is a disease that involves alterations to gene structure and gene expression at the cellular level. The role of the accumulation of mutations is well established for carcinogenesis. In this chapter we will review the structure of a gene and describe the mutations that occur during carcinogenesis.

When considering the process of carcinogenesis we must be aware that cells are equipped with defense mechanisms against mutations, such as the detection and repair of DNA damage. Detection and repair of DNA damage is particularly crucial in the time before a cell divides since errors existing during replication will be passed on to daughter cells. Pausing the cell cycle is sometimes coupled to the repair of DNA damage. Apoptosis, a more hard-line defense, can be triggered as a last resort; thus, cell suicide is the ultimate price to be paid to prevent perpetuation of DNA damage and to protect the individual from carcinogenesis (see Chapter 7). In this chapter, we will also examine how mutations in DNA occur as a consequence of exposure to carcinogens and, on the other hand, examine the DNA repair systems that are in place to maintain the integrity of the genome and suppress tumorigenesis.

2.1 Gene structure—two parts of a gene: the regulatory region and the coding region

We have 30,000 genes! They are encoded in our DNA, an impressively simplistic double-helical molecule made up of two chains of nucleotides. A nucleotide is made up of a sugar, phosphate, and a nitrogenous base (adenine, guanine, cytosine, or thymine) and it is the sequence of the bases that holds the instructional information of our genes. The central dogma of molecule biology states that DNA is transcribed into RNA and RNA is translated into protein. Gene expression refers to the transcription of a gene. For the purpose of simplicity, keep in mind that there are two distinct functional parts to a **gene** (Figure 2.1). The 5′ end of a gene contains nucleotide sequences that make up the **promoter** region, and this region is involved in regulating the expression of the gene. These 5′ nucleotide sequences interact with proteins that affect the activity of RNA polymerase and determine when and where a gene is expressed. (Note however, there are exceptions; for many genes, some regulatory regions can be located elsewhere, such as **downstream** of the gene or within introns.) The TATA box (TATAAAA) located near the start site of transcription is one of the most important regulatory elements for most genes. Binding of the TATA box-binding protein (TBP) is crucial for the initiation of transcription. A short sequence of DNA within a promoter that is recognized by a specific protein and contributes to the regulation of the gene is called a **response element** (RE). Common response elements identify genes under a common type of regulation. For example, the sequence CCATATTAGG is referred to as the serum response element (SRE) and is found in genes that are responsive to serum. Also, it is not surprising that the response element for a protein that is essential for the regulation of the cell cycle, the transcription factor E2F, is found in the promoters of the cyclin E and cyclin A genes, the products of which are major players in the cell cycle. Enhancer elements are additional regulatory DNA sequences that are position- and orientation-independent relative to a promoter and are important for tissue-specific and stage-specific expression. Downstream (the direction along the DNA molecule towards the 3′ end) of the promoter

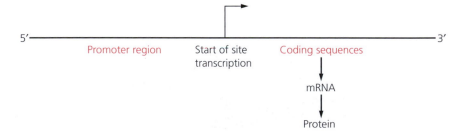

Figure 2.1 A simplistic representation: two functional parts of a gene.

are the nucleotides that will be transcribed into RNA and those coding for exons will be translated into protein. These downstream nucleotide sequences represent the coding region of the gene.

2.2 Mutations

As stated previously, most carcinogens are mutagens. These agents induce mutations either by modifying DNA (e.g. forming DNA adducts) or by causing chromosomal damage (e.g. DNA strand breaks). Several types of mutations are illustrated in Figure 2.2: transitions, transversions, insertions, deletions, and chromosomal translocations. Transitions and transversions are two types of base substitutions. A transition is the substitution for one purine for another purine and a transversion is the substitution of a purine for a pyrimidine or vice versa. Base substitutions during replication may occur for several reasons. First, DNA polymerase is not always 100% accurate. The enzyme may make an error and insert a wrong nucleotide during DNA synthesis. Also, modifications of bases due to oxidation or covalent additions and alterations of chromatin structure can cause mis-reading of the DNA template by DNA polymerase. Remember that the genetic code is a triplet code read in a sequential but non-overlapping manner. An insertion or deletion of a base can alter the reading frame (marked by a ',' in Figure 2.2) and thus can also be referred to as a frame-shift mutation. In most cases this leads to a non-functional or truncated protein product. A chromosomal translocation is the exchange of one part of one chromosome for another part of a different chromosome and results in changes of the base sequence of DNA. As we will see in later chapters, there are many examples of these types of mutations in genes regulating growth, differentiation, and apoptosis that are involved in carcinogenesis. In theory, initial mutations may occur anywhere across a particular gene but the location will determine whether some of these

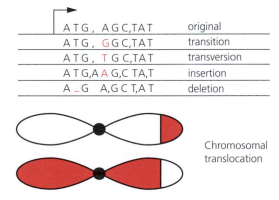

ATG, AGC,TAT	original
ATG, GGC,TAT	transition
ATG, TGC,TAT	transversion
ATG,AAG,C TA,T	insertion
A_G A,GC T,AT	deletion

Chromosomal translocation

Figure 2.2 Types of mutations.

mutations give rise to a growth advantage and contribute to carcinogenesis. For example, a mutation may alter the conformation of a cyclin protein and result in unregulated progression of the cell cycle, whereas another mutation may have no effect on protein conformation or function.

The consequence of a mutation in a gene is determined by its location with respect to the two functional parts of a gene. Mutations occurring in the promoter region may alter the regulation of the gene and affect the levels or temporal/spatial expression of the gene product. The consequence of such mutations may be over- or under-expression of the protein product or the appearance of the protein product at the wrong time or in the wrong place (i.e. the wrong cell type), respectively. Alternatively, mutations occurring in the coding region of genes may affect the structure and thus alter the function of the gene product or cause a truncation (e.g. the introduction of a stop codon) that abolishes the protein's function completely.

2.3 Carcinogenic agents

The backbone of cancer biology has been the identification of carcinogens responsible for cancer-causing mutations, and the identification of specific mutations as causative factors of carcinogenesis along with the elucidation of the pathways they affect. Several classes of carcinogens will now be described, including radiation, chemicals, infectious pathogens, and particular endogenous reactions.

Radiation as a carcinogen

Radiation is energy. There are two forms of radiation: energy traveling in waves or as a stream of atomic particles. Energy waves include gamma (γ) rays, high-energy electromagnetic radiation that is similar to X-rays. Atomic particles include alpha (α) and beta (β) particles that are emitted by radioactive atoms. (Alpha particles comprise two protons and two neutrons, while beta particles comprise electrons.)

Electromagnetic radiation is naturally occurring radiation which possesses a broad range of energies. Electromagnetic radiation moves as waves of energy, which have peaks and troughs (in a manner analogous to waves at sea). The distance between successive peaks (or troughs) is termed the wavelength. High-energy electromagnetic radiation such as cosmic radiation has a short wavelength, while low-energy radiation such as radio waves has a long wavelength. The electromagnetic spectrum spans electromagnetic radiation of varying wavelengths, as shown in Figure 2.3. The electromagnetic spectrum extends from long-wavelength radiation (not shown) to extremely short-wavelength radiation, such as

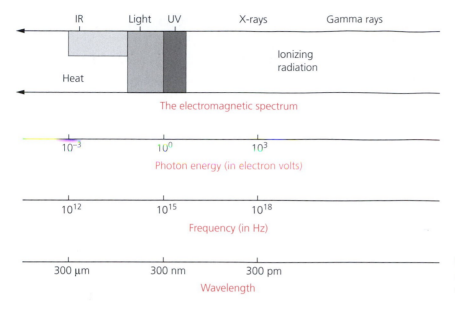

Figure 2.3 The electromagnetic spectrum and corresponding characteristics.

X-rays and gamma radiation. The visible spectrum spans those wavelengths that we can detect with our eyes as visible light. Ultraviolet (UV) radiation is emitted from the sun and has a higher energy (and so a shorter wavelength) than visible light.

Several types of radiation (including both energy waves and atomic particles) can damage DNA and act as carcinogens. The amount of energy released by a particular radiation source affects the mechanism and extent of damage to DNA. The amount of energy released by a particular radiation source and absorbed by the body tissue is measured in grays (Gy). One gray is the release to the body tissue of 1 joule (J) of energy per 1 kg of tissue. The real issue is not how much radiation is absorbed by the body tissue, however, but how much damage is done when the radiation has been absorbed. The amount of damage caused depends on the rate at which a particular radiation source releases energy. If a radiation source releases energy at a high rate, then it causes more damage than a source that releases energy more slowly.

Linear energy transfer (LET) is used to help describe the rate at which energy is released. Specifically, it describes the amount of energy released by a radiation source as it travels a fixed distance. High-LET radiation emits more energy than low-LET radiation over the same distance. Therefore, high-LET radiation (such as alpha particles) causes more biological damage than low-LET radiation (such as X-rays). The quantity and type of DNA damage caused by a particular radiation source depends on whether it is high- or low-LET radiation. Double-stranded DNA breaks are more commonly caused by high-LET radiation, and lead to chromosomal translocations and deletions.

The amount of biological damage caused by a particular source of radiation is measured in sieverts (Sv). (The numerical value of these units is determined by multiplying the gray units by a factor relating to the LET value of a particular type of radiation.)

Two classes of radiation, ionizing radiation and UV radiation, have been demonstrated to act as carcinogens and damage DNA. Let us examine both types of radiation below.

Ionizing radiation

Ionizing radiation includes both alpha and beta particles (atomic particles) and gamma rays (energy waves). When high-energy radiation, such as gamma rays, strikes molecules in its path, electrons may be displaced from atoms within the molecule. The loss of one or more electrons converts the molecule from being electrically neutral to carrying an electrical charge. The charged molecule is called an ion, and hence the radiation causing the formation of an ion is called ionizing radiation.

Ionizing radiation can damage DNA directly by causing ionization of the atoms comprising DNA, or indirectly by the interaction with water molecules (a process known as **radiolysis**) to generate dangerous intermediates called **reactive oxygen species** (ROS) (see Box 'A little lesson about ROS . . .'). These reactive oxygen species may react with DNA, or with other biomolecules, to cause damage within the cell.

A little lesson about ROS . . .

Some radiation exerts its biological effect by the generation of damaging intermediates through the interaction of radiation with water, or radiolysis. Since our body comprises between 55–60% water, radiation is most likely to strike water than any other matter. The striking of water by radiation causes it to loose an electron and become highly reactive. This sets off a chain reaction in which water is converted to oxygen, O_2, through a three-step process. Radiation interacts with a single molecule of water and thus it cannot split directly into the diatomic gases H_2 and O_2. Equation (1) below is **not** possible because this equation is not balanced.

$$H_2O \rightarrow H_2 + O_2 \tag{1}$$

The balanced equation (Equation 2) does not apply to radiation since radiation interacts with only a single molecule of water, and not the two molecules required in Equation (2):

$$2H_2O \rightarrow 2H_2 + O_2 \tag{2}$$

Instead, radiolysis results in the sequential generation of three dangerous reactive oxygen species (ROS) as an electron (e–) is lost at each step. The three ROS, formed in sequence, are the hydroxyl radical (–OH), hydrogen peroxide (H_2O_2), and the superoxide radical (O_2^-):

$$H_2O \xrightarrow{\text{e--}} \underset{\text{hydroxyl radical}}{\cdot OH} \xrightarrow{\text{e--}} \underset{\text{hydrogen peroxide}}{H_2O_2} \xrightarrow{\text{e--}} \underset{\text{superoxide radical}}{O_2^- \cdot} \xrightarrow{\text{e--}} O_2 \rightarrow$$

→ The hydroxyl radical is an extremely reactive molecule; in fact, it is one of the most reactive (and therefore dangerous) molecules known! It immediately removes electrons from any molecule in its path, turning that molecule into a free radical and so propagating a chain reaction. (A free radical is a highly unstable, reactive molecule that possesses an unpaired electron. Both the hydroxyl radical and the superoxide radical shown above are free radicals.)

Neither hydrogen peroxide nor the superoxide radical are as reactive as the hydroxyl radical. Hydrogen peroxide is actually more dangerous to DNA than the hydroxyl radical however. The slower reactivity of hydrogen peroxide (compared with the hydroxyl radical) gives the hydrogen peroxide molecule time to travel into the nucleus of a cell, where it is free to interact with and wreak havoc upon DNA.

Oxidation of DNA (the removal of electrons, by species such as the free radicals mentioned here) is one of the main causes of mutation, and explains why free radicals are such potent carcinogens. Oxidation can produce several types of DNA damage, including oxidized bases. Among the variety of oxidized nitrogenous bases observed, 8-oxoguanine is the most abundant. DNA polymerase mispairs 8-oxoguanine with adenine during DNA replication leading to a G→T transversion mutation. The presence of iron can exacerbate the consequences of H_2O_2 production. If it encounters iron and receives an electron from it, hydrogen peroxide can be reconverted into the hydroxyl radical that may attack DNA. The Fenton reaction (Equation 3) illustrates this:

$$H_2O_2 + Fe^{2+} \rightarrow OH^- + \cdot OH + Fe^{3+} \tag{3}$$

$$O_2^- \cdot + Fe^{3+} \rightarrow O_2 + Fe^{2+} \tag{4}$$

The superoxide radical is the third intermediate before the formation of oxygen. It is not very reactive but acts more as a catalyst for the generation of the other two intermediates mentioned because it helps regenerate iron (Equation 4) in the form needed for the above-mentioned Fenton reaction. Thus, the ROS intermediates affect one another.

(Lane, 2002)

People are exposed to varying amounts of ionizing radiation. Exposure to gamma rays from cosmic radiation depends on the altitude at which you live or travel. The average exposure for high-altitude flights is about $0.005–0.01$ mSv h^{-1}. A chest X-ray required for medical diagnosis of some conditions exposes patients to 0.1 mSv. The contribution of the accumulation of these varying daily exposures towards cancer risk is relatively unknown.

Studies of the victims of the atomic bombing in Japan continue to contribute to our knowledge of ionizing radiation as a carcinogen. Evidence suggests that the most important damage associated with ionizing radiation-induced carcinogenesis is double-strand DNA breaks. The Radiation Effects Research Foundation publishes periodic reports on the mortality of The Life Span Study cohort of 80,000 atomic bomb survivors (latest report Preston *et al.*, 2003). These studies have revealed three important points: (1) leukemia is the most frequent ionizing radiation-induced cancer, (2) age is an important risk factor, whereby those exposed as children are most affected, and (3) the risks of solid cancer increase with dose in a linear fashion. People exposed at 30 years of age have a risk of solid cancer that is elevated by 47% per Sv at the age of 70.

Ultraviolet radiation

Ultraviolet radiation (UV) from the sun is also carcinogenic and is a principal cause of skin cancer. Of the three types of UV light—UVA (wavelength 320–380 nm), UVB (wavelength 290–320 nm), and UVC (wavelength 200–290 nm)—UVB is the most effective carcinogen. The conjugated double bonds in the rings of the nitrogenous bases of DNA absorb UV radiation. UVB directly and uniquely causes characteristic UV photoproducts: cyclobutane pyrimidine dimers and pyrimidine–pyrimidone photoproducts (Figure 2.4a,b). Cyclobutane pyrimidine dimers are most prevalent, formed at least 20–40 times more frequently than other UV photoproducts. The formation of a pyrimidone (6–4) photoproduct mimics an abasic site (a nucleotide minus a base) and is more efficiently repaired than cyclobutane pyrimidine dimers. The formation of a pyrimidine dimer causes a bend in the DNA helix and, as a result, DNA polymerase cannot read the DNA template. Under these conditions DNA polymerase preferentially incorporates an 'A' residue. Consequently, TT dimers are

PAUSE AND THINK

Marie Curie, who worked with radioactivity all of her adult life, died of leukemia at the age of 67. The multi-stage process of carcinogenesis is manifested by the fairly long incubation periods needed to develop cancer after exposure to carcinogens.

LIFESTYLE TIP

Short-term tanning salon exposure (10 treatments in 2 weeks) results in the formation of cyclobutane pyrimidine dimers. Look at the data in Whitmore *et al.* (2001). A natural look is less taxing for your DNA!

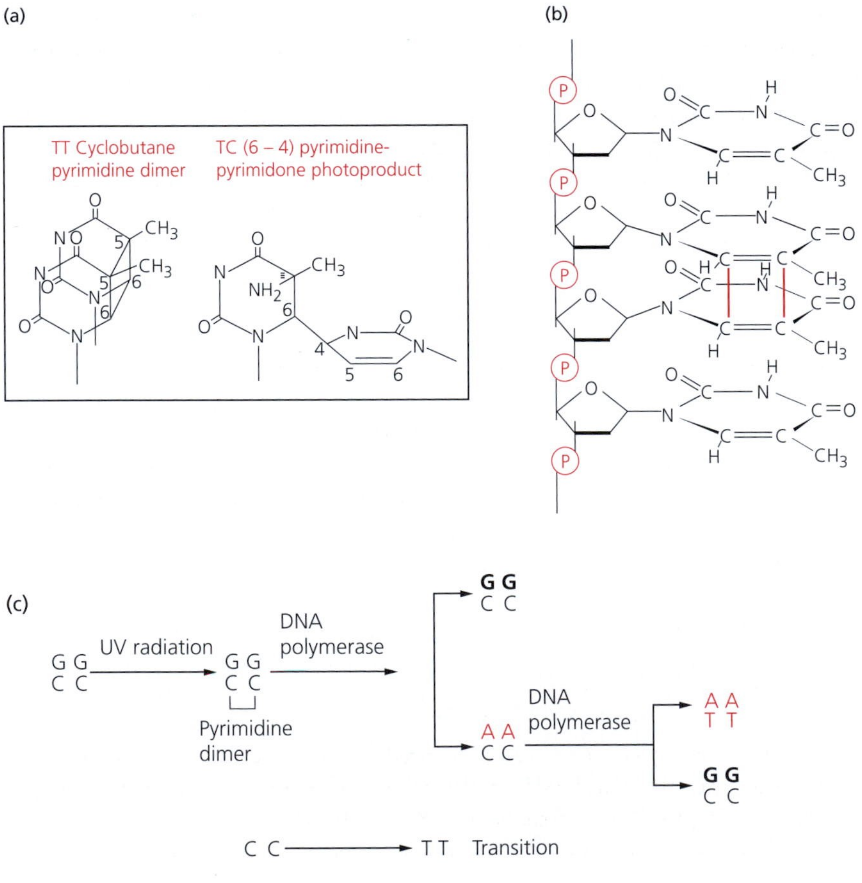

Figure 2.4 (a) UV photoproducts. (b) A pyrimidine dimer in the context of a polynucleotide chain. (c) Steps involved in UV-induced transitions.

often restored but TC and CC dimers result in transitions (TC→TT and CC→TT) (Figure 2.4c). Results from a mammalian cell system showed that cyclobutane pyrimidine dimers are responsible for at least 80% of UVB-induced mutations. The precise class of mutations resulting from pyrimidine dimers is a unique molecular signature of skin cancer (see Box 'Skin cancer')—they are not found in any other types of cancer.

UVA indirectly damages DNA via free radical-mediated damage. Water is fragmented by UVA, generating electron-seeking ROS (such the hydroxyl radical as mentioned above) that cause DNA damage (e.g. oxidation of bases). G→T transversions are characteristic of UVA damage.

Skin cancer

UV light is specifically carcinogenic to the skin because it does not penetrate the body any deeper than the skin. The skin is made up of squamous cells, basal cells, and melanocytes and skin cancers are classified by the cell type they affect: squamous cell carcinoma (SCC), basal cell carcinoma (BCC), and melanoma, respectively. The depth of transmission of each type of UV light is dependent on the wavelength: UVC only penetrates into the superficial layer of the skin, UVB penetrates into the basal level of the epidermis, and UVA penetrates into the more acellular dermis level. Sunscreens work on the basis of including UV-absorbing organic chemicals (e.g. cinnamates), inorganic zinc-containing pigments, or titanium oxides in their ingredients to minimize UV absorption by the skin. (Note that melanin formation, known to most people as tanning, is a natural defense mechanism against UV absorption.) Additional ingredients in sunscreens must be used with care as we have learned that some compounds may be photosensitized carcinogens, chemicals that can be activated by UV to become carcinogenic. Ironically, some early sunscreens included bergamot oil which contains 5-methoxy psoralen, a photosensitized carcinogen! Some drugs such as fluoroquinolone antibiotics are also photosensitized carcinogens, which explains the reasons for the precautions from doctors to stay out of the sun during their administration.

A cellular mechanism for the elimination of UV-damaged skin cells is to initiate apoptosis. This phenomenon is familiar to us as the peeling of the skin after a sunburn. The tumor suppressor p53 protein (introduced in Chapter 1 and discussed in detail in Chapter 6) is an important regulator of apoptosis. Mutation of the *p53* gene is important for the initiation of squamous cell and basal cell carcinoma, but not melanoma. The characteristic mutations (CC→TT transitions) caused only by UV and no other carcinogen were identified in the *p53* gene. Mutations in the *p53* gene which disrupt normal p53 function and provide cells with a growth advantage, may induce the formation of tumor cells. The pattern of mutation is not random but rather tends to be localized to nine places, called hot spots. This suggests that *p53* mutations are causal for skin cancer. Further investigation of why there are so few hotspots within the context of hundreds of sites with adjacent pyrimidine dimers in the *p53* gene yielded an explanation. The hot spots in *p53* are not repaired efficiently. Removal of cyclobutane pyrimidine dimers is particularly slow at these sites. The resulting loss of p53 function causes a block in apoptosis and consequently allows the proliferation of mutated *p53* cells. Thus UV radiation not only induces *p53* mutations but also selects for the clonal expansion of the *p53* mutated cells, by inducing apoptosis in normal cells with wild-type *p53*. ➔

> → Different pathways seem to be central for melanoma. The elucidation of one of these pathways was one of the first successes of the Cancer Genome Project. It identified mutations in the *BRAF* gene in 66% of malignant melanomas (Davies *et al.*, 2002). BRAF is a serine/threonine kinase that functions in the signal transduction pathway downstream of a melanocyte-stimulating hormone and may explain why there is a high frequency of *BRAF* mutations in melanoma relative to other cancers. Surprisingly, the major mutation identified (T→A) in the kinase domain is not characteristic of UV-induced mutations (CC→TT).

Chemical carcinogens

Many chemicals in our environment and in our diet play a role in human carcinogenesis. The common mechanism of action of carcinogens is that an electrophilic (electron-deficient) form reacts with nucleophilic sites (sites that can donate electrons) in the purine and pyrimidine rings of nucleic acids. Some chemical carcinogens can act directly on DNA but others become active only after they are metabolized in the body, forming what are called ultimate carcinogens, the molecules that execute the damage. A family of enzymes called the cytochrome P450 enzymes is involved in the metabolism of chemicals in the liver and is important in the activation of carcinogens to ultimate carcinogens. Genetic polymorphisms and variable expression account for differences in responses to chemical carcinogens among individuals. For example, the expression of one of the P450 enzymes called CYP1A1 (aryl hydrocarbon hydroxylase) can vary 50-fold in human lung tissue and may be responsible for the delivery of varying doses of ultimate carcinogens among smokers (Alexandrov *et al.*, 2002).

Carcinogens can be segregated into 10 groups:

(i)   polycyclic aromatic hydrocarbons

(ii)   aromatic amines

(iii)   azo dyes

(iv)   nitrosamines and nitrosamides

(v)   hyrazo and azoxy compounds

(vi)   carbamates

(vii)   halogenated compounds

(viii) natural products

(ix)   inorganic carcinogens

(x)   miscellaneous compounds (alkylating agents, aldehydes, phenolics).

Four major classes of carcinogens are described below: polycyclic aromatic hydrocarbons (PAHs), aromatic amines, nitrosamines, and alkylating agents. These carcinogens exert their effects by adding functional groups covalently to DNA. Chemically modified bases, called DNA adducts, distort the DNA helix causing errors to be made during replication. The resulting mutations initiate cell carcinogenesis.

Polycyclic aromatic hydrocarbons (PAHs)

The first demonstration that chemicals could be used to induce cancer in animals was carried out in 1915. Coal tar, containing carcinogenic PAHs, induced skin carcinomas on the ears of rabbits. Carcinogenic PAHs are derived from phenanthrene (Figure 2.5a). Additional rings and/or methyl groups in the bay region of the three aromatic rings can convert inactive phenanthrene into an active carcinogen. Benzo[a]pyrene (BP), the most well known carcinogen in cigarette smoke, and 7,12-dimethyl benz[a]anthracene (DMBA), one of the most potent carcinogens, are examples of PAHs. PAHs must be metabolized further in order to give the ultimate carcinogen that will form adducts with purine bases of DNA. The P450 enzyme, CYP1A1, is the predominant enzyme that metabolizes BP to the highly reactive mutagenic BP diol epoxides (Figure 2.5b). BP results mainly in G→T transversions.

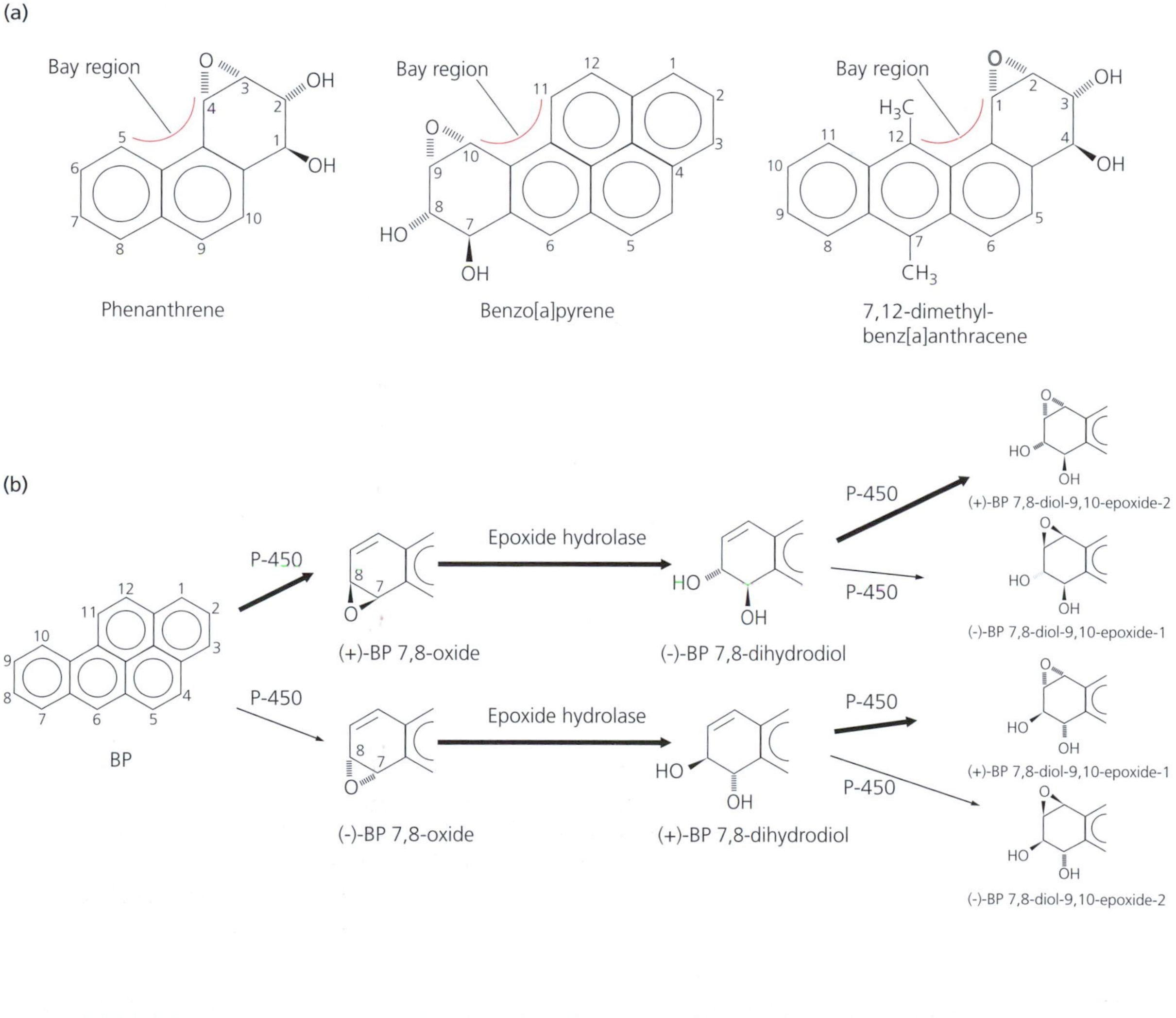

Figure 2.5 (a) Examples of polycyclic aromatic amines. (b) Metabolic activation of BP.

(a)

Phenanthrene

Benzo[a]pyrene

7,12-dimethyl-benz[a]anthracene

(b)

BP

(+)-BP 7,8-oxide

(−)-BP 7,8-oxide

(−)-BP 7,8-dihydrodiol

(+)-BP 7,8-dihydrodiol

(+)-BP 7,8-diol-9,10-epoxide-2

(−)-BP 7,8-diol-9,10-epoxide-1

(+)-BP 7,8-diol-9,10-epoxide-1

(−)-BP 7,8-diol-9,10-epoxide-2

LIFESTYLE TIP

The International Agency for Research on Cancer (IARC) has classified 81 compounds in cigarette mainstream smoke as carcinogens (Smith *et al.*, 2003). Benzo[a]pyrene (BP) ranks high in the measure of lipophilicity (a feature that allows easy entry into cells) and associated carcinogenicity. The presence of nicotine makes smoking addictive. Smoking is a cause of cancer; not smoking prevents illness. Don't choose to smoke.

A LEADER IN THE FIELD . . . of molecular carcinogenesis: Gerd Pfeifer

Gerd Pfeifer has made important contributions to determining the molecular mechanisms of cancer. Investigations into skin and lung cancer provided strong evidence that UV radiation and carcinogens in cigarette smoke are causative agents for each cancer, respectively. Gerd and his colleagues demonstrated that the mutational hotspots of the *p53* gene observed in skin cancer cells are due to low-efficiency repair of DNA at these sites as discussed in the Box 'Skin cancer' above. By mapping DNA adducts of the *p53* gene that are formed after exposure to benzo[a]pyrene diol epoxide (a potent cigarette carcinogen), Gerd and colleagues showed that the locations of these adducts matched the distribution of *p53* gene mutations in lung tumors from smokers. This seminal work, reported in *Science* in 1996, provided a direct causal link between a defined carcinogen and lung cancer.

Gerd Pfeifer received his PhD from the University of Frankfurt, Germany. He has crossed the Atlantic and is currently a Professor and Chair at the City of Hope, Beckman Research Institute in California. His research group is continuing to study the mechanisms of mutagenesis in cancer and is also currently investigating **epigenetic** mechanisms of gene regulation in cancer (discussed in Chapter 3).

Aromatic amines

Heterocyclic amines (HCAs) are carcinogens produced by cooking meat, formed from heating amino acids and proteins. About 20 HCAs have been identified. Three examples, Phe-P-1, IQ, and Mel Q, are shown in Figure 2.6. It is important to be aware of these since they illustrate an example of carcinogens to which we may be exposed daily and which are produced in our own kitchens.

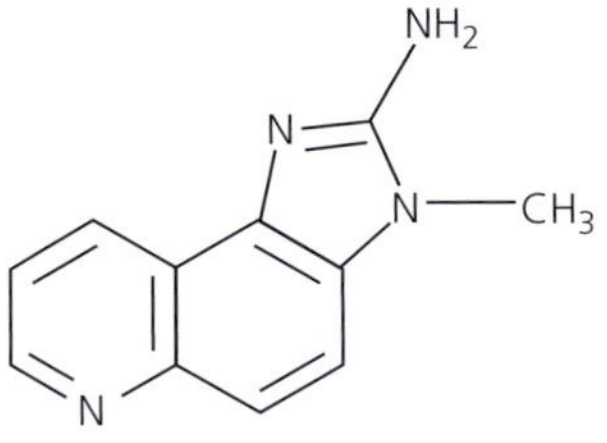

2-Amino-3 methylimidazo [4,5-f] quinoline (IQ)

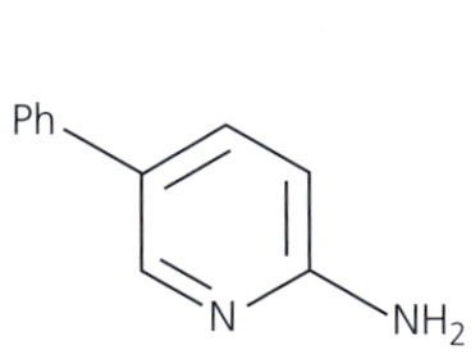

2 Amino-5 phenylpyridine (PHe-P-1)

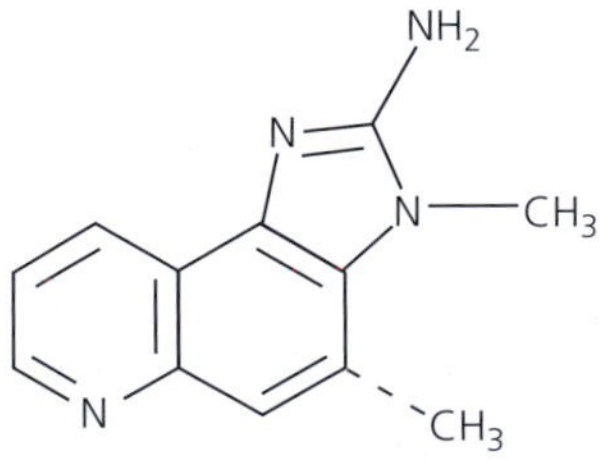

2-Amino-3,4 dimethylimidazo [4,5-f] quinoline (Mel Q)

Figure 2.6 Heterocyclic amines.

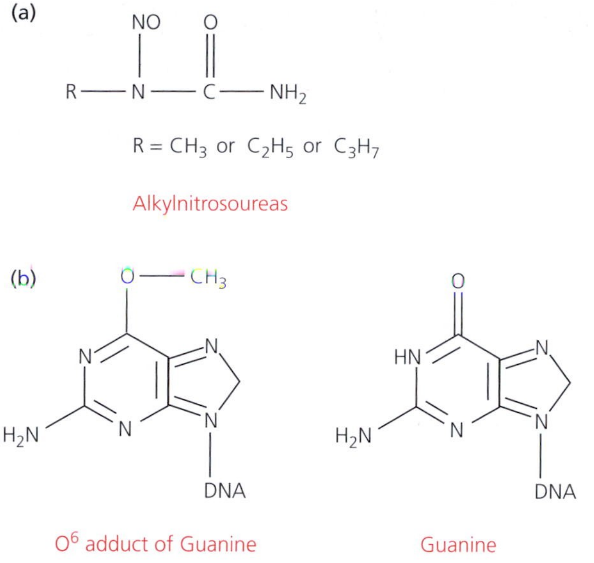

(a)

$$R - N - C - NH_2$$

with NO and O groups shown above N and C respectively.

R = CH₃ or C₂H₅ or C₃H₇

Alkylnitrosoureas

(b)

O⁶ adduct of Guanine   Guanine

Figure 2.7 (a) An example of nitrosamines: alkylnitrosoureas. (b) A potential carcinogenic product of nitrosamines: O^6 adduct of guanine. Guanine is shown for comparison.

Nitrosamines and nitrosamides

Many nitrosamines and nitrosamides are found in tobacco or are formed when preservative nitrites react with amines in fish and meats during smoking. The structure of alkylnitrosoureas, examples of nitrosamines, is shown in Figure 2.7(a). Their principal carcinogenic product is alkylated O^6 guanine derivatives, as shown in Figure 2.7(b) (guanine is depicted next to it for comparison).

Alkylating agents

Mustard gas (sulfur mustard, Figure 2.8) is the most well-known example of an alkylating agent because of its use and consequences observed during World War I. It is a bi-functional (having two reactive groups) carcinogen that is able to form intra-chain and inter-chain cross-links on DNA directly.

Fibrous minerals: asbestos and erionite

Asbestos and erionite are naturally occurring fibrous minerals that act as chemical carcinogens and mutagens. Asbestos is a group of fibrous silicate minerals that was used extensively in building materials because of its insulating properties but is now prohibited in several countries (but is still used in the developing world) due to association with several diseases of the lung, including lung cancer and mesothelioma. Erionite is a fibrous zeolite mineral formed from volcanic rock. Mechanisms of carcinogenesis include generation of ROS and induction of a chronic inflammatory response (see Chapter 10). Genetics may predispose some people to the carcinogenic effects of fibrous materials.

PAUSE AND THINK

What is the structural difference between IQ and Mel Q?

LIFESTYLE TIP

It has been suggested that changes in the way we prepare food can reduce the amounts of HCAs produced. Oven-roasting, marinading, and coating food with breadcrumbs before frying are modifications that may reduce the formation of HCAs.

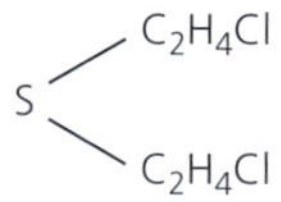

$$S \begin{matrix} C_2H_4Cl \\ C_2H_4Cl \end{matrix}$$

Figure 2.8 Structure of mustard gas.

Family pedigrees

Malignant mesothelioma is a rare cancer that is linked to fibrous minerals. It is rare in the USA and the UK; however, there is an epidemic of malignant mesothelioma in several small villages of Turkey that has been linked to exposure to erionite. Fifty per cent of all deaths in these regions are due to malignant mesothelioma! Pedigree studies of families that live in these villages uncovered a link between genetics and fiber carcinogenesis. Chemical and physical analysis, including scanning electron microscopy, mass spectrometry, and x-ray diffraction, showed that there was no difference between the type of erionite in villages that exhibited the epidemic and those that did not. However, malignant mesothelioma was prevalent in some families and absent in others and marriages between these two groups led to some offspring developing the disease. Thus the data demonstrate that a genetic predisposition can influence mineral fiber carcinogenesis.

Dogan *et al.* (2006) and family pedigree data within: available online at
http://cancerres.aacrjournals.org/cgi/reprint/66/10/5063

Infectious pathogens as carcinogens

Early in the 20th century, viruses were shown to cause tumors in animals. As we will see in Chapter 4, they have been invaluable tools for investigating the molecular events of cell transformation. Viruses that are oncogenic can be classified as DNA tumor viruses or RNA tumor viruses (also called retroviruses), depending on the nucleic acid that defines their genome. The mechanisms of carcinogenesis for these two classes of virus differ. DNA tumor viruses encode viral proteins that block tumor suppressor genes, often by protein–protein interactions (discussed in Chapter 6). Many retroviruses cause cancers in animals by encoding mutated forms of normal genes (i.e. oncogenes) that have a dominant effect in host cells (discussed in Chapter 4). Mechanisms of replication between DNA and RNA viruses also differ. Some DNA viruses, such as human papilloma and Epstein–Barr viruses, replicate strictly as episomes within host cells. Retroviruses replicate by integration of the viral genome into the host DNA and utilize the host's translational machinery to produce viral proteins. Integration may lead to deregulated gene expression.

Direct causation of cancer by specific viruses and bacteria has been demonstrated and will be discussed in detail in Chapter 10. However, a few named examples are given below. The International Agency for Research on Cancer (IARC) has classified human papillomavirus (type 16 and 18) as a human carcinogen and a causative agent of cervical cancer. In addition, Kaposi's sarcoma-associated herpesvirus (KSHV) causes Kaposi's sarcoma, hepatitis B virus is associated with liver cancer, and Epstein–Barr virus (EBV) with nasopharyngeal carcinoma. The human T-cell leukemia virus type 1 (HTLV-1) is the only retrovirus known to cause cancer in humans. It causes acute T-cell leukemia (ATL). *Helicobacter pylori*, a Gram-negative spiral bacterium, establishes chronic infection and ulcers in the stomach and alters host cell function, which is associated with carcinogenesis. The International Agency for Research on Cancer has classified *H. pylori* as a human carcinogen and one of the causative agents of gastric cancer. The typhoid pathogen, *Salmonella enterica* serovar Typhi (*S. typhi*), establishes chronic infection in the gallbladder and has been linked to hepatobiliary and gallbladder carcinoma. The molecular events behind the mechanism of bacteria-induced transformation are the subject of current studies. The promotion of host cell proliferation, the generation of oxygen free radicals and subsequent DNA damage, and the activation of oncogenes are areas of investigation (Lax and Thomas, 2002).

Endogenous carcinogenic reactions

In addition to carcinogens, endogenous cellular reactions generate mutations. Oxidative respiration and lipid peroxidation, two processes of normal cell metabolism, produce ROS that can react with DNA and lipids to produce oxidized products (e.g. 8-oxoguanine) also seen by exposure to radiation (see above). During respiration, the initiating radical, superoxide anion (O_2^-) is produced upon reduction of NADH and formation of ubisemiquinone during oxidative phosphorylation. Therefore, breathing generates the same ROS intermediates as those generated by radiation! However, the dose of these intermediates differs between the two sources: radiation produces extremely reactive hydroxy radicals immediately and randomly within a cell, while respiration produces the less reactive superoxide radical immediately and only at specific locations within the cell.

Spontaneous chemical reactions (e.g. hydrolysis of the glycosidic bond between a base and deoxyribose producing an abasic site) also contribute to the formation of mutations. Deamination of cytosine to form uracil is the most common. Errors during DNA replication and DNA recombination contribute to the formation of mutations, although the DNA polymerases used possess proofreading ability to help minimize the number of mutations caused in this way. The proofreading function is dependent on the 3′–5′ exonuclease activity of the polymerase. If an incorrect nucleotide is added to the growing 3′ end of the newly synthesized strand the DNA double helix exhibits melting; that is, the strands remain separated at this point. Melting causes the polymerase to pause and the strand is transferred to the exonuclease site. Here the incorrect nucleotide is removed, the strand is transferred back to the original polymerase binding site, and DNA synthesis reoccurs. Overall, it is estimated that 10^4 to 10^6 mutations occur in a single human cell per day. By and large, under normal circumstances, this immense error burden is successfully dealt with by the highly efficient cellular DNA repair mechanisms.

2.4 DNA repair and predispositions to cancer

DNA repair is an important line of defense against mutations caused by carcinogens and by endogenous mechanisms. If DNA lesions are not repaired before a cell replicates, they may contribute to carcinogenesis. Repair of the various types of mutation is accomplished by several different DNA repair mechanisms. Five types of DNA repair systems are described below: one-step repair, nucleotide excision repair, base excision repair, mismatch repair, and recombinational repair. Defects in most of these pathways result in a predisposition to cancer.

One-step repair

One-step repair involves the direct reversal of DNA damage. The repair enzyme alkyltransferase directly removes an alkyl group from the O^6 atom of guanine after exposure of DNA to alkylating carcinogens such as N-methylnitrosourea. In this case, a methyl group is transferred to a cysteine residue on the alkyltransferase and the alkyltransferase becomes inactive.

Nucleotide excision repair (NER)

Nucleotide excision repair is specific for helix-distorting lesions such as pyrimidine dimers and bulky DNA adducts induced by environmental agents (UVB and PAHs, respectively). This damage interferes with transcription and replication as described above. Two subpathways exist: global genome NER surveys the genome for helix distortion and transcription-coupled repair identifies damage that interferes with transcription. The lesion, along with some (24–32) adjacent nucleotides, is excised out by endonucleases, and DNA polymerase δ/ϵ is used to fill in the gap using the opposite strand as a template. Proliferating cell nuclear factor is part of the polymerase holoenzyme and physically forms a ring that encircles and binds the damaged region. Xeroderma pigmentosum (XP) is an inherited disorder characterized by a defect in NER. Affected individuals are hypersensitive to the sun and have a 1000-fold increased risk of skin cancer. Seven XP gene products (XPA–XPG) have been identified out of the 25 proteins involved in NER.

Base excision repair

Base excision repair targets chemically altered bases (e.g. 8-oxoguanine) induced mostly by endogenous mechanisms; in the absence of such repair the damage will cause a point mutation. The chemically altered bases may be small enough not to interfere with replication or transcription. For example, failure to remove a 8-oxoguanine:A base pair before replication results in a G→T transversion mutation. The first step of base excision repair is carried out by a family of DNA-damage-specific glycosylases which scan millions of base pairs per second for lesions. Glycosylases then flip the lesion outside of the helix and cleave the base from the DNA backbone, creating an abasic site. Subsequently an endonuclease cleaves the DNA strand at the abasic site and DNA polymerase β replaces the nucleotide and ligase fills the gap. Mutations in the *OGG1* gene that codes for the principal glycosylase responsible for the repair of 8-oxoguanine have not been identified in tumors to date. No inherited defects in BER had been identified in humans until recently—mutations in the *MYH* gene that encodes a DNA glycosylase responsible for the removal of mismatched adenines paired with 8-oxoguanine may be the principal cause of multiple colorectal adenoma syndrome (Al-Tassan *et al.*, 2002).

Mismatch repair

Mismatch repair corrects replication errors that have escaped editing by polymerases. It includes repair of insertions and deletions produced as a result of slippage during the replication of repetitive sequences as well as nucleotide mismatches. The molecular events can be described in brief as follows:

- recognition of the mismatch is carried out by proteins HMSH2/6 and hMSH2/3
- hMLH1/hPMS2 and hMHL1/hPMS1 are recruited
- the newly synthesized strand is identified (flagged by the replication machinery)
- endonucleases and exonucleases remove the nucleotides around and including the mismatch
- DNA polymerases resynthesize a newly replicated strand.

Hereditary non-polyposis colorectal cancer (HNPCC) is one of the most common cancer syndromes in humans. Half of all patients with HNPCC carry a germline mutation in *hMLH1* or *hMSH2*. Loss of function of the protein products encoded by these genes is responsible for complete loss of mismatch repair. Thus, cells are vulnerable to mutations.

Recombinational repair

Homologous recombination and non-homologous end-joining are two types of recombinational repair that mend double-strand DNA breaks. Homologous recombination depends on the presence of sister chromatids

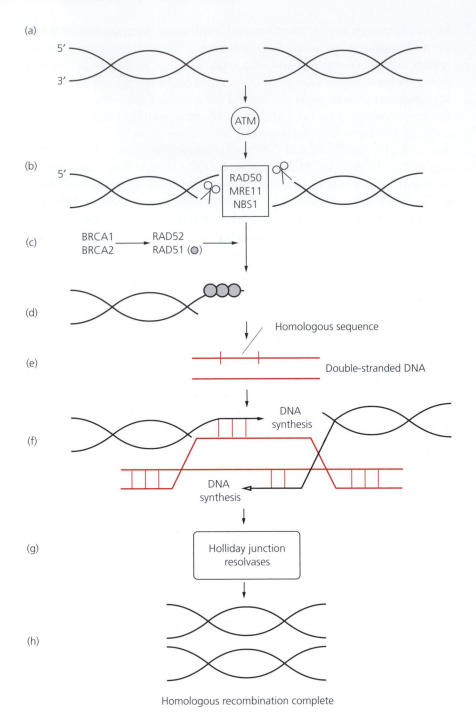

Figure 2.9 Recombinational repair.

formed during DNA synthesis as a template for recombining severed ends. Many members of the same protein family make up a complex that performs what has been nicknamed DNA gymnastics. The molecular events shown in Figure 2.9 are described in brief:

(a) A double-strand break activates the ataxia telangiectasia mutated (ATM) kinase.

(b) The RAD50/MRE11/NBS1 complex (a substrate of ATM) uses its 5′–3′ exonuclease activity (depicted by scissors in Figure 2.9) to create single-stranded 3′ ends.

(c) BRCA1/2 aids in the nuclear transport of RAD51 (shown as gray circles).

(d) RAD52 facilitates RAD51 binding to these exposed ends to form a nucleoprotein filament.

(e) RAD51 can exchange a homologous sequence from a single strand within a double-stranded molecule (shown in red; e.g. a sister chromatid), with a single-stranded sequence.

(f) The sequences from the double-stranded molecule are then used as a template sequence for repair.

(g) Resolvases restore the junctions formed as a result of homologous recombination, called Holliday junctions.

(h) Two copies of intact DNA molecules are produced with rarely any errors.

Ataxia telangiectasia is an inherited syndrome whereby patients have a mutation in the ataxia telangiectasia mutated (ATM) kinase. Patients are sensitive to X-rays and have an increased risk of lymphoma.

Suffice it to say that the other type of recombinational repair, end-joining, links non-homologous ends and is therefore error prone, and can possibly result in chromosomal translocations.

One of the main molecular players involved in carcinogenesis is p53 and should be mentioned here. p53, 'the guardian of the genome', is a protein that plays an important role in the molecular events that protect the integrity of DNA; it is central in the orchestration of DNA repair. The details of this important tumor suppressor protein will be discussed in Chapter 6.

 Therapeutic strategies

2.5 Conventional therapies: chemotherapy and radiation therapy

Conventional therapies continue to extend and save lives. It is important to understand their rationale before moving to more molecular approaches discussed later in the text. Several conventional therapies aim to induce extensive DNA damage in order to trigger apoptosis and paradoxically include agents classified as carcinogens. Other conventional therapies inhibit DNA metabolism in order to block DNA synthesis in the rapidly dividing cancer cells. DNA synthesis is essential to produce a new set of chromosomes for the daughter cells produced by cell division. Still other drugs interfere with the mechanics of cell division. Both chemotherapies and radiotherapy will be discussed.

Chemotherapy

A brief description and examples of the three main types of classical chemotherapy are given below.

Alkylating agents and platinum-based drugs

Alkylating agents and platinum-based drugs work by a similar mode of action. Alkylating agents have the ability to form DNA adducts by covalent bonds via an alkyl group. They may act during all phases of the cell cycle. Chlorambucil (Figure 2.10a) is one example of a member of the nitrogen mustard family of drugs. Its usual target is the N7 position of guanine residues. Bi-functional alkylating agents (compounds with two reactive groups) form intra-strand and inter-strand cross-links in DNA that alter the conformation of the double helix or prevent separation of the DNA strands and interfere with DNA replication. They are much more potent than monofunctional analogs, indicating that cross-linking is the basis of their function since monofunctional analogs cannot cross-link.

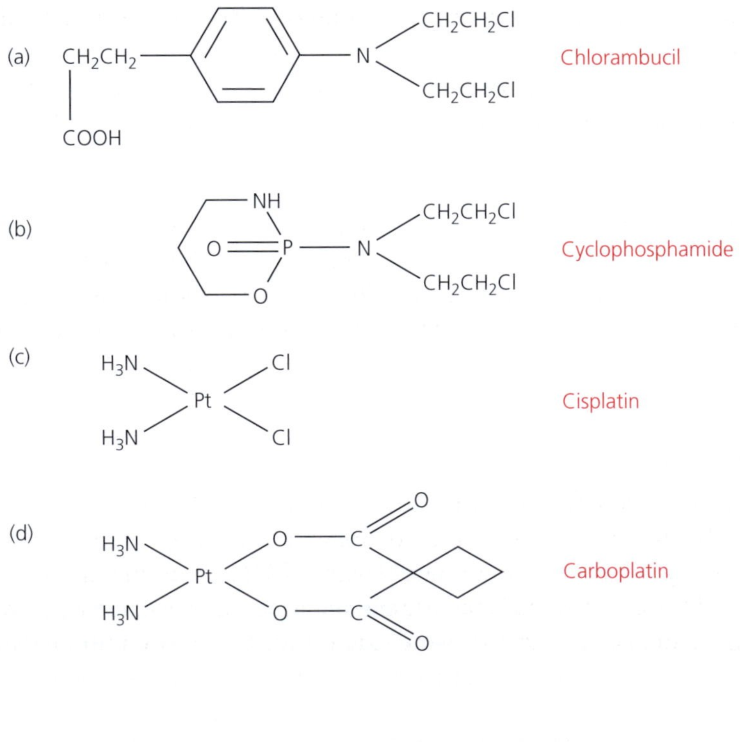

Figure 2.10 Examples of alkylating agents and platinum-based drugs.

Some drugs require metabolic activation within the body. The alkylating agent cyclophosphamide (Figure 2.10b) is one example. Oxidases in the liver produce an aldehyde form that decomposes to yield phosphoramide mustard, the biologically active molecule.

The platinum-based drugs, such as cisplatin [cis Pt(II)(NH$_3$)$_2$Cl$_2$] and carboplatin (Figure 2.10c and 2.10d, respectively), form covalent bonds via the platinum atom. Cisplatin is a water-soluble molecule that contains a Pt atom bound to four functional groups. The Pt–N bond has covalent character and is essentially irreversible, whereas that with Cl is more labile. Cl is replaced with water in the plasma and cytosol before the molecule binds to the N7 position of guanine and adenine in its DNA target. The GG, AG, and GXG (where X can be any base) adducts comprise over 90% of the total. The resulting DNA damage triggers apoptosis. Although cisplatin had a major impact on some cancers, such as ovarian cancer, it was associated with irreversible kidney damage. Later, carboplatin was identified as a less toxic platinum analog.

Antimetabolites

Antimetabolites are compounds that are structurally similar to endogenous molecules (e.g. nitrogenous bases of DNA) and therefore can mimic their role and inhibit nucleic acid synthesis. Two examples, fluorodeoxyuridylate (F-dUMP) and methotrexate, are shown alongside similar endogenous molecules, deoxyuridylate and tetrahydrofolate, respectively, in Figure 2.11. 5-Fluorouracil (5-FU) is a derivative of uracil and is converted into F-dUMP. F-dUMP competes with the natural substrate dUMP for the catalytic site of thymidylate synthase, the enzyme that produces thymidylate (dTMP) (Figure 2.12). F-dUMP forms a covalent complex with the enzyme and acts as a suicide inhibitor, generating an intermediate that inactivates the thymidylate synthase through covalent modification. As a result, the dTMP and dTTP pools are depleted, dUMP and dUTP accumulate, and DNA synthesis in rapidly dividing cells is severely compromised. Another important antimetabolite, methotrexate, targets an accessory enzyme of the same reaction. As an analog of dihydrofolate, methotrexate is a competitive inhibitor of dihydrofolate reductase, the enzyme used to regenerate tetrahydrofolate that is required in the thymidylate synthase reaction (Figure 2.12; see Chapter 11 for further discussion of tetrahydrofolate).

Organic drugs

Doxorubicin is a fungal anthracycline antibiotic that inhibits topoisomerase II, an enzyme that releases torsional stress during DNA replication, by trapping single-strand and double-strand DNA intermediates. Doxorubicin diffuses across cell membranes and accumulates in most cell types. Cardiac damage is its most severe side-effect, but new compounds (e.g.

PAUSE AND THINK

Do you recall a similar mechanism of action for any carcinogens?

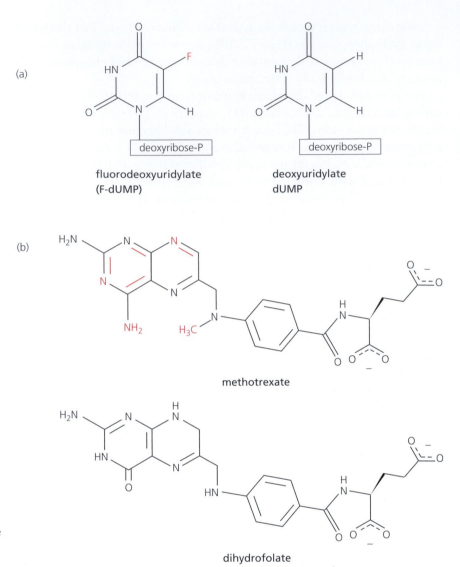

(a)

fluorodeoxyuridylate
(F-dUMP)

deoxyuridylate
dUMP

(b)

methotrexate

dihydrofolate

Figure 2.11 Antimetabolites:
(a) fluorodeoxyuridylate
(F-dUMP) and (b) methotrexate.
Structural differences between the
antimetabolite and endogenous
molecule are shown in red.

ICRF-187) that can block the cardiac toxicity are being investigated. These
drugs are primarily used to treat solid tumors (e.g. of the breast or lung).

The plant alkaloids vincristine and vinblastine (from the Madagascar
periwinkle plant) bind to tubulin and prevent microtubule assembly in
contrast to the drug paclitaxel (taxol) which binds to the β-tubulin subunit
in polymers and stabilizes the microtubules against depolymerization.
Thus two opposing strategies can be used to disrupt the mitotic spindle.

Radiation therapy

Radiation therapy, either alone or in combination with other therapies, is
received by approximately 60% of cancer patients in the USA. Ionizing

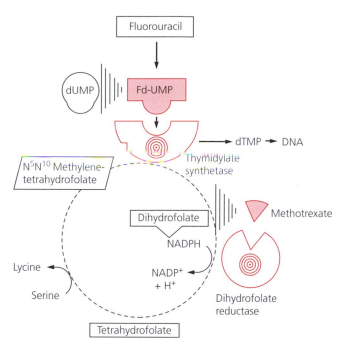

Figure 2.12 Action of antimetabolites fluorodeoxyuridylate (F-dUMP) and methotrexate (both shaded red). The enzyme thymidylate synthetase uses N^5N^{10} methylenetetrahydrofolate as a methyl donor and catalyzes the methylation of dUMP to form dTMP. The cancer drug fluorouracil is converted into the antimetabolite F-dUMP (red rectangular shape), which competes (/////) with dUMP and targets thymidylate synthetase (target symbol, ◎, shown). Methotrexate (red triangle) is an antimetabolite that competes (/////) with dihydrofolate and methotrexate targets the enzyme dihydrofolate reductase (target, ◎, symbol).

radiation is usually delivered to the tumor by electron linear accelerators. Radiation reacts with water inside cells to generate reactive oxygen species that damage DNA. Apoptosis will be induced in cells that contain large amounts of DNA damage. The supply of oxygen affects the potency of ionizing radiation and is thought to be due to the generation of ROS. Oxygen can assist in making radiation-induced damage permanent. More double-strand breaks occur in cells irradiated in the presence of oxygen than in cells irradiated in the absence of oxygen. Therefore, the number of zones of hypoxia within a solid tumor influences the outcome of radiation treatment. Targeting of the tumor has been made more precise by modern techniques such as magnetic resonance imaging (MRI) and computed tomography (CT) which produce three-dimensional images of the tumor within the body.

Heterogeneous cell sensitivity and drug resistance: obstacles to these treatments

In addition to the severe side-effects that result, there are also practical problems with conventional therapies. Cancer cells, as part of a large tumor

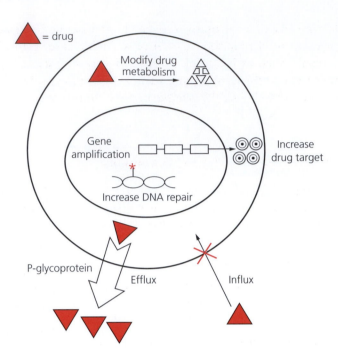

Figure 2.13 Mechanisms of drug resistance. Based on a diagram printed in *Annu. Rev. Med.* 53, Copyright (2002) by Annual Reviews (http://www.annualreviews.org/).

mass, will receive different doses of treatment depending on the location of individual cells within the mass. Cells deep within the tumor and therefore furthest from the blood supply will receive lower doses than cells on the surface of the tumor. Cells within the same tumor may have acquired different mutations and some cells may have become resistant to the drug.

Anticancer drugs impose a strong force for the selection of cells that can acquire drug resistance. There are several mechanisms that a cancer cell may utilize to become resistant to chemotherapy (Figure 2.13). Cells may become resistant by increasing the efflux of the drug, decreasing the intake of the drug, increasing the number of target molecules within the cell, or altering drug metabolism or DNA repair processes. Increasing the efflux of a drug is regulated at the cell surface. There is a family of ATP-dependent transporters that are involved in the movement of nutrients and other molecules across membranes. The multi-drug resistance gene (*MDR1*) codes for one member of this family called P-glycoprotein (P-gp) or the multi-drug transporter. This protein, normally a chloride ion efflux pump, can bind a variety of chemotherapeutic drugs including doxorubicin, vinblastine, and taxol. Upon binding, ATP is hydrolyzed and causes a conformational change of P-gp. As a result, the drug is released extracellularly. The transporter can be recycled by a second hydrolysis of ATP and continue to increase the efflux of the drug. Some drugs utilize specific transporters to enter cells. Mutations in these receptors may render them non-functional and decrease influx of the drug. Resistance to methotrexate commonly occurs by mutation of the folate transporter. An increase in the number of drug target molecules by gene amplification is another means of developing resistance against methotrexate. The *DHFR* gene is amplified in some cancer cells. An increase in the efficiency of DNA repair, such as increased alkyltransferase activity, can give rise to resistance from alkylating agents such as doxorubicin. Levels of this enzyme are found to be highly variable in different tumors.

CHAPTER HIGHLIGHTS—REFRESH YOUR MEMORY

- In simplistic terms, a gene consists of a regulatory region and a coding region. Mutations in the former may alter gene expression while mutations in the latter may affect the gene product.

- Most carcinogens are mutagens.

- Several types of mutations include: base substitutions (transitions and transversions), frameshift mutations (insertions or deletions), and chromosomal translocations.

- Mutations in the promoter region of a gene may alter its regulation.

- Mutations in the coding region of a gene may alter the function of the gene product.

- Carcinogens include radiation, chemicals, and infectious pathogens.

- Radiation can damage DNA directly or indirectly through the formation of reactive oxygen species (ROS).

- Three intermediate ROS formed from the radiolysis of water are the hydroxyl radical, hydrogen peroxide, and the superoxide radical.

- The hydroxyl radical is one of the most reactive substances.

- Many carcinogens need to be metabolized to form an ultimate carcinogen that covalently binds to DNA.

- Many chemical carcinogens add functional groups covalently to DNA.

- Both viruses and bacteria have been classified as carcinogens for specific cancers.

- One-step repair, nucleotide excision repair, base excision repair, mismatch repair, and recombinational repair are five systems for repairing damaged DNA.

- Patients with xeroderma pigmentosum have an inherited defect in NER and have a 1000-fold increased risk of skin cancer.

- Many patients with hereditary non-polyposis colorectal cancer (HNPCC) have an inherited defect in mismatch repair.

- The major types of chemotherapies are:

  alkylating agents—two examples are clorambucil and cisplatin;
  antimetabolites—two examples are 5-FU and methotrexate;
  organic drugs—two examples are vincristine and vinblastine.

- The development of drug resistance is a major problem for chemotherapy.

ACTIVITY

1. Make a list of five carcinogens and the mutations they cause. Describe the method of DNA repair used to correct each type of mutation.

FURTHER READING

Chabner, B.A. and Longo, D.L. (2001) *Cancer chemotherapy and biotherapy—principles and practice*, 3rd edn. Lippincott Williams and Wilkins, Philadelphia, PA.

David, S.S., O'Shea, V.L., and Kundu, S. (2007) Base excision repair of oxidative DNA damage. *Nature* **447**: 941–950.

Gottesman, M.M. (2002) Mechanisms of cancer drug resistance. *Annu. Rev. Med.* **53**: 615–627.

Hecht, S.S. (2003) Tobacco carcinogens, their biomarkers and tobacco-induced cancer. *Nature Rev. Cancer* **3**: 733–737.

Hoeijmakers, J.H.J. (2001) Genome maintenance mechanisms for preventing cancer. *Nature* **411**: 366–374.

Ichihashi, M., Ueda, M., Budiyanto, A., Bito, T., Oka, M., Fukunaga, M., Tsuru, K., and Horikawa, T. (2003) UV-induced skin damage. *Toxicology* **189**, 21–39.

Lane, N. (2002) *Oxygen—the molecule that made the world*. Oxford University Press, Oxford.

Lax, A.J. and Thomas, W. (2002) How bacteria could cause cancer: one step at a time. *Trends Microbiol.* **10**: 293–299.

Manning, C.B., Vallyathan,V., and Mossman, B.T. (2002) Diseases caused by asbestos: mechanisms of injury and disease development. *Int. Immunopathol.* **2**: 191–200.

Pfeifer, G.P., You, Y.-H., and Besaratinia, A. (2005) Mutations induced by ultraviolet light. *Mutation Res./Fund. Mol. Mech. Mutagenesis* **571**: 19–31.

Williams, G.M. and Jeffrey, A.M. (2000) Oxidative DNA damage: endogenous and chemically induced. *Regulatory Toxicol. Pharmacol.* **32**: 283–292.

■ SELECTED SPECIAL TOPICS

Alexandrov, K., Cascorbi, I., Rojas, M., Bouvier, G., Kriek, E. and Bartsch, H. (2002) CYP1A1 and GSTM1 genotypes affect benzo[a]pyrene DNA adducts in smokers' lung: comparison with aromatic/hydrophobic adduct formation. *Carcinogenesis* **23**: 1969–1977.

Al-Tassan, N., Chmiel, N.H., Maynard, J., Fleming, N., Livingston, A.L., Williams, G.T., Hodges, A.K., Davies, D.R., David, S.S., Sampson, J.R., and Cheadle, J.P. (2002) Inherited variants of MYH associated with somatic G:C→T:A mutations in colorectal tumors. *Nature Genet.* **30**: 227–232.

Davies, H., Bignell, G.R., Cox, C., Stephens, P., Edkins, S., Clegg, S., Teague, J., Woffendin, H., Garnett, M.J., and Bottomley, W. (2002) Mutations of the *BRAF* gene in human cancer. *Nature* **417**: 949–954.

Dogan, A.U., Baris, Y.I., Dogan, M., Emri, S., Steele, I., Elmishad, A.G., and Carbone, M. (2006) Genetic predisposition to fiber carcinogenesis causes a mesothelioma epidemic in Turkey. *Cancer Res.* **66**: 5063–5068.

Preston, D.L., Shimizu, Y., Pierce, D.A., Suyama, A., and Mabuchi, K. (2003) Studies of mortality of atomic bomb survivors. Report 13: solid cancer and noncancer disease mortality; 1950–1997. *Radiat. Res.* **160**: 381–407.

Smith, C.J., Perfetti, T.A., Garg, R., and Hansch, C. (2003) IARC carcinogens reported in cigarette mainstream smoke and their calculated log P values. *Food Chem. Toxicol.* **41**: 807–817.

Whitmore, S.E., Morison, W.L., Potten, C.S., and Chadwick, C. (2001) Tanning salon exposure and molecular alterations. *J. Am. Acad. Dermatol.* **44**: 775–780.

Chapter 3

Regulation of gene expression

Introduction

Cancer is a disease of the genome at the cellular level that may be manifested by alterations in gene expression. In this chapter we will review the molecular components involved in transcriptional regulation. As mentioned in Chapter 2, mutations in the promoter region of genes can alter the regulation of gene expression and lead to carcinogenesis. More recently, an additional mechanism of regulating gene expression called epigenetics (Greek for 'upon' the genome) has been proposed to be important for carcinogenesis. It involves alterations in inheritable information encoded by modifications of the genome and chromatin components. The structure of a gene within the context of chromatin is described below in order to elucidate how gene and chromatin structure affects gene expression. Note also that in this chapter there is a focus on DNA–protein interactions in transcriptional regulation, chromatin configuration, and telomere extension.

3.1 Transcription factors and transcriptional regulation

Transcription factors are proteins that bind to gene promoters and regulate transcription. They contain a set of independent protein modules or domains, each having a specific role important for the function of transcription factors. They include DNA-binding domains, transcriptional activation domains, dimerization domains, and ligand-binding domains.

PAUSE AND THINK

To illustrate how a domain works, let us look at an analogy in which an electrical plug represents a domain. There are many different household appliances with vastly different functions, such as a toaster, an iron, and a television. However, each appliance contains a plug that has a function independent of the rest of the appliance. It has a specific conformation that fits into an electrical socket and conducts electricity to power the appliance. A DNA-binding domain is that part of the transcription factor whose function is to recognize specific DNA promoter sequences and bind DNA. There is some variety in the structure of a domain in the same way that there are US, UK, and Continental European plugs.

Four common types of DNA-binding domains are the helix-turn-helix motif, the leucine zipper motif, the helix-loop-helix motif, and the zinc finger motif. These domains are characteristic protein conformations that enable a transcription factor to bind DNA. It is the conformation of these protein domains that facilitates binding to DNA. Take the helix-turn-helix and zinc finger domains as examples. The amino acid side-chains of the alpha helix lie in the major groove of the DNA helix and hydrogen bond to specific DNA base pairs. The zinc finger domain (approximately 30 amino acids long; Figure 3.1a) is configured around a zinc atom that links two cysteines and two histidines (shown in red) (or two cysteines and two cysteines). It consists of a simple $\beta\beta\alpha$ fold (Figure 3.1b). The side-chains of specific amino acids recognize a specific DNA sequence (about five nucleotide pairs). Transactivation domains function by binding to other components of the transcriptional apparatus in order to induce transcription by RNA polymerase, the main enzyme required for transcription. Some transcription factors work in pairs or dimers and require a dimerization domain which facilitates protein–protein interactions between them. Interactions between transcription factors are a common theme in transcriptional regulation. Some transcription factors

(a)

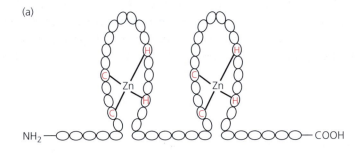

(b)

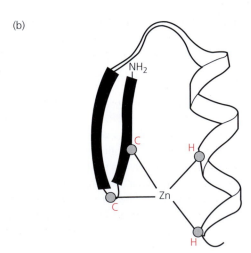

Figure 3.1 The zinc finger DNA-binding domain: (a) primary and (b) secondary structure.

only function upon binding of a ligand and therefore require a ligand-binding domain (this is analogous to the space for a coin in a pinball machine). The activity of a transcription factor can be regulated by several means: synthesis in particular cell types only, covalent modification such as phosphorylation, ligand binding, cell localization, and/or if dimeric, by exchange of partner proteins.

As we will see in the coming chapters, many oncogenic signaling pathways leading to uncontrolled growth, evasion of apoptosis, or aberrant differentiation converge on a single transcription factor that regulates a set of genes to produce a transformed phenotype. Thus, misregulation of a single transcription factor can cause cancer.

Many of the key points of transcriptional regulation can be demonstrated by two examples: the AP-1 transcription factor family and the steroid hormone receptors. The AP-1 transcription factor is important for the processes of growth, differentiation, and death and therefore plays a role in carcinogenesis. AP-1 binds either to the 12-O-tetradecanoylphorbol-13-acetate (TPA) response element or the cAMP response element in the promoter region of their target genes.

The AP-1 transcription factor is actually composed of two components and can be produced by dimers of proteins from the Jun and Fos families (Jun, Jun B, Jun D, Fos, Fos B, FRA1, and FRA 2) (Figure 3.3). Eighteen possible combinations are possible. Both Jun and Fos members contain a basic leucine zipper dimerization domain. Because the processes of growth, differentiation, and apoptosis need to be carefully regulated, AP-1 is itself

HOW DO WE KNOW THAT?

Experimental methods used to examine transcription factor binding

The interactions of transcription factors and their DNA response elements can be examined by several methods of molecular biology. These protein–DNA interactions are often first detected by gel/band shift assays (also called electrophoretic mobility shift assays or EMSAs). This assay involves the incubation of a protein, usually within a cell or nuclear extract, with a labeled DNA fragment containing the promoter sequences of interest. The products of the incubation reaction are analyzed on a non-denaturing polyacrylamide gel. DNA that has bound protein will be observed as a band that has migrated more slowly (been retarded) than unbound DNA (Figure 3.2a). Competition experiments that use irrelevant DNA fragments or known irrelevant proteins can be used to establish specificity.

Another technique that is used to examine protein–DNA interactions is DNase footprinting. DNase, an enzyme that cleaves DNA, is used to probe a promoter region. Protein bound to a DNA fragment will protect the DNA from DNase cleavage. The DNA is end-labeled and, after enzymatic treatment, is analyzed using gel electrophoresis and autoradiography. Areas of DNA that have been protected by protein binding will result in a clear region referred to as a 'footprint' (Figure 3.2b).

A third method of investigating transcription is to construct deletions or point mutations in the promoter fragment, clone them into a reporter plasmid (e.g. luciferase, whose activity can easily be detected), and examine the effects of the mutations upon transfection into cells in culture or using in vitro transcription assays (Figure 3.2c). Deletion or mutation of a promoter region that is important for transcription is indicated by a decrease in transcription.

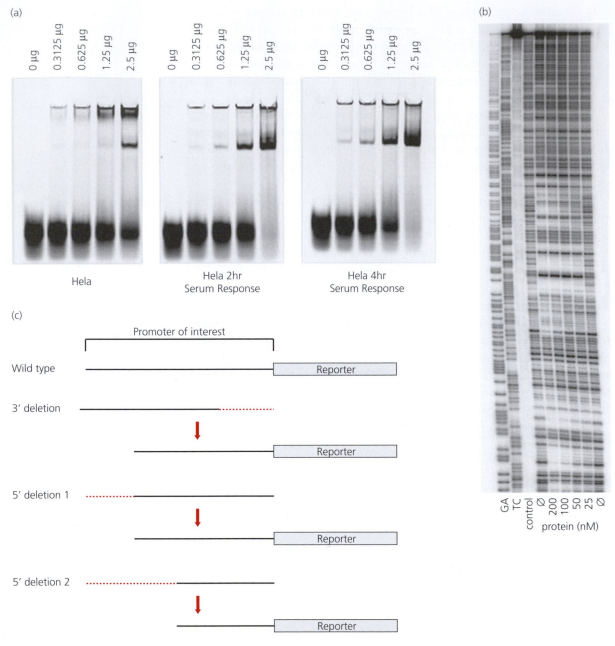

Figure 3.2 Methods used to examine transcription factor binding. (a) EMSA was used to visualize the changes in AP-1 binding following different treatments of HeLa cells: Hela (control), Hela 2hr serum response, and Hela 4hr serum response nuclear extracts were serially diluted and assayed using an infrared dye (IRDyeR700) end-labeled DNA fragment containing the AP-1 response element. Gel electrophoresis and imaging followed. Courtesy of LI-COR Biosciences. (b). A sample DNase footprinting autoradiograph. Courtesy of George P. Munson. (c) A schematic diagram of possible mutant promoter constructs linked to a reporter gene to be used for promoter analysis. The effects of promoter sequence alterations may be indicated by changes in transcriptional activity. The constructs are transfected into cells and reporter enzyme activity is used as an indicator of transcriptional activity.

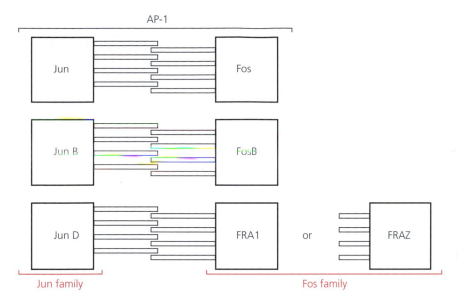

Figure 3.3 Members of the Jun and Fos transcription factor family.

activated in response to specific signals such as growth factors, ROS, and radiation. The specific combination of dimers influences the biological response. The antagonism displayed between Jun and Jun B with regard to cell proliferation in some cell types supports this: Jun acts as a positive regulator of proliferation while Jun B acts as a negative regulator in the presence of Jun.

Both the Fos and Jun family of transcription factors that make up the AP-1 complex play a role in tumorigenesis (see references in Milde-Langosch, 2005). Since TPA is a tumor promoter and the AP-1 complex binds to the TPA response element, an association of AP-1 with carcinogenesis was implicated early after this property was characterized. The first members of AP-1 identified, c-jun and c-Fos, were able to transform normal cells in culture to cancer cells and are frequently over-expressed in tumor cells.

Steroid hormones are lipid-soluble signaling molecules that exert their effects by regulating the transcription of sets of genes via specific receptors (Table 3.1). The superfamily of steroid hormone receptors act as ligand-dependent transcription factors. There are currently 48 members of the nuclear receptor family (see the Nuclear Receptor Signaling Atlas web site http://www.nursa.org/). They contain a zinc finger type of DNA-binding domain, a ligand-binding domain for a specific steroid hormone, and a dimerization domain since they activate transcription as a dimer. Each domain functions independently and in a manner that is specific for a particular steroid hormone receptor. This feature has been utilized as a molecular tool by scientists in so-called domain swap experiments which produce chimeric receptors. For example if the ligand-binding domain

Table 3.1 Examples of members of the steroid hormone receptor superfamily

Class: steroid receptors	TR/RAR/PPAR/VDR-like receptors
Androgen receptor (AR)	Peroxisome proliferator activated receptor (PPAR)
Estrogen receptor (α/βER)	Retinoic acid receptor (RAR)
Glucocorticoid receptor (GR)	Thyroid hormone receptor (TR)
Mineralocorticoid receptor (MR)	Vitamin D receptor (VDR)
Progesterone (PR)	

of the thyroid hormone receptor is swapped with the ligand-binding domain of the retinoic acid receptor, the newly formed chimeric receptor (Figure 3.4) will retain the DNA-binding domain of the thyroid hormone receptor and will activate thyroid hormone-responsive genes. However, these genes will be activated by retinoic acid via the retinoic acid ligand-binding domain, and not by thyroid hormone. Such experiments clearly demonstrate the functional independence of these domains.

Steroid hormones pass through the cell membrane and bind to their particular intracellular receptors in the cytoplasm (note: some members of the steroid hormone receptor superfamily bind to their ligands in the nucleus). Upon binding, the receptors move into the nucleus and activate transcription of their target genes through specific DNA response elements (see Figure 3.5).

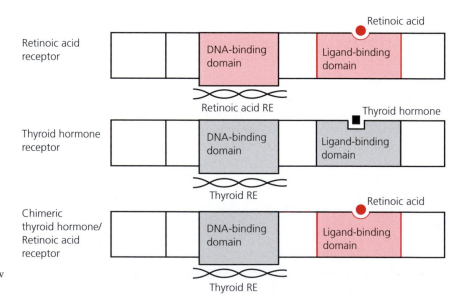

Figure 3.4 A chimeric steroid hormone receptor is shown below its two parental receptors.

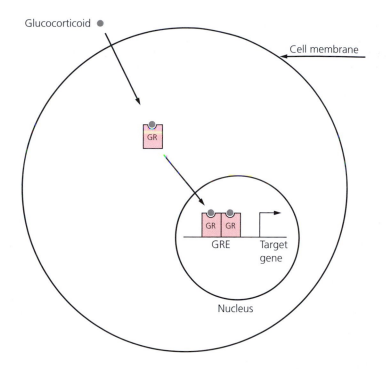

Figure 3.5 Mechanism of action of the glucocorticoid receptor (GR, red) (GRE, glucocorticoid response element).

The retinoic acid receptor (RAR), as a member of the steroid hormone receptor family, acts as a retinoic acid (RA)-dependent transcriptional regulator and is important during differentiation. Retinoic acid is derived from vitamin A. The RAR is constitutively located in the nucleus and acts as a transcriptional repressor in the absence of RA. It binds to the RA response element (RARE) in target genes as a **heterodimer** with another member of the family called RXR. Aberrant forms of RARs are characteristic of several leukemias. As we will see throughout the text, members of the steroid hormone receptor superfamily (e.g. estrogen receptor, vitamin D receptor) play an important role in many different types of cancer.

A little lesson about microRNAs

In addition to protein transcription factors that bind to DNA promoters, specialized small RNA molecules (approximately 22 nucleotides) also regulate transcription. These small non-protein-coding RNAs are called microRNAs (miRNAs). It is conservatively estimated that the human genome contains at least 300 miRNAs and most are located within introns of mRNA transcripts. Each miRNA may be able to repress hundreds of gene targets post-transcriptionally. Therefore miRNAs are abundant and very powerful regulators. They carry out this function in either of two ways: they either hybridize to protein-coding mRNA sequences and induce the RNA-mediated interference (RNAi) pathway which involves cleavage of their mRNA targets or they bind to imperfect complementary sites in the 3′ untranslated regions of their target RNAs and inhibit translation. →

→ MicroRNAs are involved in a diverse set of biological processes including growth, differentiation, and apoptosis. Not surprisingly, mutations and mis-expression of particular miRNAs are associated with cancer and are called **oncomirs**. Recent data have shown that miRNA profiles will be useful for cancer diagnosis and prognosis (Esquela-Kerscher and Slack, 2006; Yanaihara *et al.*, 2006).

3.2 Chromatin structure

Human DNA is present in the nucleus of cells in the form of 46 chromosomes. Chromosomes are made of chromatin: a thread of DNA (60%) plus associated RNA (5%) and protein (35%). It is astonishing to think that the actual length of DNA in the nucleus of a cell is over a meter when fully extended. A high level of packaging (Figure 3.6) is required to neatly organize the DNA to fit into the nucleus of a cell and to allow it to assume necessarily organized conformations for transcription and replication. Both of these processes involve denaturation of the double helix and reading of template strands.

The simplest or primary level of organization of chromatin is the wrapping of DNA around a protein 'spool' and is referred to as the 'beads on a string' array. The beads represent the nucleosome, which contains 147 base pairs (bp) of DNA wrapped 1.7 times around a core of histone proteins. The histone core is an octomer of **histones** containing two copies of histones H2A, H2B, H3, and H4. Each histone contains domains for histone–histone and histone–DNA interactions and NH$_2$-terminal lysine-rich and

PAUSE AND THINK

How would you organize long pieces of thread in a sewing box? Most thread is wrapped around a spool for orderly and easy unwinding. Few people would just leave a disorganized bunch of thread for fear of getting tangles and knots.

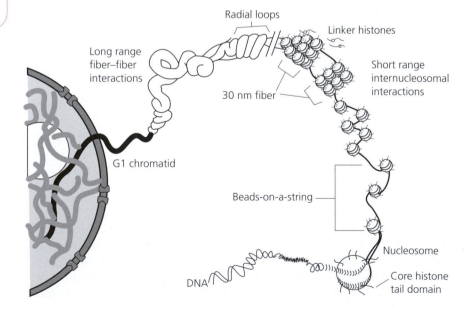

Figure 3.6 Multiple levels of chromatin structure. Reprinted, with permission, from *Annu. Rev. Biophys. Biomolec. Struct.*, 3, p. 362, Copyright 2002 by Annual Reviews (http://www.annualreviews.org).

COOH-terminal 'tail' domains which can be post-translationally modified (e.g. acetylated, methylated, or phosphorylated). Histone H1 is a linker histone and binds to DNA located outside the core. Ten to sixty base pairs of DNA separate the 'beads'. The secondary level of organization is the formation of 30 nm fibers, and these can associate to form a tertiary structure of radial loops.

Chromatin has an important role beyond being a structural scaffold. The degree of compaction or relaxation of chromatin structure can change, and it is this feature that enables it to have a regulatory role in transcription. Information about the memory and inheritance of chromatin conformation is encoded by epigenetic modifications.

3.3 Epigenetic regulation of transcription

Epigenetics refers to inheritable information that is encoded by modifications of the genome and chromatin components. These modifications affect the structure and conformation of chromatin and, consequently, transcriptional regulation. Epigenetic alterations in gene expression do not cause a change in the nucleotide sequence of the DNA and are therefore not mutations. Stable epigenetic switches are important during normal cell differentiation. (Note: it is differential gene expression that makes one cell type different from another.) Two types of epigenetic mechanisms will be discussed below: histone modifications and DNA methylation. Both can be acquired or inherited and both affect transcriptional activity by regulating the access of transcription factors to appropriate nucleotide sequences in gene promoters.

Histone modification

Histone proteins are subject to diverse post-translational modifications such as acetylation, methylation, phosphorylation, and ubiquination. The histone code hypothesis predicts that the pattern of these multiple histone modifications specifies the components and activity of the transcription regulatory molecular machinery. Let us focus on acetylation.

The acetylation pattern of histones alters chromatin structure and affects gene expression (Figure 3.7). Acetylation acts as a docking signal for the recruitment or the repulsion of chromatin-modifying factors. Histone acetyltransferases (HATs; add acetyl groups) and histone deacetylases (HDACs; ◎ remove acetyl groups) are two families of enzymes that produce the pattern. HATs acetylate specific histone-tail lysines and other non-histone proteins, including transcription factors (e.g. E2F and p53). HATs relax chromatin folding by regulating the binding of non-histone proteins and this correlates

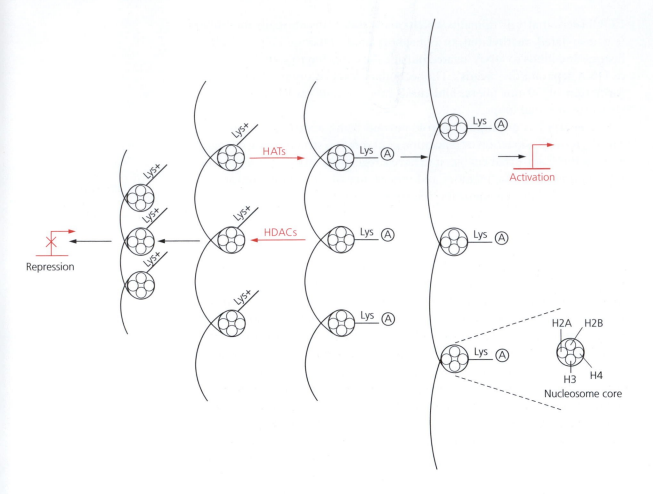

Figure 3.7 Histone acetylation affects gene expression.

PAUSE AND THINK

In general, HATs activate tran-scription and HDACs repress transcription.

with enhanced transcriptional elongation by RNA polymerase III. HDACs remove acetyl groups and restore a positive charge to lysine residues of the histone tails which stabilize chromatin compaction and higher-level packaging. This configuration of chromatin limits the accessibility of transcription factors and results in the repression of transcription.

In addition, transcriptional activators often recruit HATs and other chromatin-remodeling enzymes to the promoter region. The retinoblastoma tumor suppressor protein, mentioned as a 'molecule of fame' in Chapter 1, exerts its effects, in part, by recruiting HDACs to specific gene promoters (see Chapter 5). Thus, a signaling network seems to underlie chromatin modeling.

DNA methylation

Another epigenetic process that affects transcriptional regulation is DNA methylation. DNA methylation is the addition of a methyl group to

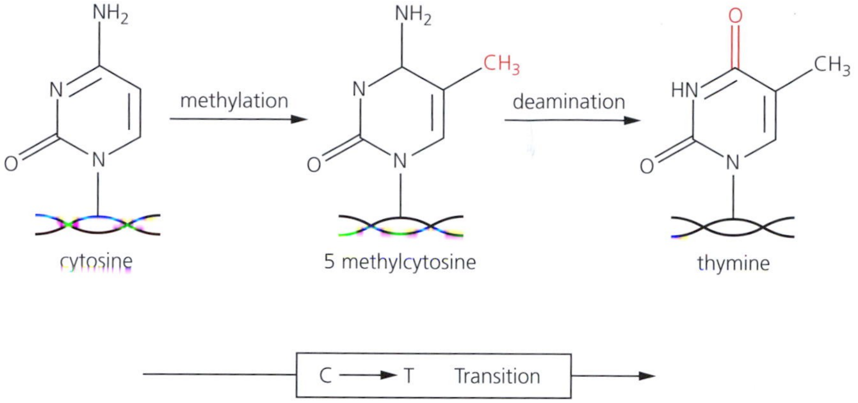

Figure 3.8 Spontaneous deamination of methylcytosine leads to a C→T transition.

position 5 of cytosine. Only 3–4% of all cytosines in DNA are methylated. Methylation only occurs at cytosine nucleotides which are situated 5′ to guanine nucleotides (CpGs). Methylcytosine deaminates spontaneously and results in C→T transitions (Figure 3.8). It is thought that evolution has selected against this dinucleotide due to the high rate of mutation, since CpG is under-represented and unequally distributed in the genome. CpG clusters, called **CpG islands**, are located in the promoter region of 50% of human genes. In general, the CpG islands found in gene promoter regions are not methylated in normal tissues and transcription may occur. Methylated cytosines are found mainly in repetitive sequences and in the CpG islands found in the promoter region of repressed genes such as X-chromosome inactivated genes, imprinted genes, and some tissue-specific genes. In these cases, methylation is a heritable signal that is associated with a compacted chromatin structure and maintains gene silencing.

Enzymes called DNA methyltransferases (DNMTs) mediate the covalent addition of a methyl group from the methyl carrier *S*-adenosyl-methionine cytosine. Three methyltransferases are known: DNMT1, DNMT3a, and DNMT3b. DNMT1 is involved in the conversion of hemi-methylated DNA to fully methylated DNA during replication. This mechanism allows methylation patterns to be inheritable; if only one strand remained methylated the signal would be lost in half of its daughter cells after replication. The other two methyltransferases are mainly involved in *de novo* methyltransferase activity (methylation of new sites).

It has been suggested that the mechanism by which methylation results in silencing is by recruiting methyl binding domain (MBD) proteins, which have been shown to interact with HDACs and chromatin-remodeling enzymes. Therefore, epigenetic regulation of transcription includes cross-talk between methylation, chromatin-remodeling enzymes and histone modification.

3.4 Evidence of a role for epigenetics in carcinogenesis

The fairly recent and still controversial proposal that epigenetic inactivation of genes is as important as the inactivation of genes by mutation during carcinogenesis has recently been put forth. A brief examination of some of the accumulating supporting evidence is described below.

Histone modification and cancer

Altered HAT or HDAC activity has been observed in several cancers. Interestingly, one gene, *EP300*, that codes for a HAT has been found to be mutated in epithelial cancers. Several of the mutations predicted a truncated protein, and inactivation of the second allele was observed in 5/6 cases, suggesting that it functions as a tumor suppressor (Gayther *et al.*, 2000).

Acute promyelocytic leukemia is characterized by a chromosomal translocation that produces a fusion protein called PML–RAR. This novel fusion protein retains the DNA-binding domain and ligand-binding domain of the RAR in addition to PML sequences. PML–RAR recruits HDAC to the promoter region of RA target genes and represses the expression of these genes. The lack of activation of RAR target genes causes the block of differentiation that characterizes the leukemia. Other tumors have also been associated with aberrant recruitment of HDACs.

Methylation and cancer

Cancer-specific changes in DNA methylation have been recognized, and many studies have focused on hypermethylation observed in normally unmethylated CpG islands of gene promoters (see Box 'Analysis of DNA methylation by sodium bisulfate treatment and methylation-specific PCR'). Gene silencing by methylation may be an important mechanism of carcinogenesis whereby critical genes normally involved in tumor suppression may be switched off. Inactivation of gene expression by methylation of the promoter regions of such genes has been observed in cancer cell lines and human tumors. For example, estrogen receptor protein is present in normal ovarian epithelial cells but is frequently lost in ovarian cancer. Hypermethylation of the estrogen receptor-α gene promoter was observed in three out of four human ovarian cell lines that lacked estrogen receptor protein (O'Doherty *et al.*, 2002). This indicates that hypermethylation may be responsible for this phenotype in ovarian tumors. As another example, the breast cancer susceptibility gene, *BRCA1*, is often mutated in a recessive manner in inherited breast cancer. Thus, the loss of function of the gene product suggests that normal BRCA1 acts to suppress breast

PAUSE AND THINK

RAR is a member of which family of transcription factors? See Section 3.1.

cancer. Mutation of *BRCA1* is very rarely observed in non-inherited breast cancer. However, interestingly, hypermethylation is associated with the inactivation of *BRCA1* in non-inherited breast cancer and therefore this may be another way of accomplishing loss of function. These findings support the view that epigenetics may be an additional mechanism for carcinogenesis. Additional examples of some key target genes affected by methylation include the *retinoblastoma* (*Rb*) gene; inhibitor of the cell cycle *p16 INK4a*; pro-apoptotic death-associated protein kinase (*DAPK*); *APC*; and the *estrogen receptor* gene. Evidence also indicates that abnormal methylation occurs in a subset of pre-malignant cells, and it has been suggested that this may 'addict' cells to altered signaling pathways and facilitate subsequent mutational events that provide the cell with a selective advantage and promote tumorigenesis.

Analysis of DNA methylation by sodium bisulfate treatment and methylation-specific PCR

Molecular biology procedures used for standard genetic analysis erase DNA methylation information, and so specialized methods for methylation analysis were developed. Sodium bisulfate treatment of genomic DNA converts unmethylated cytosine residues to uracil by deamination. 5-Methylcytosines are converted to thymine under these same conditions. Treated DNA is no longer complementary and PCR amplification requires specially designed primers. There are several possible designs for PCR amplification primers of the resulting DNA but, most commonly, primers are designed to hybridize specifically with the sodium bisulfate modified sequences. PCR that uses these types of primers is called methylation-specific PCR. Methylation-specific PCR provides information about particular methylation patterns. Analysis of many sites throughout the genome can be collected to produce a methylation profile.

The molecular mechanisms underlying specific methylation events are largely unknown. DNA methylation by itself does not directly repress transcription but requires associated proteins such as histone-modifying enzymes (described above), methyl cytosine-binding proteins, and DNMTs. These proteins collaborate to define the structure of chromatin. In addition to recruiting HDAC (discussed above), PML–RAR has also been shown to recruit methyltransferase resulting in the DNA methylation of a promoter region of a specific gene (Di Croce *et al.*, 2002). The RARβ2 gene has a RARE in its promoter and is one of the target genes of PML–RAR. It has been demonstrated that PML–RAR forms stable complexes with DNMTs at the RARβ2 promoter and that the resulting hypermethylation contributes to carcinogenesis. It has been suggested that DNMTs, in addition to mediating methylation, may act as a platform for the assembly of chromatin-modifying factors (see Pause and Think).

Since not all carcinogens are mutagens, it may be possible that some non-genotoxic carcinogens (agents that do not mutate genes) are epigenetic carcinogens. Hypermethylation has been observed in tumor-sensitive mice treated with phenobarbital, a non-genotoxic carcinogen in rodents (Watson and Goodman, 2002). The data suggest that a disruption to normal methylation patterns is related to tumor susceptibility and that non-genotoxic carcinogens may act via methylation. In addition, nutritional deficiencies (methionine, choline) seem to affect the cellular level of *S*-adenosylmethionine, an important methyl group donor. This suggests that perturbation of methylation can be produced through the diet (see Chapter 11). It has also been suggested that epigenetic gene silencing that is characteristic of normal stem cells and progenitor cells may be 'locked in' during chronic injury and inflammation (see Chapter 8 for stem cells and Chapter 10 for inflammation) and contribute to carcinogenesis. Additional direct evidence is needed to link factors that are necessary for inducing the misregulation of methylation and for inducing carcinogenesis. Or perhaps mutation is really the only culprit responsible for the misregulation of methylation? Mutation of DNA methyltransferases demonstrated in several cancers would lead directly to altered methylation, but this does not account for the specificity of tumor suppressor genes. Inversely, the role of methylation in transformation may be to promote mutation. Methylated cytosine residues have a tendency to deaminate spontaneously causing C→T transitions. This may account for the increased mutation rate observed in methylated CpG islands.

Paradoxically, the genome of a cancer cell overall can have 20–60% less methylation than a normal cell. This global hypomethylation, mainly in the coding region of genes and of repetitive DNA sequences, occurs in the cancer cell at the same time as the hypermethylation of specific genes described above. This results in the activation of genes not normally expressed. Although this phenomenon has not been vigorously studied, one report points to a causal role of DNA hypomethylation in tumor formation (Gaudet *et al.*, 2003). Mice bred to have reduced levels of DNA methyltransferase 1 exhibited genome-wide hypomethylation and developed T-cell lymphomas. Overall, epigenetics and cancer is an area where further research is obviously needed.

3.5 Telomeres and telomerase

One of the hallmarks of cancer cells is that they acquire a limitless replicative potential (see Figure 1.1). Normal cells have an autonomous program that allows for a finite number of replication cycles. This phenomenon is well known in that cells in culture only undergo a certain number of doublings before they stop dividing and enter senescence (permanent growth arrest). Telomeres, repetitive DNA sequences at the ends of chromosomes, have been shown to function as a molecular counter of the cell's replicative potential (see Verdun and Karlseder, 2007 for review). Telomeres protect the ends of chromosomes from digestion by nuclear enzymes and also prevent induction of DNA repair mechanisms that repair double-stranded breaks. Telomeres are composed of several thousand repeats of the sequence TTAGGG bound by a set of specific proteins. One set of interacting telomeric core proteins associates within a complex called the shelterin complex and functions to control telomere length and protect the chromosomal ends. Telomeres shorten by 50–200 bases with each round of DNA replication due to the limits of DNA polymerases during DNA replication (see Box 'A little lesson about DNA replication'). DNA polymerases proceed only in the 5′–3′ direction and require an RNA primer to initiate DNA synthesis. The RNA primers are removed after replication is complete. As a result, the 3′ end of the parental chromosomal DNA is not replicated and thus chromosomes progressively erode during each round of replication (Figure 3.9). When the chromosomes reach a threshold length, cells enter a stable and irreversible state of growth arrest called cellular senescence. If cells bypass this stage due to mutation and telomeres become critically short, chromosomal instability results and apoptosis (or cell transformation discussed below) is induced. Maintaining telomere length in stem cells of renewal tissue (e.g. the basal layer of the epidermis) is important for providing a longer replicative potential. Telomerase, a ribonucleoprotein containing human telomerase reverse transcriptase activity (hTERT) and a human telomerase RNA (hTR) maintain telomere length in certain cell types, such as stem cells. Reverse transcriptases are enzymes that synthesize DNA from RNA—an exception to the central dogma of molecular biology which states that RNA is synthesized from DNA. The hTR contains 11 complementary base pairs to the TTAGGG repeats and acts as a template for the reverse transcriptase to add new repeats (shown in red) to telomeric DNA on the 3′ ends of chromosomes (Figure 3.10).

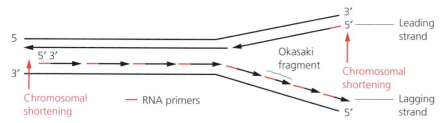

Figure 3.9 Chromosomal shortening after DNA replication.

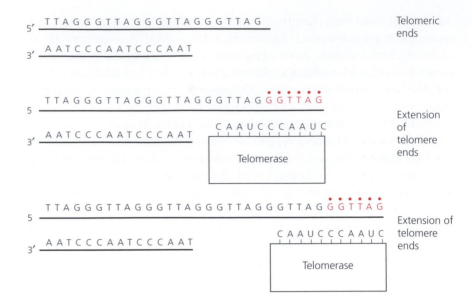

Figure 3.10 Telomere extension by telomerase.

A little lesson about DNA replication . . .

DNA replication proceeds in a semi-conservative manner: Each of the two parental strands acts as a template for the synthesis of a newly replicated strand (Figure 3.11; new DNA strand synthesis is shown in red). Each of the polynucleotide strands that make up the DNA helix has a sense of direction; that is each has a 5′ end and a 3′ end. The two strands are arranged in an antiparallel manner. Since DNA polymerases only work in a 5′–3′ direction each strand is replicated differently as the DNA helix unwinds. For one strand, the leading strand, replication proceeds in a continuous manner from the 5′–3′ end. For the other strand, the lagging strand, replication occurs in a discontinuous manner through the 5′–3′ synthesis of short Okazaki fragments. After removing the RNA primers and filling in the gaps, these fragments are ligated together by the enzyme DNA ligase to form one continuous strand. The requirement of DNA polymerase for a RNA primer and the subsequent removal of this primer causes the strands to shorten at the extreme chromosomal ends during each round of replication.

Figure 3.11 Semiconservative and semidiscontinuous DNA replication.

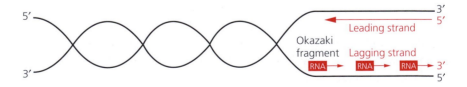

It has been shown *in vitro* that the telomere ends are not linear but rather complicated structures forming t-loops and may form four-stranded DNA conformations called G quadruplexes. It is important that chromosome ends are distinguishable from DNA double-stranded breaks. If they were not, the DNA repair processes would produce chromosomal fusions and other aberrations in an attempt to repair the damage.

Several lines of evidence have linked telomerase activity with cancer. The maintenance of telomeres seems to be important for tumor growth and approximately 90% of tumors accomplish this by upregulating telomerase. Telomerase activity was clearly a distinguishing feature in one classical study where it was detectable in cultured immortal cell lines (98 of 100) and tumor tissue biopsies (90 of 101) but undetectable in cultured normal somatic cells (22) or benign tissue samples (50). It has been found that telomerase, in addition to two oncogenes, is essential in the protocol to transform normal fibroblasts to cancer cells *in vitro*, thus providing a strong link between telomerase and tumorigenesis. Several oncogenes have been demonstrated to regulate the expression of telomerase. For example, the transcription factor c-myc (an oncogene discussed in later chapters) increases the expression of the *hTERT* gene via specific response elements in the promoter region. As mentioned above, if cells bypass the replicative senescence stage due to mutation, telomeres become critically short and chromosomal instability results. This genetic catastrophe may lead to the loss of tumor suppression mechanisms, and evasion of apoptosis. Subsequently, transformed cells emerge. Most transformed cells have upregulated telomerase activity that helps establish cell immortality.

Interestingly, modifications of the telomere hypothesis of senescence described above have recently been suggested and have strong implications for cancer. The telomere hypothesis would predict that telomeres shorten at a constant rate, yet great heterogeneity of replicative lifespan exists among cells within a clonally derived population (i.e. some cells arrest after a few divisions and some after many divisions). It has been reported that telomere shortening is accelerated by oxidative stress (von Zglinicki, 2002), which suggests that the problem of replicating the ends of chromosomes is not the only determining factor for telomere length and replicative potential. Telomeric DNA is repaired less proficiently compared with the bulk of the genome in response to oxidative damage. Unrepaired single-strand breaks accelerate telomere shortening, although the mechanism by which this occurs is unclear. These observations suggest that telomeric DNA may act as a sensor for DNA damage and may explain why there is great heterogeneity in the rate of telomeric shortening among individual cells. Therefore, telomere shortening may act as a tumor suppression mechanism by limiting replicative potential in response to genome damage.

3.6 Epigenomic and histonomic drugs

It is a fairly recent view that epigenetic silencing may be as important as mutation as a mechanism for carcinogenesis. Currently, the concept of reversing somatic mutations is difficult to envisage. However, the concept may be conceivable for epigenetic changes since these are modifications that are potentially reversible. A large number of genes known to play important roles in carcinogenesis have been shown to display hyper-methylation of their promoter regions. Since the increased methylation seen in tumor cells is not observed in normal cells, it provides a tumor-specific target for DNA methylation inhibitors. Similarly, enzymes that alter chromatin structure, such as HDACs that modify histones, provide other molecular targets. As described above, several forms of leukemia and lymphoma are associated with transcriptional repression due to recruitment of HDACs. Reversal of epigenetic silencing is an approach that may lead to new therapeutics.

DNA methylation inhibitors

Drugs that block DNA methylation are predicted to show anti-tumor effects since inactivation of tumor suppressor genes by methylation may be an important mechanism in carcinogenesis. Recall that DNA methylation occurs at position 5 on cytosine. Two 5′-modified analogs of deoxycytidine, 5-azacytidine (5-azaC) and 5-aza-2′-deoxycytidine, have been used to target DNA methyltransferases (Figure 3.12). These drugs ◎ are incorporated into DNA and/or RNA. They covalently link with DNA methyltransferases (DNMT, left red target in Figure 3.12) and sequester its action such that there is significant demethylation after several rounds

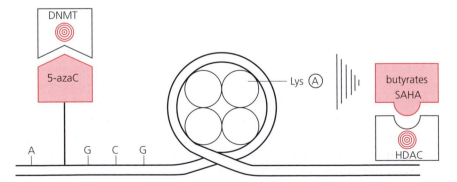

Figure 3.12 Drugs designed to target epigenetic mechanisms (shown in red).

of replication. These drugs may result in DNA instability that parallels antimetabolite chemotherapeutic agents. Another potential hindrance is that aberrant methylation and gene repression return after treatment is stopped, dictating that administration of the drug must be prolonged. Both of these drugs showed anti-leukemic activity in clinical trials but were not successful in solid tumors. 5-azaC (azacitidine; Vidaza™) has been approved by the US Food and Drug Administration (FDA) for treatment of leukemia.

Inhibitors of histone deacetylases

Histone-modifying enzymes have been targeted for the development of new cancer drugs (Figure 3.12). Recall that HDACs generally repress gene transcription and that aberrant recruitment is characteristic of some cancers such as leukemias. Reactivation of silenced genes involved in growth, differentiation, or apoptosis provides the rationale for treating such cancers with inhibitors of HDACs. Several drugs that bind to the catalytic site of HDACs (right red target in Figure 3.12) and block the binding to their substrates (acetylated lysines of histone proteins) are being tested in clinical trials: butyrates, valproic acid, the hydroxamic acid-based compounds SAHA and pyroxamide, and depsipeptide (FR901228). In general, these drugs are well tolerated and many can be administered orally. Alteration of gene expression appears to be selective. Interestingly, many HDAC inhibitors induce p21^{WAF1}, a cyclin-dependent kinase inhibitor important for growth arrest. These drugs seem to have little or no effect on normal cells. Molecular effectiveness was demonstrated by the detection of acetylated histones in particular white blood cells and tumor cells and this was associated with clinical improvement. Butyrates and SAHA (vorinostat; Zolinza™) have been approved for use in the clinic.

3.7 Telomerase inhibitors

The relatively tumor-specific expression of telomerase and its pivotal role in the ability of a cancer cell to divide indefinitely suggest that it may be a valuable molecular target for new cancer therapies. However, several parameters need to be examined when considering the inhibition of telomerase as a cancer therapy. Effectiveness may depend on initial telomere length and thus this should be assessed from tumor biopsies prior to treatment. Also the response may be slow due to the time needed for the telomeres of cancer cells to shorten enough to trigger senescence or apoptosis and long-term treatment may be necessary. In general, long-term treatment increases the probability of drug resistance. Several different strategies, targeting either the RNA component or the catalytic protein component, have been explored in pre-clinical studies. Since telomerase is dependent on its functional RNA molecule, **antisense oligonucleotides** and ribozymes have been popular agents used to target hTR. Antisense oligonucleotides are complementary to part of the target RNA and hybridize by Watson–Crick base pairing. Hybridization can inhibit function directly or trigger degradation by the recruitment of RNases. Hammerhead ribozymes contain antisense sequences for target recognition and an internal endonuclease activity that cleaves the target RNA. Reverse transcriptase inhibitors against the catalytic domain of hTERT and nucleoside analogs have also been investigated. BIBR1532 is a synthetic small molecule inhibitor that directly binds hTERT non-competitively and has been shown to induce telomere-driven senescence. G-quadruplex binding molecules that prevent interaction between the enzyme and substrate have also been developed (e.g. telomestatin). High-throughput screening has identified several natural compounds as telomerase inhibitors, such as components of mistletoe and a green tea catechin. Careful clinical trials are needed to see which, if any, anti-telomerase therapies are effective.

■ CHAPTER HIGHLIGHTS—REFRESH YOUR MEMORY

- Transcription factors recognize **DNA response elements** and are essential for the regulation of gene expression.
- Steroid hormone receptors act as ligand-dependent transcription factors.
- Chromatin has several levels of DNA packaging: the nucleosome, the 30 nm fiber, and radial loops.
- Epigenetic changes also regulate gene expression. These involve modification of nucleotides or chromatin components.
- Histone modification and methylation are two types of epigenetic mechanism.
- HATs add acetyl groups to histones and activate transcription.

- HDACs remove acetyl groups and repress transcription.
- Methylation at CpG islands represses transcription.
- Evidence is accumulating for the role of epigenetic inactivation in carcinogenesis.
- Telomeres play a role in the replicative potential of a cell.
- Telomeres shorten with each round of replication but the rate of shortening may also be influenced by oxidative stress.
- Telomerase is an enzyme that maintains telomere length.
- Telomerase activity is increased in 90% of tumors.
- Strategies for the design of new drugs target DNMTs, HDACs, and telomerase.

■ ACTIVITY

1. Formulate evidence for your view on the statement that epigenetics is as important as mutation for carcinogenesis. Include an examination of epigenetic diseases that lead to an increased risk of cancer (see Feinberg, 2007). Contribute to a class debate on this issue.

2. Look at the evidence supporting the role of oncomirs in cancer. Start with Esquela-Kerscher and Slack (2006) and Yanaihara *et al.* (2006).

■ FURTHER READING

Baylin, S.B. and Herman, J.G. (2000) DNA hypermethylation in tumorigenesis: epigenetics joins genetics. *Trends Genet.* **16**: 168–174.

Baylin, S.B. and Ohm, J.E. (2006) Epigenetic silencing in cancer—a mechanism for early oncogenic pathway addiction? *Nature Rev. Cancer* **6**: 107–116.

Brown, R. and Strathdee, G. (2002) Epigenomics and epigenetic therapy of cancer. *Trends Mol. Med.* **8**(Suppl.): S43–S48.

Esquela-Kerscher, A. and Slack, F.J. (2006) Oncomirs—microRNAs with a role in cancer. *Nature Rev. Cancer* **6**: 259–269.

Esteller, M. and Herman, J.G. (2002) Cancer as an epigenetic disease: DNA methylation and chromatin alterations in human tumors. *J. Pathol.* **196**: 1–7.

Feinberg, A.P. (2007) Phenotypic plasticity and the epigenetics of human disease. *Nature* **447**: 433–440.

Goffin, J. and Eisenhauer, E. (2002) DNA methyltransferase inhibitors—state of the art. *Ann. Oncol.* **13**: 1699–1716.

Herman, J.G. and Baylin, S.B. (2003) Gene silencing in cancer in association with promoter hypermethylation. *New Engl. J. Med.* **349**: 2042–2054.

Jones, P.A. and Baylin, S.B. (2002) The fundamental role of epigenetic events in cancer. *Nature Rev. Genetics* **3**: 415–428.

Kelland, L.R. (2001) Telomerase: biology and phase 1 trials. *Lancet Oncol.* **2**: 95–102.

Laird, P.W. (2003) The power and the promise of DNA methylation markers. *Nature* **3**: 253–266.

Marks, P.A., Richon, V.M., Breslow, R., and Rifkind, R.A. (2001) Histone deacetylase inhibitors as new cancer drugs. *Curr. Opin. Oncol.* **13**: 477–483.

Milde-Langosch, K. (2005) The Fos family of transcription factors and their role in tumourigenesis. *Eur. J. Cancer* **41**: 2449–2461.

Rezler, E.M., Bearss, D.J., and Hurley, L.H. (2002) Telomeres and telomerases as drug targets. *Current Opin. Pharmacol.* **2**: 415–423.

Schreiber, S.L. and Bernstein, B.E. (2002) Signaling network model of chromatin. *Cell* **111**: 771–778.

Shaulian, E. and Karin, M. (2002) AP-1 as a regulator of cell life and death. *Nature Cell Biol.* **4**: E131–E136.

Verdun, R.E. and Karlseder, J. (2007) Replication and protection of telomers. *Nature* **447**: 924–931.

White, L.K., Wright, W.E., and Shay, J.W. (2001) Telomerase inhibitors. *Trends Biotechnol.* **19**: 114–120.

■ WEB SITES

HDAC inhibitor in clinical trials http://www.methylgene.com
Nuclear Receptor Signaling Atlas http://www.nursa.org/

■ **SELECTED SPECIAL TOPICS**

Di Croce, L., Raker, V.A., Corsaro, M., Fazi, F., Fanelli, M., Faretta, M., Fuks, F., Lo CoCo, F., Kouzarides, T., Nervi, C., Minucci, S., and Pelicci, P.G. (2002) Methyltransferase recruitment and DNA hypermethylation of target promoters by an oncogenic transcription factor. *Science* **295**: 1079–1082.

Gaudet, F., Hodgson, J.G., Eden, A., Jackson-Grusby, L., Dausman, J., Gray, J.W., Leonhardt, H., and Jaenisch, R. (2003) Induction of tumors in mice by genomic hypomethylation. *Science* **300**: 489–492.

Gayther, S.A., Batley, S.J., Linger, L., Bannister, A., Thorpe, K., Chin, S.-F., Daigo, Y., Russell, P., Wilson, A., Sowter, H.M., Delhanty, J.D.A., Ponder, B.A.J, Kouzarides, T., and Caldas, C. (2000) Mutations truncating the EP300 acetylase in human cancers. *Nature Genet.* **24**: 300–303.

O'Doherty, A.M., Church, S.W., Russell, S.E.H., Nelson, J., and Hickey, I. (2002) Methylation status of oestrogen receptor—a gene promoter sequence in human ovarian epithelial cell lines. *Br. J. Cancer* **86**: 282–284.

von Zglinicki, T. (2002) Oxidative stress shortens telomeres. *Trends Biochem. Sci.* **27**: 339–344.

Watson, R.E. and Goodman, J.I. (2002) Effects of phenobarbital on DNA methylation in GC-rich regions of hepatic DNA from mice that exhibit different levels of susceptibility to liver tumorigenesis. *Toxicol. Sci.* **68**: 51–58.

Yanaihara, N., Caplen, N., Bowman, E., Seike, M., Kumamoto, K., Yi, M., Stephens, R.M., Okamoto, A., Yokota, J., Tanaka, T., Calin, G.A., Liu, C.-G., Croce, C.M., and Harris, C.C. (2006) Unique microRNA molecular profiles in lung cancer diagnosis and prognosis. *Cancer Cell* **9**: 189–198.

Chapter 4

Growth factor signaling and oncogenes

Introduction

One of the fundamental characteristics of cells is their ability to self-reproduce. The process of cell division (also known as cell proliferation or cell growth) must be carefully regulated and DNA replication must be precisely coordinated in order to maintain the integrity of the genome for each cell generation. As emphasized earlier in this volume, unregulated growth is a quintessential characteristic of cancer.

An extracellular growth factor stimulates cell growth by transmitting a signal into the cell, and ultimately to the nucleus, to regulate gene expression in order to produce proteins that are essential for cell division. There are four types of proteins involved in the transduction of a growth factor signal: growth factors, growth factor receptors, intracellular signal transducers, and nuclear transcription factors which elicit the mitogenic effect through the regulation of gene expression. Examining the normal mechanism of growth will allow a better understanding of the abnormalities that occur during carcinogenesis.

It is important to identify a common thread in many growth factor signal transduction pathways: many growth factor receptors are tyrosine kinases. All kinases catalyze the transfer of the γ phosphate group from ATP/GTP to hydroxyl groups on a specific amino acid in a target protein. Tyrosine kinases phosphorylate tyrosine residues in target proteins (Figure 4.1). Serine/threonine kinases phosphorylate serine and threonine residues. The addition of the phosphate group, a bulky charged molecule, may serve as a recognition site for new protein–protein interactions and/or may cause a conformational change resulting in the activation or inactivation of an enzymatic activity. Specific examples will be described below.

PAUSE AND THINK

Let us scale up from molecules to people to simplify the consequence of phosphorylation. People often use additions or accessories to increase their recognition by others; tour guides may hold up umbrellas so that their group easily recognizes them. Other additions may alter the activity of a person; the wearing of a heavy backpack may limit one's activity. The addition of phosphate residues can have analogous effects on proteins.

4.1 Epidermal growth factor signaling: an important paradigm

Epidermal growth factor (EGF) and its family of receptor tyrosine kinases serves as an important paradigm for how a signal from an extracellular growth factor can be transduced through a cell, regulate gene expression, and trigger cell proliferation. It is a model that we know a great deal about. The EGF receptor (EGFR; also known as ErbB1 or HER1), is a tyrosine kinase receptor and was the first to be discovered. Three additional family members have since been identified: ErbB2 (HER2), ErbB3 (HER3), and ErbB4 (HER4). ErbB2 does not bind to a known ligand but acts as a co-factor for the other members of the family. As members of the receptor tyrosine kinase receptor family, these receptors contain an extracellular ligand-binding domain, a single transmembrane domain, and a cytoplasmic protein tyrosine kinase domain (Figure 4.1). Getting the signal from a growth factor outside the cell to inside the nucleus where gene expression is regulated requires several steps: binding of the growth factor to the receptor, receptor dimerization, autophosphorylation, activation of intracellular transducers (including the 'star player' RAS) and a cascade of serine/threonine kinases, and regulation of transcription factors for gene expression. Each of the steps involved in the signal transduction pathway of EGF is illustrated in Figure 4.2 and described below. It is essential that you learn this model system because it will enable you to understand many other signal transduction pathways and it will be the basis for illustrating the mechanisms of carcinogenesis. Most interestingly, the components of this pathway have been targets for the design of new cancer therapeutics, some of which will be described at the end of the chapter.

Figure 4.1 Tyrosine kinase receptors phosphorylate tyrosine residues on target proteins. Phosphorylation usually results in a conformational change of the protein target.

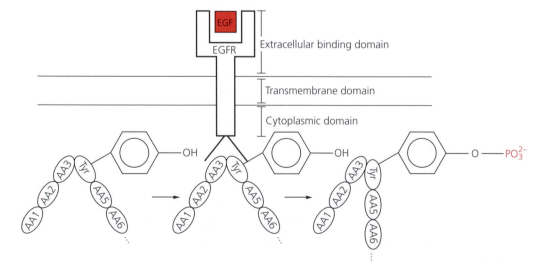

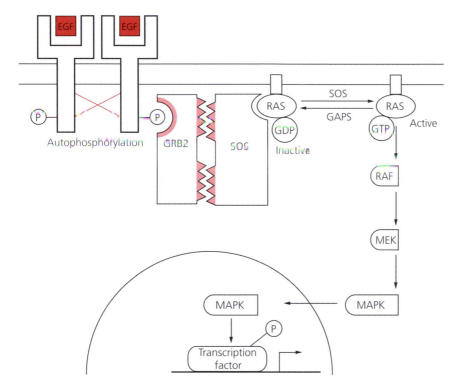

Figure 4.2 The signal transduction pathway of EGF. This pathway is characterized by the sequential steps of growth factor binding, receptor dimerization, autophosphorylation, activation of an intracellular kinase cascade, activation of transcription factors, and regulation of gene expression. Details are described in the text.

Growth factor binding

The first step in the EGF signal transduction pathway is the binding of EGF to its receptor, EGFR. Extracellular domains (I and III) of EGFR form a binding pocket for the ligand.

Dimerization

Dimerization is the process of two EGFR monomers interacting to form a dimer. The mechanism for receptor dimerization as suggested from structural studies is described below and illustrated in Figure 4.3. The binding of one EGF molecule to one receptor causes a conformational change that reveals an extracellular receptor dimerization domain (shown in red). This facilitates the binding to a similar domain in another EGF-bound receptor monomer resulting in a receptor dimer. It is important to note that EGFR can also form heterodimers with other members of the ErbB family. In general, it is assumed that receptors without a ligand are unable to dimerize, although ErbB2 may be an exception and may not have a ligand.

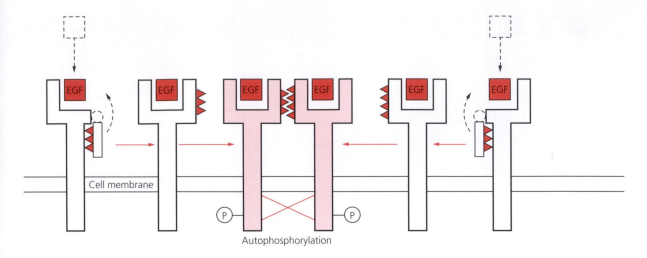

Cell membrane

P

Autophosphorylation

P

Figure 4.3 EGF receptor dimerization. Growth factor binding causes a conformational change that unmasks a dimerization domain required for receptor dimerization.

Autophosphorylation

The close proximity of two receptors, facilitated by dimerization, enables the kinase domain of one receptor of the dimer to phosphorylate the other receptor of the dimer and vice versa (see Plate 1). This intermolecular (between molecules) autophosphorylation on the cytoplasmic domain of the receptors (shown by a red 'X' in Figure 4.2) occurs at tyrosine residues in the activation loop and results in a conformational change. The change in receptor conformation permits access of ATP and substrate to the catalytic kinase domain. Autophosphorylation is also crucial for the recruitment of cytoplasmic proteins, as we will see below. At this stage a signal from outside the cell has been transduced to inside the cell.

Note that activation of the tyrosine kinase receptor needs to be turned off after a particular length of time. Mechanisms for the termination of kinase activity include additional phosphorylation triggering a conformational change that inhibits extracellular ligand binding and kinase activity, dephosphorylation of regulatory phosphorylated tyrosine residues by tyrosine phosphatases, binding of negative regulators (e.g. RALT) to the kinase domain, and receptor endocytosis and degradation. However, recent data suggest that internalization of the receptor may also play a role in the transport of the receptor to the nucleus and the induction of specific genes (see Linggi and Carpenter, 2006).

Translocation of specific proteins to the membrane

Activation of the tyrosine kinase catalytic domain facilitates further phosphorylation. Some phosphorylated tyrosine residues create high-affinity binding sites for proteins that contain Src homology 2 (SH2) domains and act as docking sites for the recruitment of specific intracellular proteins.

SH2 domains (approximately 100 amino acids long) and Src homology 3 (SH3) domains (approximately 50 amino acids long) mediate protein–protein interactions in pathways activated by tyrosine kinases. SH2 domains recognize and bind to distinct amino acid sequences (1–6 residues) C-terminal to the phosphorylated tyrosine residue and SH3 domains recognize and bind to proline and hydrophobic amino acid residues. Both SH2 and SH3 domains are frequently found in the same protein. Proteins mentioned later in the text that contain SH2 and SH3 domains include SRC, ABL, Grb2, and PI3-K.

Grb2, an intracellular protein that contains SH2 and SH3 domains, recognizes the phosphorylated receptor via its SH2 domains and facilitates the recruitment of specific proteins to the membrane via its SH3 domains. Specifically, the two SH3 domains of Grb2 interact with the exchange protein SOS (son of sevenless), which facilitates the activation of the pivotal intracellular transducer RAS. Thus, the activator of RAS is translocated from the cytoplasm to the membrane in response to growth factor stimulation.

RAS activation

The RAS proteins are 'star players' in regulating cell growth because of their position in the signal transduction pathway; they act as a pivotal point for the integration of a growth factor signal initiating from the membrane with a number of crucial signaling pathways that carry the signal through the cytoplasm and into the nucleus. N-, H-, and K-RAS are the three members of the family. They are GTP-binding proteins such that when they are bound to GTP they are activated and when they are bound to GDP they are inactivated. Nucleotide exchange factors, such as SOS mentioned above, catalyze the exchange of GTP for GDP. GTPase activating proteins (GAPs) catalyze the hydrolysis of GTP to GDP to terminate the signal, although RAS proteins possess some intrinsic GTPase activity which allows for self-regulation.

In the EGFR pathway, the protein–protein interactions facilitated by the SH3 domains of Grb2 with the SH3 domains of SOS bring SOS to the membrane where RAS is located, and this results in RAS activation. RAS proteins undergo a series of post-translational modifications that direct their trafficking in the cell. Farnesylation, the addition of the C15 farnesyl isoprenoid lipid to the C-terminal CAAX motif (where C represents cysteine, A represents an aliphatic amino acid, and X represents any amino acid), is one modification that is required for localizing RAS to the cell membrane (Figure 4.4). It is interesting to note that it has recently been demonstrated that endogenous RAS is capable of activating downstream signaling pathways from subcellular membrane compartments (ER and Golgi) upon EGF stimulation (Hingorani and Tuveson, 2003).

> **PAUSE AND THINK**
>
> Remember that a domain is a part of a protein with a specific configuration that has a specific function analogous to an electrical plug (see Chapter 3).

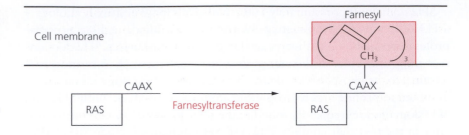

Figure 4.4 Localizing RAS to the cell membrane by farnesylation.

This adds a new dimension to our knowledge since it was previously thought that localization to the plasma membrane was essential for RAS activity. Furthermore, it has been demonstrated that RAS can transform cells from their subcellular compartments as well as from the membrane. These new observations must be considered in the rationale for designing new cancer therapies.

Raf activation

RAS–GTP binds to and contributes to the activation of the serine/ threonine kinase Raf, one of its main effectors. The recruitment of Raf to the cell membrane is necessary for its activation by RAS-GTP. Activated Raf phosphorylates mitogen-activated protein kinase kinase (MAPKK, MEK).

> **A little lesson about the MAP kinase family: MAP kinase kinase kinases, MAP kinase kinases, and MAP kinases**
>
> The nomenclature may seem confusing at first but it is due to the fact that a series of phosphorylation steps is necessary for enzyme activation: a kinase (MAPKKK) phosphorylates another kinase (MAPKK), which itself phosphorylates yet another kinase (MAPK). Raf is a MAPKKK. A unique feature of MAP kinase activation is that it requires both tyrosine and threonine phosphorylation. MAPKK is a dual-specificity kinase that phosphorylates both tyrosine and threonine residues.

The MAP kinase cascade

The activated MAPKKs go on to phosphorylate another family of serine/ threonine kinases, the mitogen-activated protein kinases (MAPKs) (also known as extracellular signal-regulated kinases; ERKs). The MAPKs are a family of serine/threonine kinases that provide the cytoplasmic link between the activated RAS on the plasma membrane and regulation of gene expression, since activated MAPKs can enter the nucleus. The activity of many transcription factors is regulated by phosphorylation and thus MAPKs can affect the activity of transcription factors via phosphorylation.

Although this discussion focuses on MAPK, there are actually three distinct but parallel MAP kinase pathways: MAPK, JNK, and p38. As noted in this section, MAPK is activated by growth factors. JNK and p38 are activated by a various environmental stress signals such as ultraviolet and ionizing radiation. The JNK and p38 pathways usually trigger apoptosis. Thus all three MAPK pathways act as a common mechanism that serves multiple signaling pathways and results in various cellular responses.

Regulation of transcription factors

The AP1 transcription factor is an important target of the MAPK cascade. As a transcription factor, it binds to DNA and regulates the expression of genes involved in growth, differentiation, and death. One mechanism, whereby AP-1 induces cell cycle progression, is by binding to and activating the cyclin D gene, a critical regulator of the cell cycle. AP-1 is not a single protein but rather is made up of the products of two gene families, *jun* and *fos*. These proteins contain basic leucine zipper domains that facilitate their binding as dimers to either the cAMP response element (CRE) or the 12-O-tetradecanoylphorbol-13-acetate (TPA) response element in a target gene. AP-1 activity is induced by two mechanisms. First, direct phosphorylation of members of the Fos family by MAPK affects their DNA-binding activity. Secondly, MAPK phosphorylation and subsequent activation of other transcription factors increases the expression of both *fos* and *jun* genes. As a result, AP1 activity increases and subsequent transcriptional regulation proceeds.

The Myc family of transcription factors (Myc, Max, Mad, Mxi) can dimerize in different ways and lead to distinct biological effects of growth, differentiation, and death. Several seem to be targets of MAPKs. Myc is a short-lived protein that promotes proliferation by regulating the expression of specific target genes. Gene targets of myc include *N-Ras* and *p53*, but the identification of additional targets is the subject of ongoing research. Myc requires the constitutively expressed family member Max to function. Myc and Max form heterodimers via basic helix-loop-helix leucine zipper domains and bind to a regulatory sequence called the E-box in their target genes. Heterodimer formation and DNA binding are crucial for the oncogenic, mitogenic, and apoptotic effects of Myc. Other heterodimers, such as Max and Mad/Mxi, are inhibitory for Myc function. They can also bind to the E-box in gene promoters but they repress transcription. Thus, the Myc family of transcription factors forms a network of interacting basic helix-loop-helix leucine zipper proteins and the identity of the members within a heterodimer determines the biological effect elicited.

Self-test Close this book and try to redraw Figure 4.2. Check your answer. Correct your work. Close the book once more and try again.

PAUSE AND THINK

The three-letter language of molecular terms sounds peculiar at first but with practice will become familiar and allow you to build your molecular vocabulary.

Good! Now let us backtrack to illustrate how you can build levels of complexity on the foundation you have learned. RAS has been noted to be a 'major player' for the integration of a growth factor signal with a number of crucial signaling pathways. In fact, all receptor tyrosine kinases activate RAS. Raf was described above as one effector protein that leads to the activation of the MAPK cascade but there are several other effector proteins of RAS activation. Phosphatidylinositol 3-kinase (PI3K), a lipid kinase, is another effector protein downstream of RAS that can be introduced at this point (see Pause and Think).

Crystal studies have shown that RAS interacts directly with the catalytic structure of PI3K. Production of the second messenger, PIP3, recruits the serine/threonine kinase PDK-1 to the membrane. Akt, another serine/threonine kinase, is also recruited to the membrane where it is phosphorylated and activated by PDK-1. Activated Akt is translocated into the nucleus where it phosphorylates nuclear substrates, including transcription factors. Activated Akt is also involved in anti-apoptotic and survival roles by phosphorylating distinct target proteins.

Self test Draw a diagram of a growth factor signal transduction pathway including two effector proteins of RAS activation. Check your answer with Figure 4.5. Correct your work.

The effect of cell signaling on cell behavior

We have seen above that growth factor signaling can lead to cell proliferation via signaling to the nucleus. In addition, cell signaling can have effects on cell behavior. This is clearly demonstrated by the intracellular tyrosine kinase SRC (the gene *src* is discussed below). In addition to having a role in cell proliferation, SRC plays an important role in the regulation of cell adhesion, invasion, and motility upon EGF receptor activation. SRC is a phosphoprotein which contains SRC homology domains, including a SH2 and SH3 domain. It also contains a negative regulatory domain near the carboxy-terminus. When Tyr530 in this negative regulatory domain is phosphorylated, it binds to the internal SRC SH2 domain and results in an intramolecular association which represses the kinase domain and keeps SRC in an inactive state (Figure 4.6). One way in which SRC can be activated is via receptor tyrosine kinases, such as the EGF receptor. Upon stimulation of the EGF receptor by growth factor, the autophosphorylated receptor can interact with the SH2 domain of SRC, disrupting its negative regulatory intramolecular conformation. The activated kinase phosphorylates a wide range of target proteins, including focal adhesion proteins (e.g. focal adhesion kinase, FAK), adaptor proteins, and transcription factors. The regulation of focal adhesion proteins within the dynamic

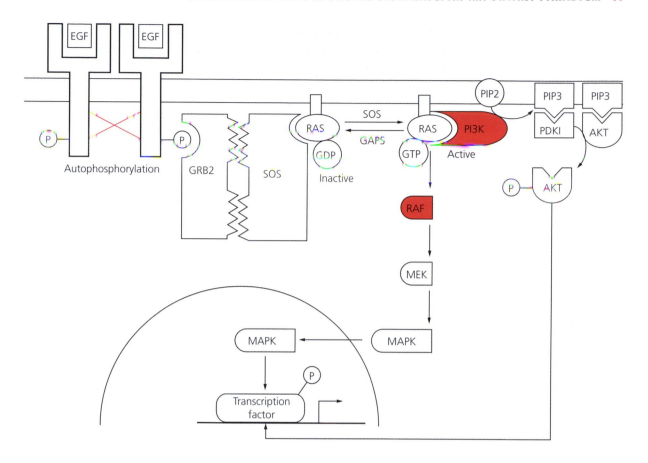

subcellular structures called focal adhesions is particularly important for adhesion and motility. These structures associate with cytoskeletal fibers that ultimately control cell shape and motility. Assembly of focal adhesions facilitates cell adherence while disassembly facilitates motility. Activation of SRC leads to disassembly of focal adhesions and thereby permits increased motility. SRC also regulates cell invasion by inhibiting E-cadherin (see Chapter 9).

Figure 4.5 The EGF signal transduction pathway showing two effectors of RAS (shown in red).

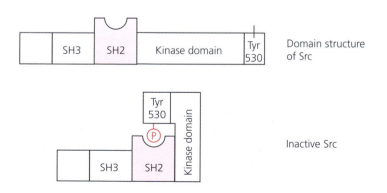

Figure 4.6 The protein domains of SRC and a negative regulatory intramolecular interaction.

Thus, the effects of growth factor cell signaling through tyrosine kinase receptors are indeed manifold, as is illustrated by the many downstream effects that occur upon SRC activation.

4.2 Oncogenes

Cancer arises from mutations in genes that are involved in growth, differentiation, or death. There are two major classifications of mutated genes that contribute to carcinogenesis: oncogenes and tumor suppressor genes. A general description of an oncogene is a mutated gene whose protein product is produced in higher quantities or whose altered product has increased activity and therefore acts in a dominant manner. A mutation in only one allele is sufficient for an effect. Tumor suppressor genes (see Chapter 6), on the other hand, are genes in which the mutation has caused a loss of function, and therefore most are recessive in nature because both alleles must be mutated. More than 100 oncogenes and at least 15 tumor suppressor genes have been identified.

Studies of retroviruses

Studies of retroviruses have led to great insights into cancer biology and have become the foundation of our knowledge of oncogenes. Several landmark experiments were performed based on the early observation that viruses could cause cancer in animals and the results pointed to the discovery of oncogenes. In 1911, Peyton Rous prepared a cell-free filtrate from a chicken sarcoma and demonstrated that he could induce sarcomas in healthy chickens with this filtrate. The causative agent was identified as the Rous Sarcoma Virus. Many decades later, oncogenic transformation by this virus was found to be due to an 'extra' gene contained in its genome that was not required for viral replication. The first so-called 'oncogene' was identified as *v-src* (pronounced 'v sark'). The oncogene product was characterized as a 60 kDa intracellular tyrosine kinase.

A LEADER IN THE FIELD . . . of oncogenes: Joan Brugge

Joan Brugge has been a personal influence in my own career. Although she was never one of my official mentors, she created an extremely encouraging atmosphere at the State University of New York at Stony Brook while I was carrying out my PhD research. Her style in carrying out research was always natural, enthusiastic, and genuinely inquisitive. She is a model scientist. Joan's own motivation for carrying out cancer research stemmed from the loss of a family member to cancer. Joan made great strides early in her career. ➔

→ Working with Ray Erikson at the University of Colorado during her post-doctoral tenure, she carried out pioneering work on the first retroviral oncogene product, the SRC protein.

Joan received her BA in biology from Northwestern University and her PhD in virology from Baylor College of Medicine. In addition to the State University of New York at Stony Brook, she was on the faculty at the University of Pennsylvania and is currently Acting Chair of the Department of Cell Biology at Harvard Medical School. In between her academic appointments she was the Scientific Director of ARIAD Pharmaceuticals, Inc. in Cambridge, MA. Joan has recently been awarded a Research Professorship from the American Cancer Society, the Society's most prestigious research award, for her significant contributions to cancer research. She is currently investigating the initiation and progression of breast cancer using three-dimensional cellular models.

In 1976, a startling discovery was made. Bishop and Varmus found that there was a gene with a homologous sequence to *v-src* in uninfected chickens. Moreover, upon further investigation this gene could be found in organisms from fruitflies to humans. Following further examination, a fundamental principle of cancer biology was revealed: almost all known oncogenes are altered forms of normal genes or proto-oncogenes.

● Exception: some protein products of DNA tumor viruses behave like oncogenes but are not viral versions of cellular oncogenes. They act by blocking the activity of tumor suppressor proteins. See Chapters 6 and 10.

The name proto-oncogene is sometimes used in cancer biology to distinguish the normal cellular (c) gene (e.g. *c-src*) from the altered form transduced by retroviruses (v) (e.g. *v src*). The *v-src* sequence lacks the carboxy-terminal negative regulatory domain present in *c-src* and has point mutations throughout the gene.

A LEADER IN THE FIELD . . . of oncogenes: Harold Varmus

Harold Varmus, along with J. M. Bishop, received the Nobel Prize in Physiology or Medicine in 1989 for studies carried out at the University of California, San Francisco, that laid down the foundation for the role of mutations in carcinogenesis. They discovered that some genes of cancer-causing viruses were mutated forms of normal cellular genes. As we see in this chapter, this was the birth of the concept of proto-oncogenes and of the molecular biology of cancer.

Harold Varmus is a native of Long Island, NY (like myself). He obtained a Master's Degree in English from Harvard University and is a graduate of Columbia University's College of Physicians and Surgeons. →

→ Varmus was named by President Clinton to serve as the Director of the National Institutes of Health, a position he marked with many advancements during his 6 years' service. He has acted as an advisor to the Federal Government and as a consultant for several pharmaceutical companies and academic institutions. He is currently the President and Chief Executive Officer of Memorial Sloan-Kettering Cancer Center in New York City. His current research includes the development of mouse models for human cancer.

At this point a short review of the retroviral life cycle is necessary. The life cycle of retroviruses brands them as intracellular parasites in that they rely on their host cell for energy and to synthesize viral proteins. After injecting their infectious nucleic acid (RNA) into a host cell, the viral RNA is first reverse transcribed into DNA. This provirus DNA is integrated randomly into the host chromosome, where it will be replicated, transcribed, and translated as host DNA. The translation of viral RNA then produces viral proteins for the synthesis of new viral particles. During evolution, the virus can acquire fragments of genes from the host at integration sites and this process may result in the creation of oncogenes. The Rous Sarcoma Virus acquired a truncated form of *c-src*. Alternatively, and depending on the integration site, viral DNA may be translated as a fusion protein in conjunction with cellular DNA resulting in a novel fusion protein, or host genes may fall under the regulation of viral regulatory sequences. The resulting disruptions to host gene expression are other mechanisms of virus-induced oncogenesis. This knowledge aids our general understanding of the mechanisms of carcinogenesis, because although viruses are not the major cause of human cancers, the mechanism of oncogenic activation of proto-oncogenes is similar. For example, chromosomal translocations may have the same consequence as the integration of a virus into a host chromosome; a crucial gene may come under the influence of novel regulatory sequences and result in abnormal quantities of the gene product. The new gene configuration may serve as an oncogene.

It is important to become familiar with examples of oncogenes to bolster the lesson learned from viral studies: almost all known oncogenes are altered forms of normal genes.

There are examples of oncogenes for every type of protein involved in a growth factor signal transduction pathway. Several examples are described below.

Growth factors

The first evidence for the role of proto-oncogenes came from analysis of the viral oncogene *v-sis*. Its protein product was cytoplasmic and was found to be a truncated version of a growth factor normally secreted by platelets, called platelet-derived growth factor (PDGF). Thus, the identity of the product of the proto-oncogene or cellular gene *c-sis*, is PDGF. It is a component of a wound response and its normal role is to stimulate epithelial cells around the wound edge to proliferate and repair the damage. The significance of the oncogenic form may be its aberrant location (cytoplasmic rather than secreted) and the subsequent activation of the PDGF signal pathway at inappropriate times (e.g. other than in response to a wound), leading to unregulated growth.

Growth factor receptors

The oncogene *v-erbB* was originally identified from (and named after) the avian erythroblastosis leukemia virus. It is a truncated form of the epidermal growth factor receptor whereby the extracellular domain is deleted. Thus, the identity of the product of the proto-oncogene or cellular gene *c-erbB*, is EGFR. The mutated receptor triggers cell division in the absence of EGF. Point mutations that accomplish the same effect of interfering with growth factor binding and inducing constitutive activation have been identified in human cancers. Increasing the amount of normal *c-erbB* product by gene amplification is another mechanism that contributes to carcinogenesis, particularly breast cancer. Gene amplification involves multiple duplications of a DNA sequence due to errors at DNA replication forks.

The proto-oncogene *ret*, another growth factor tyrosine kinase receptor, heterodimerizes with cell-surface receptors GFR-α1–4 in order to transduce the signal for glial-derived neurotrophic factor (GDNF). It plays an important role in kidney development and neuronal differentiation. Papillary thyroid carcinoma cells often carry somatic chromosomal re-arrangements involving the amino-terminal parts of numerous genes and the sequences of *ret* that code for the tyrosine kinase domain. The fusion protein products display kinase activity that is independent of GDNF signaling.

Germline mutations are associated with three familial tumor syndromes: multiple endocrine neoplasia 2A (MEN2A), MEN2B, and familial medullary thyroid carcinoma. The mutations that have been identified illustrate different mechanisms for oncogenic activation. Almost all MEN2A patients have mutations in conserved extracellular cysteines. Resulting intermolecular disulfide bonds cause constitutive Ret dimerization and aberrant activation. In MEN2B patients, oncogenic activation is achieved by altering the substrate-binding pocket of the tyrosine kinase domain. A conserved Met is characteristic of the substrate-binding domain of receptor tyrosine kinases whereby Thr is conserved for cytoplasmic tyrosine kinases. The characteristic mutation of MEN2B is a substitution mutation, whereby Thr replaces this conserved Met residue (Met918Thr). This results in altered substrate access leading to increased kinase activity and altered substrate specificity that is characteristic of cytoplasmic tyrosine

PAUSE AND THINK

What types of genes are usually involved in inherited predispositions to cancer? Although tumor suppressor genes are most often involved, here we see an unusual example of an oncogene (*ret*) playing a role in cancer predisposition.

kinases instead of receptor tyrosine kinases. Thus, the signal transduction pathways are highly disrupted.

Oncogenic activation of receptor tyrosine kinases occurs through specific mutations that lead to constitutive ('always on') tyrosine activation or dimerization.

Intracellular signal transducers

The oncogenic activation of *ras* is observed in about 30% of human tumors. The majority of mutations are located in codons 12, 13, and 61. The consequence of each of these mutations is a loss of GTPase activity of the RAS protein, normally required to return active RAS–GTP to inactive RAS–GDP. The effect is constitutive activation of RAS protein, even in the absence of mitogens. Some specific mutations in the *ras* gene are characteristic for specific cancers. A point mutation within codon 12 that results in the substitution of valine (GTC) for glycine (GGC) is characteristic of bladder carcinoma, while substitution of serine (AGC) is common in lung cancer.

HOW DO WE KNOW THAT?

Transformation assays and mutational analysis

The early classical paper by Reddy *et al.* (1982) illustrates fundamental experimental methods that were used to identify oncogenes and their genetic alterations. The ability of the *ras* oncogene (identified in a 6.6 *Bam*H1 fragment of T24 DNA) to transform cells was demonstrated in a prototypical (original) *in vitro* cell transformation assay, Figure 4.7a (see Section 1.2). This assay is based on the characteristic that cancer cells grow as foci against a monolayer of normal cells. To identify a smaller fragment of the gene that contained the genetic alteration, a series of deletion mutants were transfected into NIH3T3 cells and assayed for formation of foci (transforming activity is indicated by a +/− sign next to each deletion construct shown in

Figure 1 of Reddy *et al.* (1982)). The research team then used comparative sequence analysis of the small fragment identified by deletion analysis to identify a single point mutation within the small fragment in human bladder carcinoma cells. The method of sequence analysis was according to the procedures of Maxam and Gilbert (see Figure 4.7).

In vivo experiments supported the role of the *ras* oncogenes in carcinogenesis. Cells transfected with a plasmid capable of expressing high levels of *c-ras* showed the ability to form tumors in mice (Chang *et al.*, 1982) and a *ras* knock-out mouse exhibited decreased tumor formation during skin carcinogenesis (Ise *et al.*, 2000).

PAUSE AND THINK

Classify each type of evidence above according to the 'show it', 'block it', 'move it' criteria discussed in Section 1.2.

Genes that code for cytoplasmic tyrosine kinases such as SRC, serine/threonine kinases such as RAF and MAPK, and nuclear kinases such as ABL, can also undergo oncogenic activation. As discussed above, intramolecular associations normally regulate c-SRC kinase activity; the SRC SH2 domain binds a carboxy-terminal phosphorylated tyrosine residue (Tyr530) and results in a conformation that blocks the SRC kinase active site. Repression of SRC kinase activity can be relieved by dephosphorylation of Tyr530, or by the binding of the SH2 domain to specific activated

(a) Cell transformation assay

(b) Maxam–Gilbert sequencing

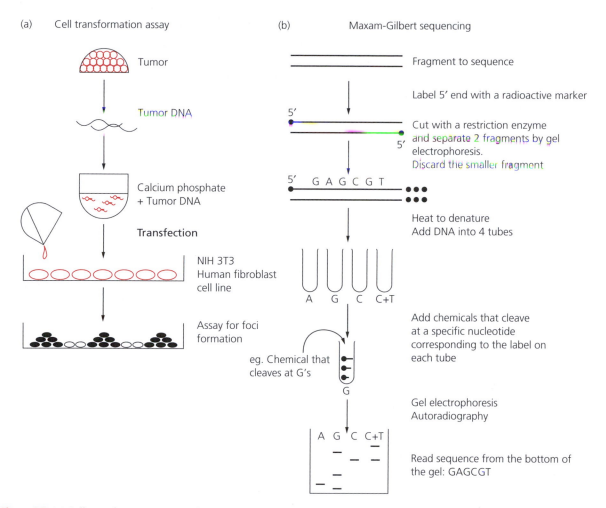

Figure 4.7 (a) Cell transformation assay, (b) DNA sequencing by the Maxum–Gilbert method. Chemicals are used to cleave an end-labeled DNA segment at specific nucleotides and fragments are analyzed by gel electrophoresis and autoradiography. Note that there is not a specific enzyme that cuts only at Ts but instead cuts at Cs + Ts. Thus if there is a band in both the C lane and the C + T lane, the nucleotide is a C; if there is a band only in the C + T lane, the nucleotide is a T.

tyrosine kinase receptors (see Pause and Think). In colon cancer, the protein product of oncogenic *src* is characterized by a truncation at Tyr530. This aberrant protein is unable to adopt the inactive conformation described above and therefore kinase activity is constitutive ('always on').

PAUSE AND THINK

How does this interaction described above compare with that of the SH2 domain of Grb2 and a receptor tyrosine kinase? In both cases, the SH2 domain recognizes a phosphotyrosine residue. The SH2 domain of SRC regulates intramolecular interactions but the SH2 domain of Grb2 regulates intermolecular interactions between itself and receptor tyrosine kinases.

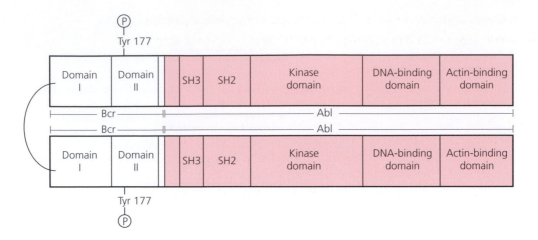

Figure 4.8 The BCR–ABL fusion protein.

Let us look at *abl* as another example. *c-abl* is a gene whose product is a nuclear tyrosine kinase that plays a role in DNA damage-induced apoptosis. It is normally activated by ionizing radiation and particular drugs via the serine/threonine kinase ATM. Oncogenic activation occurs through the chromosomal translocation t(9;22), whereby *abl* becomes juxtaposed to a breakpoint cluster region, *bcr*. Thus DNA sequences that are normally not next to each other are now fused and, upon transcription, give rise to a fusion protein with novel features (Figure 4.8). Translocated Bcr retains domains I and II (shown in white) while ABL retains the SH3 and SH2 domains, the kinase domain, the DNA-binding domain, and the actin-binding domain (shown in red). BCR–ABL molecules associate with each other forming homo-oligomeric complexes, mediated by the coiled-coil motif in domain I of Bcr. Oligomerization permits autophosphorylation at Tyr177 within domain II, and this triggers activation of the ABL tyrosine kinase. The fusion protein BCR–ABL is maintained in the cytoplasm. Consequently, a nuclear kinase is activated in the cytoplasm and has access to a range of novel substrates, interfering in the normal signal transduction pathways of the cell.

Transcription factors

It is not surprising that the transcription factor AP-1, which is an important regulator of cell growth, differentiation, and death, is also involved in transformation. Components of AP-1, Jun and Fos, are encoded by proto-oncogenes *c-jun* and *c-fos* and several mechanisms of oncogenic activation of these genes exist. Normally *c-fos* mRNA is short lived so that the response to a mitogen is transient. Truncation of the 3′ end of *v-fos* eliminates a motif involved in mRNA instability (ATTTATTT) and produces a mRNA with a longer half-life. The aberrant expression of *v-fos* mRNA results in an increase in *v-fos* gene product and an inappropriate increase in the transcription of AP-1-regulated genes. Oncogenic activation may also involve the deletion of a regulatory promoter sequence, the serum response element, such that transcription of the *fos* gene occurs even in the absence of serum mitogens.

Oncogenic activation of *c-myc* occurs from constitutive and over-expression of the c-Myc protein. Chromosomal translocation of *myc* (chromosome 8) to a location that falls within the regulation of the strong promoter of immunoglobulin genes (chromosome 14) increases the amount of expression from the *myc* gene. This mechanism of oncogenic activation of *c-myc* is commonly observed in Burkitt's lymphoma. The increase of Myc protein results in an inappropriate increase in the transcription of Myc-regulated genes.

Remember that steroid hormone receptors act as ligand-dependent transcription factors. In addition to *v-erbB* discussed above, another onco-gene, *v-erbA*, was originally identified from (and named after) the avian erythroblastosis leukemia virus. The identity of the product of the proto-oncogene or cellular gene *c-erbA* is the thyroid hormone (triiodothyronine, T3) receptor. Oncogenic activation is achieved by mutations that pre-vent thyroid hormone binding and inhibit transcriptional activation. This type of mutation is referred to as a **dominant negative** mutation because the product of this mutation codes for receptors that can bind to DNA and block access of wild-type receptors, including other steroid hormone receptor family members that may form heterodimers with thyroid receptors at their response elements. Since the product of *v-erbA* can form **homodimers** (note that the product of the proto-oncogene *erbA* homodimerizes poorly), it is thought that the homodimers mediate the dominant negative effect on the response elements. Most mutations of thyroid hormone receptors identified in human cancers result in dominant negative products, suggesting that they may be involved in human cancers, but this is an issue that needs further investigation (Gonzalez-Sancho *et al.*, 2003) (see Pause and Think).

PAUSE AND THINK

In the discussion above regarding three specific transcription factors, you will notice that AP-1 and Myc activity increase in some cancers while thyroid hormone receptor activity decreases in some cancers. What can you postulate about the target genes of these transcription factors? The target genes for AP-1 and Myc are likely to code for proteins that promote growth while the target genes of thyroid hormone receptor are likely to inhibit growth.

Mechanisms of oncogenic activation

As can be seen from the above, several mechanisms can be used to activ-ate proto-oncogenes to become oncogenes (Figure 4.9). Point mutations

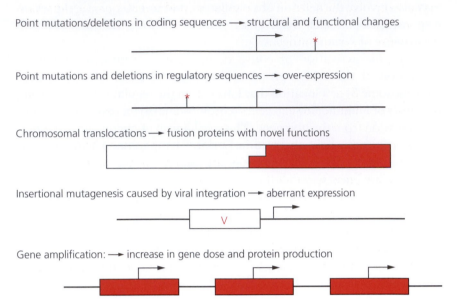

Figure 4.9 Mechanisms that activate proto-oncogenes to become oncogenes.

and deletions in the coding region are a common mechanism and often change the structure and/or function of the proto-oncogene product. Both mechanisms of oncogene activation were described for the *EGFR* gene. Mutations in the gene promoter region can lead to over-expression of a proto-oncogene. Chromosomal translocations as well as insertional mutagenesis cause the juxtaposition of sequences not normally next to each other, and often this configuration can cause altered expression. The translocation involving *c-myc* and immunoglobulin regulatory sequences mentioned above is one example . Alternatively, fusion proteins can have novel characteristics. The Philadelphia chromosome relocates the nuclear kinase, c-Abl, to the cytoplasm where it encounters novel substrates. Gene amplification is another mechanism for activation of *erbB2* and is observed in breast cancer.

◎ Therapeutic strategies

Knowledge of the molecular details of the EGFR signal transduction pathway and related pathways has led to the launch of many new cancer therapeutics targeting individual components. There has been great success for some and valuable lessons from others. The future is hopeful as we continue to unravel the molecular biology of signal transduction pathways and move forward in the design of additional new therapeutics. The strategies of some new therapeutics aimed at molecular targets within these pathways are described below.

4.3 Kinase inhibitors

Many types of kinases, including transmembrane tyrosine kinases, cytoplasmic kinases, and nuclear kinases, are implicated in cancer, as we have seen above. Therefore they have become an important target for the design of new cancer therapeutics. In theory, one may predict that designing drugs with great specificity to a subset of kinases would be difficult because the structure of the catalytic domains of different kinases is very similar when the kinases are in the active state. However, the synthesis of specific kinase inhibitors has clearly been demonstrated and examples are described below and illustrated in Figure 4.10.

Anti-EGFR drugs

The *ErbB2* gene, a member of the EGFR family, is amplified in 30% of breast cancer patients. Over-expression of this gene in cell culture

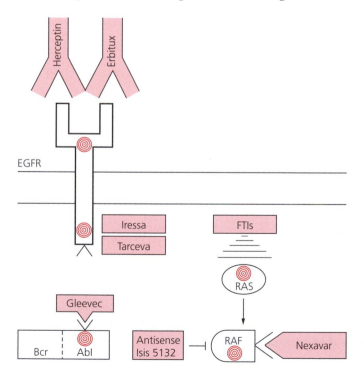

Figure 4.10 Therapeutic strategies that target kinases and RAS. Molecular targets are indicated with a target symbol (◎) and therapeutic agents are shaded in red.

experiments and in transgenic mice (see Box 'Analysis of gene function using transgenic mice') results in cell transformation and the induction of breast cancer, respectively. This suggests that ErbB2 has a causal role in breast cancer. Several small-molecule kinase inhibitor drugs directed against the tyrosine kinase activity of EGFR family members have been developed, including Iressa (ZD1839), Tarceva, and ABX-EGF. Iressa and Tarceva have been approved for the treatment of advanced non-small cell lung cancer (see Pao *et al.*, 2004 and Section 12.4 for further discussion).

Analysis of gene function using transgenic mice

One strategy for investigating the function of a gene is to put it in a place where it is not normally located or remove it from where it normally resides and observe any changes. Transgenic mice contain an additional or altered gene in all of their cells. Transgenic mice can be created by the direct injection of DNA into a fertilized egg. More commonly, foreign DNA is introduced into embryonic stem cells in culture prior to their transplantation into an early embryo (blastocyst). A series of breeding stages must follow to generate fully **homozygous** transgenic mice, since the founder animal is chimeric (not all cells of the organism contain the altered DNA) rather than transgenic. The cell culture step allows for selection and analysis of DNA integration to take place prior to the creation of a mouse. To create a knock-out mouse, a vector is designed so that it will insert into a specific gene location by homologous recombination (see Section 2.4) and disrupt the endogenous gene such that gene function is repressed. Complex transgenic experiments may use tissue-specific or inducible promoters to induce the expression of the foreign gene in a particular location or specific time.

A different approach has also proved successful. Instead of targeting the tyrosine kinase domain of the ErbB2 receptor, the unique extracellular domain was targeted using monoclonal antibodies. Herceptin (trastuzumab) is a humanized (produced with human recombinant immunoglobulin genes) monoclonal antibody that binds the extracellular domain of ErbB2 with high affinity. Herceptin functions through a combination of mechanisms of action including enhanced receptor degradation, inhibition of angiogenesis and recruitment of immune cells, resulting in antibody-dependent cellular cytotoxicity. Herceptin was approved by the US Food and Drug Administration in 1998 for treatment of metastatic breast cancer whose tumors over-express ErbB2 and thus it is the first genomics-based therapy administered selectively, based on the molecular profile of the tumor. Erbitux (cetuximab) is a chimeric antibody directed against EGFR which has also been approved (Switzerland 2003, USA 2004). Genomic characterization of tumor DNA is elucidating subsets of molecularly distinct tumor types within a class of cancer (e.g. breast cancer) that will respond differently to targeted treatments. This is a significant step towards individually tailored treatment, whereby treatment is matched to the molecular make-up of the patient's tumor and promises to increase the success rate of a given drug.

Strategies against Raf

Since 20% of all tumors have activating mutations in *ras*, targeting downstream effectors could prove valuable as a cancer treatment. Several strategies to target the serine/threonine kinase Raf, one of the main effectors of RAS, have been developed. One strategy has been to synthesize anti-sense oligonucleotides that can bind to raf RNA. The RNA hybrids are most likely targeted for degradation or block translation and result in a reduction of Raf protein. The reagent ISIS5132 (Isis Pharmaceuticals) is one such agent that has entered clinical trials. Phase I trials showed the reagent to be non-toxic. Phase II trials were disappointing because a reduction in Raf levels was not observed and no efficacy was observed in patients with non-small cell lung carcinoma.

Another strategy commonly used to target other kinases has also been applied to the serine/threonine kinase Raf. A kinase inhibitor directed towards the ATP-binding site of Raf, called Nexavar (sorafenib; previously called BAY43-9006), was approved for treatment of advanced renal cell carcinoma (USA 2005, Switzerland and Mexico 2006; Wilhelm *et al.*, 2006). In order to investigate whether there was modulation of the defined molecular target, Raf, the phosphorylation of Raf targets was monitored. Data demonstrated a reduction in downstream MAPK phosphorylation in the blood of patients receiving the well-tolerated oral treatment. Note that it is important to monitor molecular endpoints (MAPK activity), in addition to clinical endpoints (anti-tumor activity). Nexavar also blocks several receptor tyrosine kinases (VEGFR1, -2, and -3, PDGFRb, c-Kit, and RET and is therefore a multikinase inhibitor. Since these molecular targets are involved in tumorigenesis and angiogenesis, further clinical studies may reveal that treatment with Nexavar can be applicable for other cancers.

Imatinib (Gleevec™; STI571)

Chronic myelogenous leukemia (CML) accounts for 15–20% of all leukemias. Bone marrow transplantation is the only hope for a cure but is not feasible for a variety of reasons (including donor matching) for the majority of patients. Interferon-α, accompanied by severe side-effects, was until recently the standard treatment. The knowledge of the molecular biology of the disease has led to successful specific molecular targeting and the development of a most successful drug. Most CML patients (95%)

carry the Philadelphia chromosome, the product of the chromosomal translocation t(9;22)(q34;q11) generating the BCR–ABL fusion protein. As a result of this translocation, the tyrosine kinase activity of ABL is constitutive and is retained in the cytoplasm rather than the nucleus. As a result of aberrant kinase signaling, there is abnormal proliferation of white blood cells, the hallmark of leukemia. Transformation is dependent on the BCR–ABL kinase activity and therefore provides the perfect therapeutic target.

Imatinib (Gleevec™), a small-molecule tyrosine kinase inhibitor, has been successful in the treatment of CML, resulting in remission in 96% of early stage patients. It is a paradigm for targeted cancer therapy, having flown through clinical trials and approval (2001) within 3 years (discussed further in Chapter 12). The compound was modeled and synthesized after related lead compounds (compounds that shows a desired activity, e.g. kinase inhibition) called phenylaminopyrimidines, identified from high-throughput screens of chemical libraries. The compound was originally optimized for inhibiting PDGF-R tyrosine kinase activity but was later found to inhibit ABL and c-kit as well. Gleevec binds to the ATP-binding pocket within the catalytic domain, but the fairly narrow specificity of the compound seems to be due to preferential binding of the drug to the inactive state of the kinase as evidenced by analysis of crystal structures (Schindler et al., 2000). Gleevec recognizes the autoinhibitory conformation of the activation loop of the protein that regulates the kinase activity. The structure of the inactive state is distinctive between different kinases. The drug has a half-life of approximately 15 h and conveniently allows daily oral administration.

Pre-clinical data demonstrated inhibition of proliferation in cultured cells and in cells from CML patients with the Philadelphia chromosome as well as tumor regression in mice. This evidence allowed progression to clinical trials. The threshold dose for significant therapeutic efficacy was found to be 300 mg in Phase I trials. Parameters of how well the drug works, efficacy endpoints, were measured by the degree of cytogenetic (chromosomal) and hematologic (blood count) response. A complete cytogenetic response was defined as 0% Philadelphia chromosome-positive cells in metaphase (partial, 1–35%, minor, 36–65%, minimal, 66–95%, or no response >95%, were additional parameters used). Hematologic response is simply graded by white blood cell counts. Importantly, molecular target inhibition was also analyzed. Quantification of the levels of phospho-CRKL, a BCR–ABL substrate found in neutrophils, allowed for the assessment of the inhibition of kinase activity and aided in the determination of effective dosage. As mentioned above, it is important to monitor the modulation of the defined molecular target (BCR–ABL).

Note that the CML has three disease phases: chronic (lasting 3–5 years), accelerated (lasting from 3–9 months), and blast crisis (lasting 3–6 months). Due to an increase of cell proliferation, the number of white blood cells increases as the disease progresses. The effectiveness of Gleevec decreases with advanced disease phase (53% response in accelerated phase and 30% response in blast crisis). Although only 9% of early stage patients relapsed, 78% of late-stage patients relapsed. The mechanism for the majority of these cases is due to reactivation of the kinase activity due to mutation or *Bcr–Abl* amplification. Analysis of clinical samples showed that six out of nine patients had a single amino acid substitution at a contact residue identified in the crystal structure (Gorre *et al.*, 2001). These mechanisms suggest that the initial chromosomal translocation is not only important for initiation but also for maintenance of the cancer phenotype and supports the concept of oncogene addiction: the dependence of a cancer cell on a specific oncogene for its maintenance. STI-571 has also been approved to target c-kit in gastrointestinal stromal tumors and additional studies are investigating its use against PDGF-R in glioblastomas (see Pause and Think).

> **PAUSE AND THINK**
>
> What is the difference between the types of molecular targets described above? They include three different types of kinases: a transmembrane receptor tyrosine kinase, a cytoplasmic serine/threonine tyrosine kinase, and a nuclear tyrosine kinase, respectively.

4.4 RAS-directed therapies

As mentioned above, *ras* is often oncogenically activated during carcinogenesis. The enzyme farnesyltransferase is crucial in the post-translational processing of RAS and its subsequent localization to the plasma membrane and thus was seen as a rational target for new cancer drugs. The major strategy was to design compounds called farnesyltransferase inhibitors (FTIs) that would compete with the carboxy-terminal CAAX motif of RAS (see Figure 4.10). Although results were promising in pre-clinical trials performed on mouse models, those in human clinical trials were not as positive. The discrepancy appears to be due to species differences in enzymatic activities: two members of the RAS family, K-RAS and N-RAS, can be modified by another enzyme, geranylgeranyltransferase (GGT) in the absence of farnesyltransferase so that a type of enzymatic 'redundancy' is present in humans but not in mice. However, despite the reporting of 'no effect' for many farnesyltransferase inhibitor clinical trials, results from leukemia trials are more encouraging, although the mechanism of action is not known. Mutational analysis has suggested that farnesylation of RAS is required for biological functions other than membrane targeting, since it is also important for RAS signaling from subcellular compartments. Therefore, further investigations of the role of farnesyltransferase in carcinogenesis are needed.

Conclusion

Cancer is a disease characterized by uncontrolled growth. Therefore a clear understanding of growth regulation has helped to reveal the mechanisms of carcinogenesis. This was illustrated by the elucidation of the existence of oncogenes, which include altered versions of normal genes involved in growth. Oncogenes often play a role in growth factor signal transduction. The knowledge of the intricacies of growth factor signal transduction pathways have been and will be essential to the design of successful, low-toxicity cancer therapeutics designed against molecular targets.

■ CHAPTER HIGHLIGHTS—REFRESH YOUR MEMORY

- Growth factors, growth factor receptors, intracellular signal transducers, and nuclear transcription factors play a role in growth factor signal transduction.

- Many growth factor receptors are tyrosine kinases. Kinases phosphorylate specific amino acid residues in target proteins.

- Phosphorylated proteins can be recognized by specific protein domains (e.g. SH2) and thus can serve as a recruitment platform.

- RAS plays a pivotal role in the EGFR pathway; it links activation of tyrosine kinase receptors with downstream signaling pathways.

- Raf, a serine/threonine kinase activated by RAS initiates a cascade of phosphorylations by the MEK and MAP kinases.

- One ultimate destination of signaling initiated by growth factors is the regulation of transcription factors in the nucleus. Another is affecting cell behavior.

- Retroviruses have been instrumental in the elucidation of oncogenes.

- Most oncogenes are altered versions of normal genes.

- Constitutive kinase activation is a common consequence of oncogenic mutations of tyrosine kinase receptors.

- Aberrant subcellular localization is another consequence of oncogenic activation.

- Many molecular components of growth factor signal transduction pathways have been targets for new cancer therapeutics.

- Different domains of tyrosine kinase receptors have been targeted for the development of new cancer therapies.

- The testing of new therapeutics should include an assay for the modulation of the defined molecular target.

■ ACTIVITY

1. A new oncogene called 'gre' has been discovered. It is a tyrosine kinase receptor. Propose a likely mechanism of its oncogenic activation. Describe the components of the signal transduction pathway it may activate, drawing upon your knowledge of other known tyrosine kinase receptors. Suggest a therapeutic strategy for designing a new anticancer drug for this new target.

2. Discuss the importance of protein–protein interactions in growth factor signal transduction pathways.

■ **FURTHER READING**

Bennasroune, A., Gardin, A., Aunis, D., Cremel, G., and Hubert, P. (2004) Tyrosine kinase receptors as attractive targets of cancer therapy. *Crit. Rev. Oncol. Hematol.* **50**: 23–38.

Blume-Jensen, P. and Hunter, T. (2001) Oncogenic kinase signaling. *Nature* **411**: 355–365.

Downward, J. (2003) Targeting ras signalling pathways in cancer therapy. *Nature Rev. Cancer* **3**: 11–22.

Druker, B.J. (2002) STI571 (Gleevec) as a paradigm for cancer therapy. *Trends Mol. Med.* **8**: S14–S18.

Krause, D.S. and Van Etten, R.A. (2005) Tyrosine kinases as targets for cancer therapy. *New Engl. J. Med.* **353**: 172–187.

Linggi, B. and Carpenter, G. (2006) ErbB receptors: new insights on mechanisms and biology. *Trends Cell Biol.* **16**: 649–656.

Sawyers, C.L. (2002) Rational therapeutic intervention in cancer: kinases as drug targets. *Current Opin. Genet. Dev.* **12**: 111–115.

Schlessinger, J. (2000) Cell signaling by receptor tyrosine kinases. *Cell* **103**: 211–225.

Schlessinger, J. (2002) Ligand-induced, receptor-mediated dimerization and activation of EGF receptor. *Cell* **110**: 669–672.

Yeatman, T.J. (2004) A renaissance for Src. *Nature Rev. Cancer* **4**: 470–480.

Zandi, R., Larsen, A.B., Andersen, P., Stockhausen, M.-T., and Poulsen, H.S. (2007) Mechanisms for oncogenic activation of the epidermal growth factor receptor. *Cell Signal.* **19**: 2013–2023.

Zwick, E., Bange, J., and Ullrich, A. (2002) Receptor tyrosine kinases as targets for anticancer drugs. *Trends Mol. Med.* **8**: 17–23.

■ **WEB SITE**

Tarceva. Download 'How Tarceva works' http://www.tarceva.net/

■ **SELECTED SPECIAL TOPICS**

Chang, E.H., Furth, M.E., Scolnick, E.M., and Lowy, D.R. (1982) Tumorigenic transformation of mammalian cells induced by a normal human gene homologous to the oncogene of Harvey murine sarcoma virus. *Nature* **297**: 479–483.

Gonzalez-Sancho, J.M., Garcia, V., Bonilla, F., and Munoz, A. (2003) Thyroid hormone receptors/THR genes in human cancer. *Cancer Lett.* **192**: 121–132.

Gorre, M.E., Mohammed, M., Ellwood, K., Hsu, N., Paquette, R., Nagesh Rao, P., and Sawyers, C.L. (2001) Clinical resistance to STI-571 cancer therapy caused by BCR-ABL gene mutation or amplification. *Science* **293**: 876–880.

Hingorani, S.R. and Tuveson, D.A. (2003) Ras redux: rethinking how and where Ras acts. *Curr. Opin. Genet. Dev.* **13**: 6–13.

Ise, K., Nakamura, K., Nakao, K., Shimizu, S., Harada, H., Ichise, T., Miyoshi, J., Gondo, Y., Ishikawa, T., Aiba, A., and Katsuki, M. (2000) Targeted deletion of the *H-ras* gene decreases tumor formation in mouse skin carcinogenesis. *Oncogene* **19**: 2951–2956.

Pao, W., Miller, V.A., and Kris, M.G. (2004) 'Targeting' the epidermal growth factor receptor tyrosine kinase with gefitinib (Iressa) in non-small cell lung cancer (NSCLC). *Semin. Cancer Biol.* **14**: 33–40.

Reddy, E.P., Reynolds, R.K., Santos, E., and Barbacid, M. (1982) A point mutation is responsible for the acquisition of transforming properties by the T24 human bladder carcinoma oncogene. *Nature* **300**: 149–152.

Schindler, T., Bornmann, W., Pellicena, Miller, W.T., Clarkson, B., and Kuriyan, J. (2000) Structural mechanism for STI-571 inhibition of Abelson tyrosine kinase. *Science* **289**: 1938–1942.

Wilhelm, S., Carter, C., Lynch, M., Lowinger, T., Dumas, J., Smith, R.A., Schwartz, B., Simantov, R., and Kelley, S. (2006) Discovery and development of sorafenib: a multikinase inhibitor for treating cancer. *Nature Rev. Drug Discovery* **5**: 835–844.

Chapter 5

The cell cycle

Introduction

Cancer is characterized by abnormal cell proliferation. Cell proliferation involves the reproduction of a cell to form two daughter cells. Each daughter cell can reproduce to form two daughter cells, and so on; thus cell reproduction is cyclic. The sequence of stages through which a cell passes between one cell division and the next is called the **cell cycle** (Figure 5.1) and is made up of four stages: G_1, **S phase**, G_2, and **M phase**. G_1, S, and G_2 make up the part of the cycle called interphase. The genetic material of a cell is replicated in S phase (DNA synthesis). M phase involves the partitioning of the cell to produce two daughter cells and includes **mitosis** and cytokinesis. G_1 and G_2 are 'gaps' preceding the S and M phases during which time the cell prepares for the next phase.

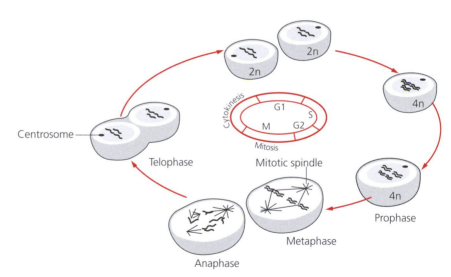

Figure 5.1 The cell cycle. The four phases, G_1, S, G_2 and M phase (including cytokinesis), are shown in the center of the diagram. Cells are illustrated around the phases of the cell cycle and their chromosome content in relation to the four phases of the cell cycle is depicted. Cells in different phases of the cell cycle have different DNA content: G_1:2n (two copies of every chromosome); S: begins with 2n and becomes 4n; G_2: 4n; M: begins with 4n and produces 2n daughter nuclei. Figure from *The Cell Cycle: Principles of Control* by David O Morgan with the permission of Oxford University Press.

In the last chapter we examined the molecular mechanisms involved in growth factor signal transduction pathways. We mentioned that the pathway culminates by regulating the expression of target genes, including the induction of genes whose products are essential in cell proliferation. In this chapter we will introduce the cyclins and cyclin-dependent kinases, main players in the cell cycle, some of which are encoded by genes regulated by growth factor signaling pathways. We will also examine the molecular mechanisms of the cell cycle and specific mutations that affect the cell cycle and play a role in carcinogenesis. Lastly we will discuss therapeutic strategies that target molecules of the cell cycle.

5.1 Cyclins and cyclin-dependent kinases (cdks)

The average length of the cell cycle is 16 h (15 h for interphase and 1 h for mitosis) as shown in Figure 5.2, but note that this can vary depending on the cell type. Cells in interphase can be distinguished microscopically from cells in mitosis because chromosomes are not visible in interphase and can only be observed during mitosis due to chromosome condensation.

Starting from the beginning of G_1 (Figure 5.2, top), progression of the cell cycle is illustrated in a clockwise manner. Most cells in an adult are not in the process of cell division. They are quiescent and enter an inactive period called G_0, a phase outside of the cell cycle. **Mitogens** or growth factors can, however, induce cells in G_0 to re-enter the cell cycle and pass

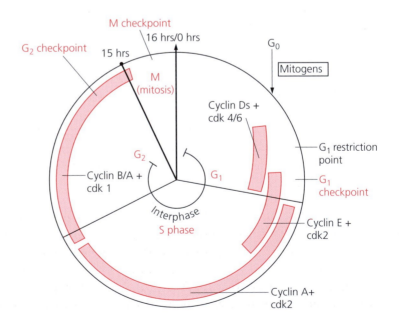

Figure 5.2 The pattern of cyclin–cdk activity during the cell cycle (shown by red bars) and the cell cycle checkpoints (G_1, G_2, and M).

a control point called the G_1 restriction point (find this point in Figure 5.2). Before the passage of the restriction point, cell division is dependent on mitogens; afterwards cells are irreversibly committed to progress through the cycle without the need for growth factors. The passage of the cell through the different phases of the cell cycle is coordinated and regulated by a set of proteins called cyclins and their associated cyclin-dependent kinases (cdks). Cyclins were so named because of the cyclical changes in their concentrations that occur over a series of cell divisions. The concentration of cyclin protein is dependent on the transcription of its gene and by subsequent regulated protein degradation. The pairing of cyclins to the cdks is highly specific. Cyclins are regulatory subunits of their cdks. Upon binding of a cyclin to its cdk partner, cyclin induces a conformational change in the catalytic subunit of the cdk revealing its active site. Note that the concentration of cdks does not fluctuate during the cell cycle.

Different cyclin–cdk complexes are present at specific points in the cell cycle and are important regulators of irreversible phase transitions (depicted by the red bars in Figure 5.2). In the last chapter we saw that the cyclin D gene is one of the final targets of the EGF signaling pathway. This is an important molecular link between growth factors and how they actually stimulate cell proliferation. Cyclin D is the first cyclin to be synthesized and, together with cdks 4/6 drives progression through G_1. As we will see below, cyclin D plays a role in the regulation of expression of the cyclin E gene, whose product is important for the G_1 to S phase transition. Cyclin A–cdk2 is important for S phase progression. Cyclins A, B–cdk1 directs G_2 and the G_2 to M phase transition.

Cell cycle checkpoints (see Figure 5.2), a series of biochemical signaling pathways that sense and induce a cellular response to DNA damage, are important for maintaining the integrity of the genome. The G_1 checkpoint leads to the arrest of the cell cycle in response to DNA damage, ensuring that DNA damage is not replicated during S phase. The G_2 checkpoint leads to the arrest of the cell cycle in response to damaged and/or unreplicated DNA to ensure proper completion of S phase. The M checkpoint leads to the arrest of chromosomal segregation in response to misalignment on the mitotic spindle. The components of the checkpoints are proteins that act as DNA damage sensors, signal transducers, or effectors. Disruption of checkpoint function leads to mutations that can induce carcinogenesis.

The cyclin–cdk complexes exert their effect by phosphorylating target proteins. As we saw in Chapter 4, phosphorylation is an important mechanism for regulating the activity of proteins. The targets include a diverse set of proteins including transcriptional regulators, cytoskeletal proteins, nuclear pore and envelope proteins, and histones. Specific examples include condensins, nuclear lamins, GM130 of the Golgi apparatus, the famous transcriptional regulator, retinoblastoma protein (RB or pRB), and transcription factors E2F and Smad 3. Consequently, essential events of the cell cycle including chromosomal condensation, nuclear breakdown, fragmentation of the Golgi apparatus, regulated gene expression, and mitotic spindle assembly are facilitated. Note that dephosphorylation is an important mechanism for resetting the cell for another round of the cell cycle.

HOW DO WE KNOW THAT?

Protein cross-linking and immunopurification (see Sanchez and Dynlacht, 2005)

There are several approaches that can help identify the substrates of cdks. One common method is to cross-link proteins, carry out immunopurification of protein kinases, and use mass spectroscopic analysis to identify associated proteins. The identification of RB as a cdk substrate was demonstrated by the immunoprecipitation of RB using a cdk2 antibody.

Another method for identifying cdk substrates is to screen cDNA expression libraries using a solid-phase phosphorylation assay. Bacterial expressed cDNA libraries are transferred to filters and probed with a solution of a functionally active cdk of interest and labeled ATP. Proteins are produced from the cDNA libraries, some of which interact with cdk. When cdk phosphorylates a target protein using the labeled ATP, a radioactive signal is generated. The signal is visualized by autoradiography at the position of proteins phosphorylated during the assay.

Candidate molecules must be validated by several criteria including: (i) the phosphorylation state must be the same *in vitro* and *in vivo*; (ii) phosphorylation must be shown to be cell cycle dependent; (iii) phosphorylation should have a functional consequence in the cell cycle.

LEADERS IN THE FIELD . . . of the cell cycle: Tim Hunt, Lee Hartwell, and Paul Nurse

The award of the Nobel Prize in Physiology or Medicine in 2001 to Tim Hunt, along with Lee Hartwell and Paul Nurse, indicates the great contributions that these men have made to science. The prize was received for studies on the regulation of the cell cycle during which the cyclins were discovered. Each of these three scientists worked independently on three different model systems: Hunt worked on sea urchins, Hartwell on budding yeast, and Nurse on fission yeast. One early experiment seemed to serve as the foundation for future work on the cell cycle: the discovery that the cytoplasm of a hormone-treated frog oocyte was able to induce maturation (including the first meiotic division) in a recipient untreated oocyte. The substance in the cytoplasm was termed maturation-promoting factor (MPF). It was later identified in mitotic cells and was then also called mitosis-promoting factor. Similarities between MPF and cyclins–cdks uncovered by these scientists led to the discovery that MPF was in fact a cyclin–cdk complex. The mechanism by which the cell cycle is regulated, as elucidated by the work of Hunt, Hartwell, and Nurse, offered new insights into the molecular biology of cancer.

Tim Hunt completed his PhD in Biochemistry in Cambridge and a post-doctoral fellowship at the Albert Einstein College of Medicine, New York. He is currently a Principal Scientist at Cancer Research, UK where he continues his research and teaching. I heard Tim give a talk at the Royal Society in London. He opened the lecture with a scan of a tumor from his mother-in-law to illustrate the devastating results of the deregulation of the →

→ cell cycle. He is a scientist who is skilled at communicating the mechanics of molecular science in relation to the human state of disease. Lee Hartwell earned his PhD at MIT, Massachusetts, and is the President and Director of the Fred Hutchinson Cancer Research Center where he applies his knowledge towards the development of new cancer therapies. Paul Nurse obtained his PhD at the University of East Anglia, UK and is currently the President of Rockefeller University in New York.

5.2 Mechanisms of cdk regulation

In an adult more than 25 million cells undergo cell division per second. The magnitude of this number suggests the need for precise regulation. Cdks are serine/threonine kinases that, sequentially, regulate progression through the phases of the cell cycle via phosphorylation. Therefore, the regulation of cdk activity is crucial for precise cell reproduction.

There are four mechanisms of cdk regulation: association with cyclins, association with cdk inhibitors, addition of phosphate groups that activate cdk activity, and addition of phosphate groups that inhibit cdk activity (Figure 5.3). Because of the precise window of time for which regulators

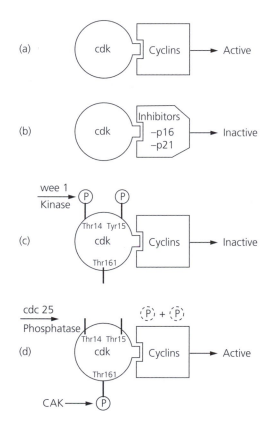

Figure 5.3 Mechanisms of cdk regulation: (a) association with cyclins activates cdks; (b) association with inhibitors inactivates cdks; (c) inhibitory phosphorylation at Thr14 and Tyr15 by wee1 kinase inactivates cdks; (d) the removal of inhibitory phosphates by cdc phosphatase and activating phosphorylation by cdk-activating kinases (CAK) activates cdk.

of the cell cycle are required, the 'disappearance' of a factor is as important as its appearance. That is, precise protein degradation also plays an important role in the control of the cell cycle (Reed, 2003). The mechanisms of cdk regulation are discussed below.

Association with cyclins

The binding of cyclins to their partner cdk causes a crucial conformational change in the cdk that allows binding of a protein substrate and correct positioning of ATP. The inactive cdk molecule has a conformation that blocks the binding of the protein substrate and correct alignment of ATP. Some cyclins are also involved in increasing the affinity of cdks to specific substrates. As mentioned above, the amounts of cyclin protein vary through the cell cycle. Protein levels are modified by transcriptional regulation of the cyclin genes and by protein degradation. As we saw in the last chapter, the signaling pathway for the growth factor EGF results in the transcriptional activation of the cyclin D gene and allows progression through the restriction point. Degradation of cyclin proteins is carried out by the proteasome, a complex of proteases. The covalent addition of ubiquitin, a small polypeptide, to the lysine amino acids of the cyclin flag the protein for degradation by the proteasome. The enzyme that catalyzes the transfer of ubiquitin to the target protein is called a ubiquitin-protein ligase. Ubiquitin-mediated proteolysis of cyclins prevents constitutive activity of cdks. Note that ubiquitination is also important in stem cell maintenance and angiogenesis and will be discussed in Chapters 8 and 9.

Association with inhibitors

Two families of inhibitors are involved in regulating cyclin–cdk activity: the $p16^{ink4a}$ (INK) family and the p21 (Cip/Kip) family. Members of the $p16^{ink4a}$ family include $p16^{ink4a}$, $p15^{ink4b}$, $p18^{ink4c}$, and $p19^{ink4d}$. The INK proteins bind cdks 4/6 and interfere with the binding of cdks 4/6 to cyclin D. The p21 family members include $p21^{cip1}$, $p27^{kip1}$, and $p57^{kip2}$. These inhibitors interact with both cyclins and their associated cdks (mainly with cdk2 and cyclin E) and block the ATP-binding site, thus disabling kinase activity. Upon mitogenic stimulation and subsequent cyclin D synthesis, cyclin D-dependent kinases sequester inhibitors of the Cip/Kip family, facilitating cyclin E–cdk2 activation. Again, ubiquitin-mediated degradation of inhibitors ensures that the inhibitors are present during a defined window of time during the cell cycle.

Regulation by phosphorylation

Regulation of cdk activity by phosphorylation involves both activation and inhibition. Two phosphorylation sites on the amino-terminal end are inhibitory when phosphorylated. The tyrosine kinase, wee1, phosphorylates Thr14 and Tyr15. These amino acids are located deep within the ATP-binding site of the cdk and phosphorylation of these sites physically interferes with ATP binding. Two steps are required for cdks to become active: dephosphorylation of the inhibitory phosphate groups by cdc25 phosphatases and phosphorylation of a central threonine residue, Thr161, by cdk-activating kinase (CAK). Note that complete activation of cdks requires phosphorylation at this site and that association with cyclins alone does not lead to full activation. In addition, this phosphorylation event is not temporally regulated with respect to the phases of the cell cycle as CAK activity is constant throughout the cycle.

5.3 Progression through the G₁ checkpoint

A key substrate of the cyclin D–cdk 4/6 complex is the RB protein (discussed further in the next chapter). RB serves as a molecular link for the G_1–S phase transition. RB does not bind to specific DNA sequences but instead regulates the activity of the E2F transcription factor family, which is crucial for the expression of genes needed for S phase. It does this by physically interfering with the transactivation domain of E2Fs. Note that to date there are eight E2Fs and two associated subunits (called DP). The activity of RB is regulated by sequential phosphorylation events by cyclin–cdks. Let us examine the details of the RB protein below.

Structure of the RB protein

The nuclear RB protein, along with two other related proteins, p107 and p130, is a member of the 'pocket proteins' and contains conserved structural and functional domains that bind to various cell proteins. The pocket comprises the A domain and the B domain joined by a linker region. The binding of the two main cellular effector proteins, histone deacetylase (HDAC) and the E2F transcription factor, to the pocket region (Figure 5.4) is important for its function. HDACs contain the LXCXE motif, an amino acid sequence that is required to bind to the B domain of the pocket of the RB protein. E2F and its associated subunit DP can bind to the pocket of RB simultaneously with HDAC because E2F and DP recognize a different conserved sequence at the interface of the A and B domains of the pocket. The next question to examine is how binding of HDAC and E2F contributes to the function of RB.

Molecular mechanisms of the effects of RB

The major point of control for RB protein is the transition from the G_1 phase of the cell cycle to S phase (see Figure 5.2). It executes this control

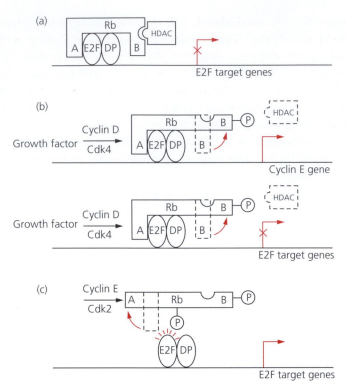

Figure 5.4 Structure and function of the RB protein. (a) Hypophosphorylated RB sequesters E2F/DP and HDAC. Transcription is repressed. (b) Partial phosphorylation of RB by cyclin D–cdk4 causes a conformational change, and release of HDAC but not E2F/DP. Repression is relieved for some genes such as cyclin E (top) but not for E2F target genes (bottom). (c) Additional phosphorylation by cyclin E–cdk2 causes an additional conformational change, release of E2F/DP, and transcription of E2F target genes.

by its interactions with the transcription factor E2F and HDACs. (Recall that HDACs regulate gene expression via an epigenetic mechanism; see Chapter 3.) The interactions between RB and E2F and HDACs are regulated by serine/threonine phosphorylation. In the absence of a growth signal, RB is in a hypophosphorylated state (i.e. it does not have many phosphates attached) and binds to both E2F and HDAC (Figure 5.4a). By binding to E2F, RB sequesters it and blocks its transactivation domain, preventing E2F from interacting with the general transcription factors (e.g. TATA-binding protein). RB also inhibits the expression of E2F target genes by recruiting HDACs, enzymes that deacetylate histones and increase chromatin compaction. Thus, the trimeric complex of RB with HDAC and E2F regulate transcription and consequently cell cycle progression; genes such as *cyclin E*, *cyclin A*, and *cdk 2*, whose products are required for progression through the cell cycle, are not expressed.

It is the cyclin D and E families and their cdks that phosphorylate RB in a progressive manner, in response to a growth signal. Figure 5.4 shows how phosphorylation leads to conformational changes in the RB protein and causes the sequential release of HDAC and E2F. HDAC is no longer localized to repress transcription and the transcription factor E2F is free to activate genes necessary for proliferation. Phosphorylation of RB is carried out in two steps. First, cyclin D–cdk4 phosphorylates carboxy-terminal residues of RB upon growth factor stimulation. The increase in negative charge causes intramolecular interactions with lysine residues (positively charged amino acids) near the LXCXE domain. The resulting conformational change releases HDAC, a LXCXE-bound protein, but not E2F (Figure 5.4b). RB-mediated transcriptional repression of some genes, and not others, is relieved in the absence of HDAC. The cyclin E gene (Figure 5.4b, top), but not E2F target genes (Figure 5.4b, bottom), is expressed upon the release of HDAC from RB. The cyclin E–cdk2 complex then phosphorylates additional amino acid residues of RB, including Ser567 close to the linker region. This results in a conformational change of the RB pocket domain causing the release of E2F and subsequent expression of its target genes, such as cyclin A, thymidylate synthase, and dihydrofolate reductase, that are important for S phase (Figure 5.4c).

In conclusion, the sequential action of these two cyclin–cdk complexes is important. Phosphorylation of RB by cyclin D–cdk4 is a prerequisite for cyclin E–cdk2 phosphorylation in that it induces the expression of the *cyclin E* gene and uncovers cyclin E–cdk2 phosphorylation sites. Subsequent phosphorylation of RB by cyclin E–cdk causes the release of E2F. It is speculated that additional cyclin–cdk complexes may also be involved. Note that there are many phosphorylation sites within RB which are involved in its regulation but the Figure 5.4 is a simplified version used to illustrate the concept of sequential phosphorylation. For example, recently phosphorylation of the carboxy-terminal domain has been demonstrated to be involved in the release of E2F (Rubin *et al.*, 2005).

Self test Close this book and try to redraw Figure 5.4. Check your answer. Correct your work. Close the book once more and try again.

5.4 The G$_2$ checkpoint

The G$_2$ checkpoint blocks entry into M phase in cells that have incurred DNA damage in previous phases or have not correctly completed S phase. DNA damage activates either of two kinases, ATM or ATR. These kinases then phosphorylate and activate Chk1 and Chk2 kinases. One target of these checkpoint kinases are the Cdc25 tyrosine phosphatases (mentioned above) that regulate cdk activity by removing inhibitory phosphates. Specific Cdc25s (type B and C) are important in the G$_2$–M phase transition. Activation of the G$_2$ checkpoint results in the inhibition of Cdc25s by Chk1/2.

PAUSE AND THINK

Try to draw a diagram that illustrates this pathway. Compare your diagram with Figure 5.5.

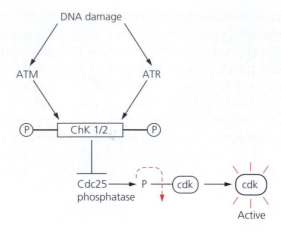

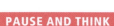

PAUSE AND THINK

One of the types of classical chemotherapies discussed in Chapter 2 targets topoiso-merase II. Can you remember the name of this drug? The answer is doxorubicin, a fungal anthracycline antibiotic.

There is also a decatenation G_2 checkpoint that is involved in detangling intertwined daughter chromatids after DNA synthesis. This process enables chromatid separation during anaphase of mitosis. Topo-isomerase II, an enzyme that can release torsional stress by making double-strand DNA breaks to allow unwinding, is key in the decatenation G_2 checkpoint.

5.5 The mitotic checkpoint

The mitotic checkpoint (also known as the spindle assembly checkpoint) is a signaling cascade that ensures correct chromosomal segregation during mitosis and the production of two genetically identical nuclei.

A little lesson about the stages of mitosis . . .

There are four stages of mitosis: prophase, metaphase, anaphase, and telophase (see Figure 5.6 and Plate 2).

Prophase is marked by the appearance of the chromosomes due to condensation, nuclear membrane breakdown, separation of duplicated centrosomes, and assembly of mitotic checkpoint proteins at the centromeres.

Metaphase is characterized by the aligning of the chromosomes on the metaphase plate and the assembly of microtubules to form the mitotic spindle. Microtubule capture of both centromere regions of a chromatid pair results in checkpoint silencing. When the last pair is attached to the spindle metaphase is completed and anaphase begins.

Anaphase is marked by the spindle pulling apart and separating chromatid pairs.

Telophase includes the accumulation of chromosomes at their respective poles, re-forming of the nuclear membrane, chromosome decondensation, and cytokinesis (separation into two separate cells).

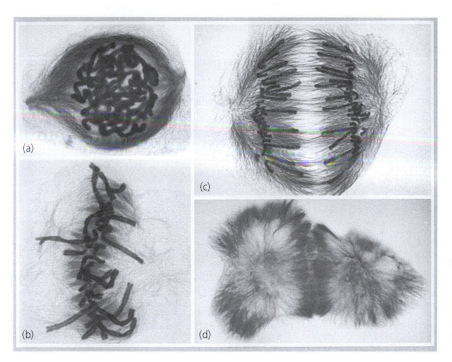

Figure 5.6 Cells in the four stages of mitosis: (a) prophase, (b) metaphase, (c) anaphase, (d) telophase (all magnified about 2700 times). Courtesy of www.micro.utexas.edu. See color plate.

Spindle microtubules attach to the centromere regions of chromosomes during metaphase such that sister chromatids can be pulled to opposite poles during anaphase. Unattached chromatid pairs recruit several checkpoint proteins that produce inhibitors of the anaphase-promoting complex. This complex functions as a ubiquitin-protein ligase and targets specific proteins for degradation in order for anaphase to begin. After each chromatid pair is attached to the spindle, the inhibition of the anaphase-promoting complex stops. One crucial target protein of the anaphase-promoting complex is securin, and upon its degradation, the protease separase is activated. Separase cleaves a protein link between sister chromatids and this allows them to separate during anaphase. Cyclins are also targets of the anaphase-promoting complex. Thus the mitotic checkpoint plays an important role, preventing mis-segregation of single chromosomes.

Aurora kinases

The Aurora kinases (A, B, and C) regulate important aspects of mitosis, including chromosome segregation and the spindle checkpoint. (Note that Aurora kinase A, B, and C are also known as STK15, STK12, and STK13, respectively.) They are serine/threonine kinases that phosphorylate target proteins, many of which play a role in chromosome structure and spindle assembly. Histone H3 is one such target. The activities of the Aurora

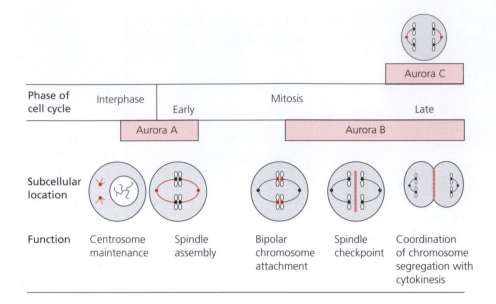

Phase of cell cycle	Interphase		Mitosis		

Figure 5.7 Subcellular location of Aurora kinase A, B, and C (illustrated in red) in relation to the cell cycle. Implicated functions are noted.

kinases are coordinated to specific cellular locations and events of the cell cycle (Figure 5.7). Aurora kinase A localizes to centrosomes during interphase. It is upregulated at the beginning of mitosis and relocates to the spindle poles and spindle microtubules, suggesting a role in centrosome maturation and assembly of the spindle apparatus. Aurora kinase B activity is highest later in mitosis and localizes first with centromeres, then with the middle of the spindle, and later between the dividing cells, suggesting a role in bipolar spindle attachment to chromosomal centromeres, and the spindle checkpoint and monitoring of chromosomal segregation and cytokinesis. Aurora kinase C is active during late mitosis and localizes to spindle poles. The precise temporal regulation of the Aurora kinases is regulated by phosphorylation, protein inhibitors, and targeted degradation.

5.6 The cell cycle and cancer

Genes encoding cell cycle regulators are frequently mutated in human tumors, suggesting that aberrant regulation of the cell cycle can lead to carcinogenesis. Recall from Chapter 1 that growth signal autonomy is one of the six hallmarks of cancer. Mutations in genes of the molecular components of the growth factor signaling pathway (Chapter 4) and in genes that code for regulation of the cell cycle can lead to growth signal autonomy.

Mutations found in cancer include over-expression of cyclin (e.g. cyclin D and E) and cdk genes (e.g. cdks 4/6) by gene amplification. DNA amplification of the cyclin D gene occurs in 1 in 6 breast cancers (about 15%). One study reported 20% of squamous cell carcinomas of the skin contain additional cyclin D gene copies.

HOW DO WE KNOW THAT?

Fluorescent *in situ* hybridization (FISH) (see Utikal *et al.*, 2005)

FISH is used to detect gene amplification. Serial sections of tissue or cells in culture are placed on a microscope slide and incubated at a high temperature in a solution that causes the DNA strands to separate. A single-stranded DNA probe that consists of a section of the sequence that is being searched for is either directly fluorescently labeled or labeled with a small molecule (usually biotin) and allowed to hybridize to the chromosomal DNA within the tissue. Molecules that have not hybridized are washed away. Directly labeled fluorescent probes may be viewed immediately under a fluorescence microscope. Alternatively, a fluorescently labeled molecule that binds biotin (e.g. avidin and/or antibodies) may be used to 'visualize' the DNA of interest. Fluorescence can be used to quantify gene copy number. Controls may include unaffected healthy tissue and probes to additional unrelated genes. An example of cells analyzed by FISH is shown in Plate 3. When looking at this image one can see that there is a higher number of cyclin D gene copies (red) in relation to the number of centromeric regions of chromosome 11 (green) in many of the nuclei of the carcinoma.

Deletion of the gene coding for the inhibitor p16^{ink4a} (frequent in mesothelioma, a cancer linked to asbestos exposure and pancreatic carcinomas) is also common. Experimental findings from p16^{ink4a} knock-out mice demonstrated that loss of p16^{ink4a} results in increased incidence of spontaneous and carcinogen-induced cancers (Sharpless *et al.*, 2001). Mutations in RB will be discussed in Chapter 6.

Cyclin D mRNA and protein levels are over-expressed in 50% of breast cancers. Experimental evidence, including the induction of hyperplasia and adenocarcinoma of the breast in transgenic mice, suggests that the gene for cyclin D is a proto-oncogene. Both oncogenes, such as EGFR, and estrogen exert their mitogenic effect by transcriptional activation of cyclin D. The cyclin D gene does not contain an estrogen response element in its promoter region and thus the estrogen receptor (ER) may act as a transcriptional co-activator (Chapter 3). However, the mechanism by which cyclin D exerts its oncogenic effects is not clear and may even involve a cdk-independent mechanism (Roy and Thompson, 2006). Cyclin D enhances estrogen receptor-mediated transcription by binding to the hormone-binding domain of ER and increasing protein interactions with ER's co-activators.

Defects in the decatenation G$_2$ checkpoint are associated with chromosome breakage and may lead to genetic instability. This has been supported by evidence from cancer cell lines [see references within Kaufmann (2006) such as the work of Doherty *et al.* (2003) and Nakagawa *et al.* (2004)].

It is a current debate about whether aneuploidy, the condition of having an abnormal chromosome number and content, facilitates or drives tumorigenesis. Whatever the answer, aneuploidy is the most common characteristic of human solid tumors. Aneuploidy may be caused by defects in centrosomes, the organizers of the mitotic spindle, or in cytokinesis. Aberrations of the mitotic checkpoint may also lead to aneuploidy. The mitotic checkpoint is not all or none but rather can be weakened by depleted individual components. This is because many proteins are involved, so a deletion of one component may allow the mitotic checkpoint to function, albeit at a reduced efficiency. Large numbers of mis-segregated chromosomes leads to cell death, but a weakened checkpoint may lead to some abnormal number of chromosomes that is not sufficient to induce cell death.

Evidence suggests that mutations in genes that code for components of the mitotic spindle are not common in human tumor cells. However, a decreased quantity of the mitotic checkpoint proteins has been observed in aneuploid tumor cells with an aberrant mitotic checkpoint. Tumor suppressors or oncoproteins may transcriptionally regulate these proteins, causing a decrease in protein levels. A rare recessive disorder called mosaic variegated aneuploidy, caused by mutations in a gene encoding one of the checkpoint proteins, is characterized by aneuploidy and an increased risk of childhood cancers. The evidence described supports a link between a weakened mitotic checkpoint and the process of carcinogenesis.

The Aurora kinases are frequently amplified in several types of tumors. The gene encoding for Aurora A has been demonstrated to be a cancer-susceptibility gene (Ewart-Toland *et al.*, 2003). Researchers found that there is a genetic variant involving an amino acid substitution that modifies cancer risk, perhaps by causing aneuploidy. They suggest that the variant form modifies the interactions of Aurora A with associated regulatory proteins in humans. Additional data from other laboratories show that over-expression of this gene leads to centrosome amplification, chromosomal instability, and transformation. Over-expression of this gene has been reported in 94% of invasive ductal breast adenocarcinomas, characterized in early stages by genetic instability.

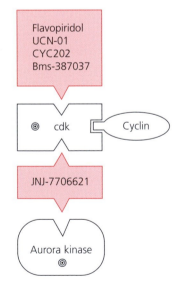

Figure 5.8 Cyclin-dependent kinase inhibitors. Inhibitors are shown in red. JNJ-7706621 is a dual inhibitor of cdks and Aurora kinase.

◎ Therapeutic strategies

Therapeutic strategies that target components of the cell cycle are in development, and several are in clinical trials. Because kinases play a central role in the cell cycle, and have been implicated in carcinogenesis, identification of kinase inhibitors is an important drug strategy. Proteins involved in the mitotic spindle are other important drugs targets. Several strategies are discussed below and are illustrated in Figure 5.8.

5.7 Cyclin-dependent kinase inhibitors

As we have seen above (Section 5.1), phosphorylation by cdks is a key step in the regulation of the cell cycle. These serine/threonine kinases are over-expressed and/or amplified in some cancers, making them possible molecular targets for cancer therapies. A semi-synthetic flavonoid called flavopiridol acts as a competitive inhibitor of all cdks tested, by targeting their ATP-binding site (Senderowicz, 2003). Interestingly, it is related to a compound isolated from a plant found in India that is known to have medicinal properties. Flavopiridol induces cell cycle arrest at G_1/S and G_2/M phases. It also affects cdk family members that have a role in transcriptional control and inhibits gene expression of cyclin D1 and D3. Flavopiridol was the first cdk inhibitor to be tested in clinical trials. Due to its poor oral bioavailability, it is administered intravenously. Anti-tumor activity was demonstrated in some patients with lymphoma but, in general, flavopiridol failed to demonstrate significant clinical activity as a single agent for many solid tumors in Phase II studies. However, investigations into its potential in combination with existing chemotherapeutic agents is ongoing. In light of the increasing complex roles of the cdk family (such as in transcriptional regulation and neuronal function), potential side-effects of the drug will require careful evaluation. UCN-01, CYC202 (R-roscovitine; Cyclacel Ltd), and BMS-387032 are other cdk inhibitors in clinical trials (Figure 5.8). New semi-selective cdk inhibitors (e.g. paullones, oxindoles) are also being developed. PD0332991 is a selective inhibitor of cdks 4/6 and has shown promising pre-clinical results.

5.8 Other cell cycle kinase targets

Cell cycle checkpoint kinase inhibitors (e.g. against CHK1 and CHK2) are also being identified and used as an anticancer strategy. These agents prevent cell cycle arrests and may potentiate the effects of classical chemotherapeutics that cause DNA damage and subsequent apoptosis.

A dual inhibitor of cdks and Aurora kinase, called JNJ-7706621, has been developed (Emanuel et al., 2005; Johnson and Johnson Pharmaceuticals) (Figure 5.8). As a strong inhibitor of cyclin B–cdk1, JNJ-7706621 functions primarily by inducing G_2/M arrest, although additional mechanisms occur. Pre-clinical studies have demonstrated anti-proliferative activity against a range of human cancer cell lines (with a ten-fold lower activity against normal cells) and anti-tumor activity in xenograft mouse models. This suggests that this drug may have a wider therapeutic index in clinical trials and warrants further studies.

5.9 Inhibitors of the mitotic spindle

As discussed under therapeutic strategies in Chapter 2 (see Organic drugs), some conventional chemotherapies interfere with microtubule formation and spindle formation. Paclitaxel/taxol stabilize microtubules while the vinca alkaloids (vinblastine, vincristine) inhibit microtubule assembly. These drugs result in chromatid pairs that are not attached to spindle fibers and thus activate the mitotic checkpoint. It is thought that the mechanism of action of these drugs is cytostatic, but induction of apoptosis may also be a consequence. A molecule called KSP, an ATP-dependent microtubule-motor protein, is required for spindle pole separation and is a new molecular target for the development of cancer therapies. A small-molecule inhibitor of KSP called ispinesib (Cytokinetics) also leads to chronic mitotic checkpoint activation (and possibly subsequent apoptosis) and is currently being tested in Phase I and II trials.

■ **CHAPTER HIGHLIGHTS—REFRESH YOUR MEMORY**

- The cell cycle is made up of four phases: G_1, S, G_2, and M.

- There are three cell cycle checkpoints: the G_1, G_2, and M checkpoints.

- The progression of a cell through the different phases of the cell cycle is highly regulated by cyclins and cyclin-dependent kinases (cdks).

- Cdks are regulated by association with cyclins, inhibitors, and by activating and inhibitory phosphorylation.

- Proteolysis is important for regulating the activity of key regulators of the cell cycle.

- The retinoblastoma (RB) protein is an important target of cyclin D–cdks 4/6 and a key regulator of the G_1 to S phase transition.

- RB exerts its effects by protein–protein interactions with the E2F transcription factor and HDACs.

- The activity of RB is regulated by phosphorylation via different cyclins–cdks.

- Hypophosphorylated RB inactivates E2F and recruits HDACs.

- Phosphorylated RB releases E2F and HDACs, which facilitates transcription and cell cycle progression into S phase.

- The G_2 checkpoint is induced by DNA damage and aberrant DNA synthesis and blocks entry into M phase.

- The mitotic checkpoint prevents mis-segregation of chromosomes during anaphase.

- Aurora kinases are important for centrosome and mitotic spindle function.

- Aberrant regulation of the cell cycle can lead to cancer.

- Cyclin D amplification often occurs in breast cancer and squamous cell carcinoma.

- Several cdk inhibitors have entered clinical trials.

- Several conventional chemotherapies exert their effects by activating the mitotic checkpoint.

■ **ACTIVITY**

1. Critically discuss your views on whether you would carry out research on cdk inhibitors, and if so what strategy would you use. Support your view with pre-clinical and clinical evidence.

2. It has been stated in this chapter that ubiquitin-mediated proteolysis is crucial for regulation of the cell cycle. Find evidence that supports the statement that unregulated proteolysis in the cell cycle can lead to cancer. Begin with the paper by Reed (2003).

■ **FURTHER READING**

Adams, P.D. (2001) Regulation of the retinoblastoma tumor suppressor protein by cyclin/cdks. *Biochim. Biophys. Acta* **1471**: M123–M133.

Classon, M. and Harlow, E. (2002) The retinoblastoma tumor suppressor in development and cancer. *Nature Rev. Cancer* **2**: 910–917.

Collins, I. and Garrett, M.D. (2005) Targeting the cell division cycle in cancer: CDK and cell cycle checkpoint kinase inhibitors. *Curr. Opin. Pharmacol.* **5**: 366–373.

DiCiommo, D., Gallie, B.L., and Bremner, R. (2000) Retinoblastoma: the disease, gene and protein provide critical leads to understand cancer. *Semin. Cancer Biol.* **10**: 255–269.

Fischer, P.M. and Gianella-Borradori, A. (2003) CDK inhibitors in clinical development for the treatment of cancer. *Exp. Opin. Invest. Drugs* **12**: 955–970.

Kaufmann, W.K. (2006) Dangerous entanglements. *Trends Mol. Med.* **12**: 235–237.

Kops, G.J.P.L., Weaver, B.A.A., and Cleveland, D.W. (2005) On the road to cancer: aneuploidy and the mitotic checkpoint. *Nature Rev. Cancer* **5**: 773–785.

Malumbres, M. and Barbacid, M. (2001) To cycle or not to cycle: a critical decision in cancer. *Nature Rev. Cancer* **1**: 222–231.

Massague', J. (2004) G1 cell-cycle control and cancer. *Nature* **432**: 298–306.

Meraldi, P., Honda, R., and Nigg, E.A. (2004) Aurora kinases link chromosome segregation and cell division to cancer susceptibility. *Curr. Opin. Genet. Dev.* **14**: 29–36.

Shah, M.A. and Schwartz, G.K. (2006) Cyclin dependent kinases as targets for cancer therapy. *Update Cancer Ther.* **1**: 311–332.

Swanton, C. (2004) Cell-cycle targeted therapies. *Lancet Oncol.* **5**: 27–36.

Weaver, B.A.A. and Cleveland, D.W. (2005) Decoding the links between mitosis, cancer and chemotherapy: the mitotic checkpoint, adaptation, and cell death. *Cancer Cell* **8**: 7–12.

Zhu, L. (2005) Tumour suppressor retinoblastoma protein Rb: a transcriptional regulator. *Eur. J. Cancer* **41**: 2415–2427.

■ **SELECTED SPECIAL TOPICS**

Emanuel, S., Rugg, C.A., Gruninger, R.H., Lin, R., Fuentes-Pesquera, A., Connolly, P.J., Wetter, S.K., Hollister, B., Kruger, W.W., Napier, C., Jolliffe, L., and Middleton, S.A. (2005) The *in vitro* and *in vivo* effects of JNJ-7706621: A dual inhibitor of cyclin-dependent kinases and aurora kinases. *Cancer Res.* **65**: 9038–9046.

Ewart-Toland, A., Briassouli, P., de Koning, J.P., Mao, J.-H., Yuan, J., Chan, F., MacCarthy-Morrogh, L., Ponder, B.A.J., Nagase, H., Burn, J., Ball, S., Almeida, M., Linardopoulos, S., and Balmain, A. (2003) Identification of Stk6/STK15 as a candidate low-penetrance tumor-susceptibility gene in mouse and human. *Nature Genet.* **34**: 403–412.

Reed, S.I. (2003) Ratchets and clocks: the cell cycle, ubiquitylation and protein turnover. *Nature Rev. Mol. Cell Biol.* **4**: 855–864.

Roy, P.G. and Thompson, A.M. (2006) Cyclin D1 and breast cancer. *The Breast* **15**: 718–727.

Rubin, S.M., Gall, A.-L., Zheng, N., and Pavletich, N.P. (2005) Structure of the Rb C-terminal domain bound to E2F-DP1: A mechanism for phosphorylation-induced E2F release. *Cell* **123**: 1093–1106.

Sanchez, I. and Dynlacht, B.D. (2005) New insights into cyclins, CDKs, and cell cycle control. *Semin. Cell Dev. Biol.* **16**: 311–321.

Senderowicz, A.M. (2003) Small-molecule cyclin-dependent kinase modulators. *Oncogene* **22**: 6609–6620.

Sharpless, N.E., Bardeesy, N., Lee, K.H., Carrasco, D., Castrillon, D.H., Aguirre, A.J., Wu, E.A., Horner, J.W., and De Pinho, R.A. (2001) Loss of p16Ink4a with retention of p19Arf predisposes mice to tumorigenesis. *Nature* **413**: 86–91.

Sherr, C.J. (2000) The Pezcoller Lecture: cancer cell cycles revisited. *Cancer Res.* **60**: 3689–3695.

Utikal, J., Udart, M., Leiter, U., Kaskel, P., Peter, R.U., and Krahn, G. (2005) Numerical abnormalities of the Cyclin D1 gene locus on chromosome 11q13 in non-melanoma skin cancer. *Cancer Lett.* **219**: 197–204.

Chapter 6

Growth inhibition and tumor suppressor genes

Introduction

The human body has mechanisms exerted by tumor suppressor genes that normally 'police' the processes that regulate cell numbers and ensure that new cells receive DNA that has been precisely replicated. Recall from Chapter 1 that the balance between cell proliferation, differentiation, and apoptosis maintains appropriate cell numbers. Many tumor suppressor gene products act as stop signs to uncontrolled growth and therefore may inhibit the cell cycle, promote differentiation, or trigger apoptosis. If both copies of a tumor suppressor gene become inactivated by mutation or epigenetic changes, the inhibitory signal is lost, and the result may be unregulated cell growth, a hallmark of cancer. Other tumor suppressor gene products are involved in DNA repair. If inactivated, DNA repair may be defective and failure to repair DNA may give rise to mutations that lead to cancer. Two alleles of every gene are present in the human genome (except those on sex chromosomes) and, in most cases, loss of tumor suppressor gene function requires inactivation of both copies. This often happens by mutation in one copy and loss of the remaining wild-type allele (**loss of heterozygosity**, LOH).

6.1 Definitions of tumor suppressor genes

Hereditary syndromes that predispose individuals to cancer can be explained by the inheritance of a germline mutation (passed on from egg/sperm DNA and thus present in all cells of an individual) in one tumor suppressor allele and the acquisition of a somatic mutation or other inactivating alteration in the second allele later in life. This was first proposed by Knudson and is known as Knudson's two-hit hypothesis. It states a strict definition of a tumor suppressor gene: a gene in which a germline mutation predisposes an individual to cancer. Although this hypothesis describes the mechanism by which mutation of most tumor

Table 6.1 Tumor suppressor genes. From Macleod, K. (2000) Tumor suppressor genes. *Curr. Opin. Genet. Dev.* **10**: 81–93, Copyright (2000). Reprinted with permission from Elsevier

Tumor suppressor gene	Human chromosomal location	Gene function	Human tumors associated with sporadic mutation	Associated cancer syndrome	Tumor phenotype of knock-out mouse mutants (hetero/homozygote)
RB1	13q14	Transcriptional regulator of cell cycle	Retinoblastoma, osteosarcoma	Familial retinoblastoma	MTC, pituitary adenocarcinoma, pheochromocytomas
Wt1	11p13	Transcriptional regulator	Nephroblastoma	Wilms tumor	None
p53	17q11	Transcriptional regulator/ growth arrest/apoptosis	Sarcomas, breast/brain tumors	Li–Fraumeni	Lymphomas, sarcomas
NF1	17q11	Ras-GAP activity	Neurofibromas, sarcomas, gliomas	Von Recklinghausen neurofibromatosis	Pheochromocytomas, myeloid leukemia, neurofibromas in DKO chimeras
NF2	22q12	ERM protein/cytoskeletal regulator	Schwannomas, meningiomas	Neurofibromatosis type 2	Sarcomas: metastases on p53 background
VHL	3p25	Regulates proteolysis	Hemangiomas, renal, pheochromocytoma	Von–Hippel Lindau	None
APC	5q21	Binds/regulates β-catenin activity	Colon cancer	Familial adenomatous polyposis	Intestinal **polyps** in Apc^{Min}
INK4a	9p21	p16^{Ink4a} cdki for cyclin D–cdk (4/6); p19^{ARF} binds mdm2, stabilizes p53	Melanoma, pancreatic	Familial melanoma	Lymphomas, sarcomas
PTC	9q22.3	Receptor for sonic hedgehog	Basal cell carcinoma, medulloblastoma	Gorlin syndrome	Medulloblastomas
BRCA1	17q21	Transcriptional regulator/DNA repair	Breast/ovarian tumors	Familial breast cancer	None
BRCA2	13q12	Transcriptional regulator/DNA repair	Breast/ovarian tumors	Familial breast cancer	None
DPC4	18q21.1	Transduces TGF-β signals	Pancreatic, colon, hamartomas	Juvenile polyposis	Cooperates with Apc^{Δ716} in colorectal carcinoma
FHIT	3p14.2	Nucleoside hydrolase	Lung, stomach, kidney, cervical carcinoma	Familial clear cell renal carcinoma	Not reported
PTEN	10q23	Dual-specificity phosphatase	Glioblastoma, prostate, breast	Cowden syndrome, BZS, Ldd	Lymphoma, thyroid, endometrium, prostate
TSC2	16	Cell cycle regulator	Renal, brain tumors	Tuberous sclerosis	Not reported
NKX3.1	8p21	Homeobox protein	Prostate	Familial prostate carcinoma	Not reported
LKB1	19p13	Serine/threonine kinase	Hamartomas, colorectal, breast	Peutz–Jeghers	Not reported
E-Cadherin	16q22.1	Cell adhesion regulator	Breast, colon, skin, lung carcinoma	Familial gastric cancer	Dominant negative, promotes invasion/metastasis
MSH2	2p22	*mut S* homolog, mismatch repair	Colorectal cancer	HNPCC	Lymphoma, colon/skin carcinoma
MLH1	3p21	*mut L* homolog, mismatch repair	Colorectal cancer	HNPCC	Lymphoma, intestinal adenoma/carcinoma
PMS1	2q31	Mismatch repair	Colorectal cancer	HNPCC	None
PMS2	7p22	Mismatch repair	Colorectal cancer	HNPCC	Lymphoma, sarcoma
MSH6	2p16	Mismatch repair	Colorectal cancer	HNPCC	Lymphoma, intestinal adenomas/carcinomas

This table does not include the susceptibility genes associated with ataxia telangiectasia (*ATM/ATR*), xeroderma pigmentosum (nucleotide excision repair genes), Bloom's syndrome (*BLM*), Werner's syndrome (*WRN*), or Fanconi's anemia (*FAA, FAC, FAD*), although mutation of these genes is associated with cancer predisposition. Nor does it include putative tumor suppressor genes which are subverted by chromosomal translocation, for example *PML*. Genes such as *MADR2*, *TGF-β receptor 2*, *IRF-1*, *p73*, *p33^{ING1}*, *PPAR*γ, *BUB1*, and *BUBR1* have been shown to be mutated in certain human tumors but are not included here because germline mutation of these genes is not yet associated with any hereditary human cancer syndrome.

BZS, Bannayan–Zonana syndrome; HNPCC, Hereditary non-polyposis colorectal cancer; Ldd, Lhermitte–Duclos syndrome.

suppressor genes has an effect, exceptions and additional complexities exist and will be mentioned later. Examples of tumor suppressor genes that fit this definition are shown in Table 6.1.

Let's look at the breast cancer susceptibility genes *BRCA1* and *BRCA2* as an example. Some families are prone to increased risk of developing breast and ovarian cancers. The hereditary breast and ovarian susceptibility genes *BRCA1* and *BRCA2* are well-known tumor suppressor genes that play a role in this hereditary syndrome, which make up about 5–10% of all breast cancer cases. The mechanism of these tumor suppressors follows Knudson's hypothesis in that one germline mutation predisposes individuals to breast and ovarian cancer. The mutated genes most often produce a truncated protein and therefore cause loss of function. Breast and ovarian tumors that develop in these individuals exhibit loss of heterozygosity. In some cases of **sporadic** (non-hereditary) breast cancer, BRCA1 protein levels are reduced, not due to mutation but rather to epigenetic mechanisms. Both BRCA proteins are involved in homologous recombination and double-strand break repair (see Figure 2.9) and therefore help maintain the integrity of the genome. They also have a role in the regulation of transcription and chromatin structure. Note, however, that there is no clear homology between BRCA1 and BRCA2. One proposal of how mutations in the *BRCA* genes cause cancer suggests that defective recombination destabilizes the genome and leads to chromosomal rearrangements and mutation. Another proposal regarding a role for BRCA proteins in estrogen signaling is discussed in Chapter 11.

Historically, tumor suppressor genes were called 'anti-oncogenes' since some of them seemed to 'undo' pathways of oncogene activation. Although the term is no longer used, it can be a helpful tool for illustrating the function of some tumor suppressor genes. The role of aberrant phosphorylation by kinases during carcinogenesis was emphasized in Chapter 4.

PAUSE AND THINK

Since kinases are enzymes that phosphorylate, what types of enzymes 'undo' kinases? Phosphatases are enzymes that remove phosphate groups.

It is therefore predictable that some genes that encode phosphatases which antagonize kinase activity, could act as 'anti-oncogenes'. Inactivation of these phosphatase genes by mutation removes the inhibitory signal and the kinase activity becomes unregulated.

One gene encoding a phosphatase that is frequently mutated in many cancers is *PTEN* (phosphatase and tensin homolog on chromosome 10). *PTEN* codes for a phosphatase with dual specificity: it can act as both a protein and lipid phosphatase. Its role as a lipid phosphatase in oncogenesis is best known. PTEN dephosphorylates the membrane lipid PIP3 (phosphatidyl-inositol-3 phosphate) to form PIP2. This antagonizes (shown by the reversed red arrow) the PI3 kinase pathway (Figure 6.1).

PAUSE AND THINK

Recall that stimulation of cell membrane receptors recruits PI3 kinase to the membrane where it phosphorylates PIP2 to generate PIP3, a potent second messenger that activates a cascade of proteins important for cell division and inhibition of apoptosis. This signal must be tightly regulated to prevent uncontrolled growth.

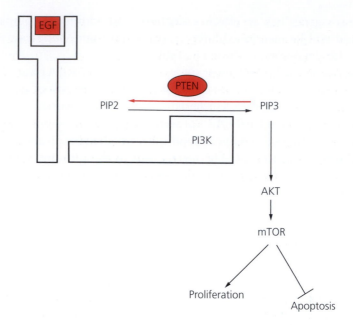

Figure 6.1 PTEN antagonizes the PI3 kinase pathway.

Loss of the inhibitory dephosphorylation activity of PTEN in the *PTEN* mutant phenotype results in a constitutively active PI3 kinase pathway, involving activation of protein kinases Akt and mTOR (mammalian target of rapamycin). The net result is the inhibition of apoptosis and induction of cell proliferation. This favors oncogenesis. Note that this gene also fits the tumor suppressor definition above since a germline mutation of *PTEN* causes Cowden syndrome which predisposes patients to cancer.

Another protein-tyrosine phosphatase, PTPN1, encoded by the *PTPN1* gene, regulates tyrosine kinase receptor signaling by dephosphorylating EGFR and PDGFR. Accelerated development of lymphomas has been reported upon analysis of *PTPN1* knock-out mice. Several other protein-tyrosine phosphatases also act as tumor suppressor genes.

HOW DO WE KNOW THAT?

Enzyme kinetics and cell growth assays (see data reported in Wang *et al.*, 2004)

Mutations in several protein-tyrosine phosphatase genes were identified in human colorectal tumors. This was done by amplifying the exons of 87 different protein-tyrosine phosphatase genes from tumor genomic DNA and sequencing these exons. DNA from normal tissue of matching patients was used as a control to identify somatic (tumor-specific) mutations. Biochemical analysis demonstrated that these mutations gave rise to proteins that had reduced phosphatase activity. This was done by expressing mutant protein-tyrosine phosphatase catalytic domains in bacteria. After purification, enzyme kinetics were studied. The rate of substrate hydrolysis was plotted against substrate concentration and the Michaelis–Menton equation was used to determine K_m and K_{cat}. Growth of cells in culture was suppressed by transfection of the wild-type protein but not upon transfection of the mutant proteins. Growth was examined by staining cells with crystal violet 2 weeks post-transfection and colonies were counted. This genetic, biochemical, and cellular evidence demonstrates that these protein-tyrosine phosphatase genes are mutated in tumors and produce loss-of-function proteins, suggesting that they act as tumor suppressors.

Note that not all kinases are oncogenic and not all phosphatases are tumor suppressors. Ataxia telangiectasia mutated (ATM) kinase functions in DNA repair as mentioned in Chapter 2, and plays a role in tumor suppression. Many other examples exist. The role of different protein-tyrosine phosphatases as either oncogenes or tumor suppressor genes is reviewed in Ostman *et al.* (2006).

An examination of two 'star players' in the world of tumor suppressor genes, the retinoblastoma (*Rb*) gene (also discussed in Chapter 5) and the *p53* gene, is central to this chapter. The roles of both gene products during carcinogenesis are described below.

6.2 The retinoblastoma gene

Retinoblastoma is a rare childhood cancer with a worldwide incidence of 1 in 20,000. There are two forms of the disease, a familial (inherited) form and a sporadic form (Figure 6.2). About 40% of all retinoblastoma cases are familial and about 60% are sporadic. In the familial form of the disease, one germline mutation in the *Rb* gene is passed to the child and is present in all cells. A second mutation is acquired in a particular retinoblast that consequently gives rise to a tumor in the retina. One inherited mutated gene results in a sufficiently high probability that a second mutation may occur. It has been suggested that the first mutation generates genomic instability resulting in the high probability of a second mutation, and this is sometimes referred to as a mutator phenotype. In sporadic

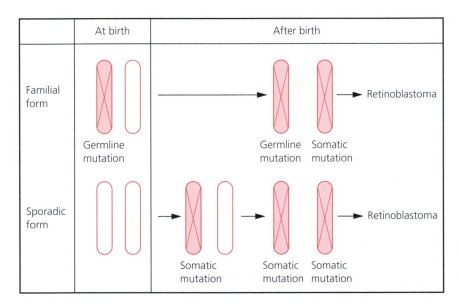

Figure 6.2 The familial and sporadic forms of retinoblastoma: germline versus somatic mutations.

retinoblastoma, both mutations occur somatically in the same retinoblast. Since there are approximately 10^8 retinoblasts in the retina there is a low chance that sporadic retinoblastoma will occur more than once in an individual; hence sporadic cases usually only affect one eye while familial cases are often bilateral. The disease demonstrates Knudson's two-hit hypothesis: two separate mutations—one in each of the two retinoblastoma alleles—are needed to inactivate the two copies of the *Rb* allele and prevent expression of the RB protein. A mutation in one *Rb* allele is insufficient to knock out functional RB and so cancer-causing mutations are recessive. An understanding of the molecular mechanisms of the gene product underlying this disease elucidates important principles about tumor suppressor proteins.

The retinoblastoma protein (RB, sometimes called pRB) is the product of the retinoblastoma tumor suppressor gene (*Rb*). As we discussed in Chapter 5, its main role is to regulate the cell cycle by inhibiting the G_1 to S phase transition. Cell proliferation is dependent on the transcription of a set of target genes to produce proteins that are needed for cell division (e.g. thymidylate synthase; dihydrofolate reductase). RB is an indirect regulator of transcription for specific gene expression that affects cell proliferation and differentiation. Protein–protein interactions facilitate the function of RB as a transcriptional regulator; RB binds to and modulates the activity of a critical transcription factor (E2F) and chromatin remodeling enzymes (see Figure 5.4).

PAUSE AND THINK

As a tumor suppressor protein, do you suppose RB inhibits or activates the transcription factors needed for cell proliferation? It inhibits the transcriptional activity of factors needed for cell cycle progression. Therefore, target genes important for cell growth are not expressed. On the other hand, loss of the tumor suppressor protein RB results in the loss of inhibition and consequently uncontrolled cell cycle progression and division. Think about the role of RB in differentiation. Do you suppose it inhibits or activates transcription factors that are responsible for turning on cell-type specific genes? As a tumor suppressor it stimulates the activity of transcription factors, such as Myo D, that activate genes involved in differentiation. Loss of RB leads to an increase in cell number and to the failure of differentiation.

6.3 Mutations in the RB pathway and cancer

Retinoblastoma is initiated by the loss of both *Rb* alleles. The types of mutations identified are mostly deletions, frameshift, or **nonsense mutations** that result in the abrogation of RB function as would be predicted from Knudson's two-hit hypothesis. In addition, **missense mutations** that lie within the pocket domain have been reported. It is of interest that mutations of Ser567 (described above) have been found in human tumors because, normally, phosphorylation of this amino acid causes the release of E2F. Mutation of Ser567 may disrupt the regulation usually observed at this site. Since the RB pathway is central in cell cycle regulation, tumor initiation may be induced via any mutation that blocks RB function and causes E2F to be available to activate transcription regardless of the presence or absence of a growth signal. Although the *Rb* gene is expressed in all adult tissues, only retinoblastoma and a very few other types of cancer are initiated by loss of RB. Yet this pathway is still inactivated in most human tumors and is targeted by human tumor viruses (see Section 6.6). These observations suggest that we have more to learn about the different roles of RB and the requirements of different cell types. For example, early studies suggest that RB may have a role in differentiation as well as cell cycle progression in the developing retina.

6.4 The p53 pathway

The *p53* gene was the first tumor suppressor gene to be identified and, since its discovery, scientists have found that the p53 pathway is altered in most human cancers. Two *p53* homologs, *p73* and *p63*, have also been identified but mutations in cancer cells are rare. Its protein product, p53, is at the heart of the cell's tumor suppressive mechanism and thus has been nicknamed the 'guardian of the genome'. In the absence of cellular stress, low levels of p53 induce antioxidant activity which decreases the levels of reactive oxygen species (ROS) and subsequent DNA damage (Sablina *et al.*, 2005). As mentioned in Chapter 2, normal cell metabolism produces ROS that can react with DNA. It has been estimated that endogenous ROS modify approximately 20,000 bases of DNA per day in a single cell (Sablina *et al.* 2005). p53 accomplishes this by upregulating genes whose products have antioxidant functions such as glutathione peroxidase 1 and sestrins, proteins involved in hydrogen peroxide metabolism. This antioxidant activity guards against mutation and may help prevent cancer.

Many types of 'danger signals', such as cell stress and DNA damage, can activate p53 and trigger several crucial cellular responses that suppress tumor formation (Figure 6.3). Upstream stress activators include radiation-, drug-, or carcinogen-induced DNA damage, oncogenic activation, hypoxia and low ribonucleotide pools. These conditions may nurture tumor initiation. In response to these stress signals p53 can elicit downstream cellular effects including cell cycle arrest, apoptosis, DNA repair, and inhibition of angiogenesis. The ability to cause the cell cycle to pause allows

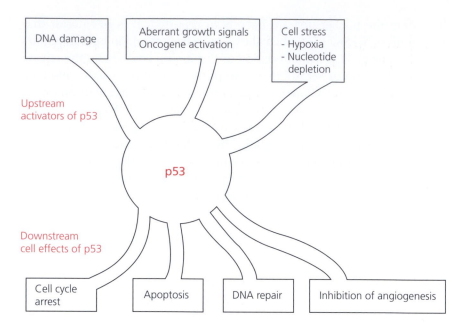

Figure 6.3 Upstream activators and downstream effects of p53.

for repair of DNA mutations and prevents their propagation within the genome. Apoptosis is another means of preventing propagation of mutations; cell suicide benefits the organism as a whole if DNA damage cannot be repaired. Mutated cells are better dead. Apoptosis is the critical biological function mediating the tumor suppressor function of p53. It should be mentioned that p53 may also play a pro-oxidant role under certain stress conditions that may contribute to the cellular effect of apoptosis.

Self test   Close this book and try to redraw Figure 6.3. Check your answer. Correct your work. Close the book once more and try again.

The overall regulation of the p53 pathway possesses an extraordinary complexity that compels us to try to unravel each layer. Let us begin by examining the structure of the p53 protein and its interactions with its inhibitors, and then move on to dissecting how its activity is switched on and how it exerts its effects.

Structure of the p53 protein

The *p53* gene, located on chromosome 17p13, contains 11 exons that encode a 53 kDa phosphoprotein. The p53 protein is a transcription factor containing four distinct domains: the amino-terminal transactivation domain, the DNA-binding domain containing a Zn^{2+} ion, an oligomerization domain, and a carboxy-terminal regulatory domain (Figure 6.4). The

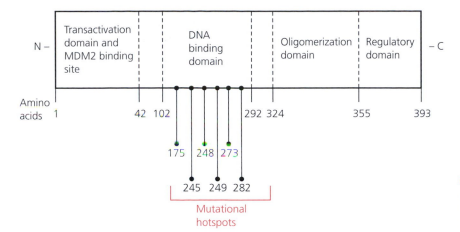

Figure 6.4 Domains of the p53 protein and location of mutational hotspots (marked in red).

p53 protein binds as a tetramer to a DNA response element containing two inverted repeats of the sequence 5′-PuPuPuC(A/T)-3′ (Pu symbolizes either purine base A or G) in order to regulate transcription of its target genes. Oligonucleotide array experiments have demonstrated that p53 binds to approximately 300 different gene promoter regions, thus suggesting that p53 has a powerful regulatory role. Several of these specific target genes and the mechanism of how they exert their effect will be discussed later in the chapter.

Regulation of p53 protein by MDM2

Normally, the level of p53 protein in a cell is low. The activity of p53 in a cell is regulated at the level of protein degradation, not at the level of expression of the *p53* gene. The MDM2 protein, a ubiquitin ligase, is its main regulator. Ubiquitin ligases are enzymes that attach a small peptide called ubiquitin to proteins, flagging it for **proteolysis** (enzymatic protein degradation involving cleavage of peptide bonds) in proteosomes. MDM2 modifies the carboxy-terminal domain of p53, and thus targets it for degradation by proteosomes in the cytoplasm. In addition, MDM2 modifies the activity of p53 since it binds to and inhibits the p53 transactivation domain at the amino-terminal and transports the protein into the cytoplasm, away from nuclear DNA. Thus the activity of p53 as a transcription factor is out of reach. The binding of MDM2 to p53 is part of an autoregulatory feedback loop (Figure 6.5, shown by red arrows) since the MDM2 gene is a transcriptional target of p53. Therefore, p53 stimulates the production of its negative regulator MDM2 that causes the degradation of p53. Small amounts of p53 will reduce the amount of MDM2 protein and this will result in an increase of p53 activity, thus completing the loop.

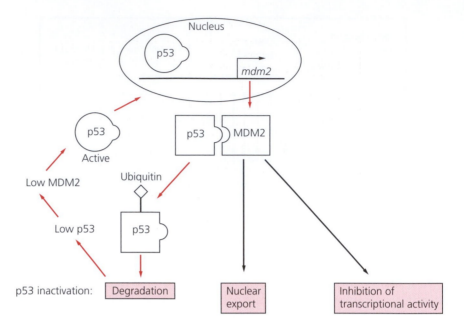

Figure 6.5 Regulation of p53 by MDM2. See text for details.

Upstream: molecular pathways of p53 activation

The mechanism by which p53 becomes activated depends on the nature of the stress signal. Stress is 'sensed' by cellular proteins, many of which are kinases that convey the danger signals to p53 via phosphorylation. Disruption of the p53–MDM2 interaction is fundamental to the activation of p53 by its upstream factors.

The upstream activators of p53 utilize three main independent molecular pathways to signal cellular distress (Figure 6.6). DNA damage caused by ionizing radiation is signaled by two protein kinases. The first kinase, ATM, stimulated by DNA double-strand breaks, phosphorylates and activates a second kinase Chk2. Both ATM and Chk2 kinases phosphorylate amino-terminal sites of p53 and this phosphorylation interferes with binding of MDM2. A second molecular pathway that signals cellular distress to p53 is executed by two different kinases, ATR and casein kinase II. These also phosphorylate p53 and disrupt its interaction with MDM2. Lastly, activated oncogenes, such as Ras, induce the activity of the protein p14arf, another modulator of the p53–MDM2 complex. P14arf is one of two translational products of the *INK4a/CDKN2A* gene (p16, a cyclin kinase inhibitor, is the other product). P14arf does not bind to the interface of p53–MDM2, but functions by sequestering MDM2 to the nucleolus of the cell. All three pathways prevent degradation of p53 by MDM2.

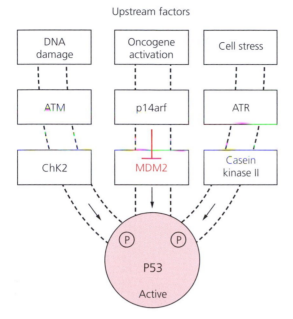

Upstream factors

Figure 6.6 Upstream activators of p53. The first and the last pathways involve kinases and result in the phosphorylation of p53 (shown as P). All pathways disrupt the interaction of p53 with MDM2.

Downstream: molecular mechanisms of p53 cellular effects

The main mechanism by which p53 exerts its tumor suppressing effects is by inducing the expression of specific target genes. Let us examine how the resulting network of proteins triggers these responses (Figure 6.7).

Inhibition of the cell cycle

One of the central functions of p53 is to cause cell cycle arrest in response to DNA damage so that there is an opportunity to repair the damage prior to the next round of replication; thus damaged DNA will be prevented from being replicated and passed on to daughter cells and maintenance of the genome will be facilitated. The molecular mechanism responsible for this cellular response involves the transcriptional induction of the *p21* gene. Its product, the p21 protein, inhibits several cyclin–cdk complexes and causes a pause in the G_1 to S (and G_2 to M) transition of the cell cycle (see Pause and Think).

PAUSE AND THINK

Why would an inhibitor of cyclin–cdk complexes cause a pause in the G_1–S transition? Recall the role of cyclin–cdk complexes in the cell cycle; importantly they act as kinases. As kinases they phosphorylate. What do they phosphorylate? RB. Failure of the cdk complex to phosphorylate RB prevents the release of the transcription factor E2F and blocks the transition into S phase.

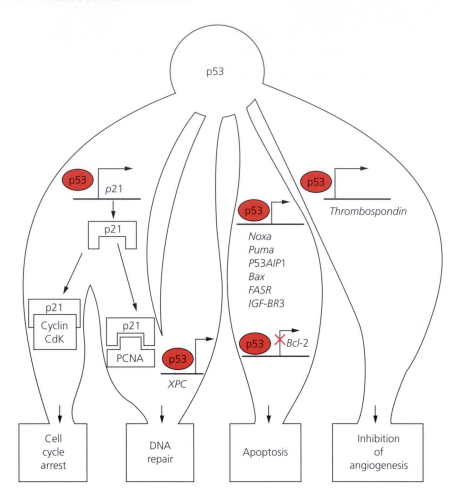

Figure 6.7 Downstream effects of p53. p53 exerts many of its effects by regulating target genes as shown.

In addition, p21 also binds PCNA (proliferating cell nuclear antigen), a protein that has a role in DNA synthesis and DNA repair. The interaction with p21 is such that it inhibits PCNA's role in DNA replication but not in DNA repair. Therefore, p21 is an important part of the molecular mechanism that facilitates the ability of p53 to bring about a pause in the cell cycle and at the same time allow DNA repair.

Apoptosis

The expression of several mediators of apoptosis is transcriptionally regulated directly by p53 (Table 6.2). The targets include genes that code for proteins involved in two apoptotic pathways that respond to external and internal signals, respectively. (Apoptosis will be described in Chapter 7.) In general, genes encoding proteins that promote apoptosis, pro-apoptotic proteins, are induced while genes encoding proteins that antagonize apoptosis, anti-apoptotic proteins, are repressed. The mitochondrial pro-apoptotic proteins NOXA, PUMA, and p53AIP1, that cause

Table 6.2 p53-inducible apoptotic target genes

Gene	Location of gene product
Bax	Intrinsic pathway
NOXA	Intrinsic pathway
PUMA	Intrinsic pathway
P53AIP1	Intrinsic pathway
FAS	Extrinsic pathway
IGF-BP3	Extrinsic pathway
DR5	Extrinsic pathway
PIDD	Extrinsic pathway
PERP	Endoplasmic reticulum

the release of cytochrome c and activate the apoptosome, are induced. Also, p53 tips the balance regulated by the Bcl-2 protein family towards apoptosis by inducing gene expression of the pro-apoptotic protein Bax and repressing the expression of anti-apoptotic protein Bcl-2. Fas receptor (FASR) is a transmembrane receptor that receives extracellular stimuli to stimulate apoptosis. Expression of the *Fas receptor* gene is induced by p53. Apoptosis is also triggered when survival signaling is blocked by p53's induction of IGF-BP3 (insulin-like growth factor-binding protein 3). IGF-BP3 blocks the signaling of IGF-1 to its receptor. Activation of these different pathways in concert is required for a full apoptotic response. Transcription-independent mechanisms for the induction of apoptosis by p53 also exist and will be discussed in Chapter 7.

DNA repair and angiogenesis

Both DNA repair and angiogenesis are covered in depth elsewhere in this volume (Chapters 2 and 9, respectively). In general, a role for the transcriptional regulation of important genes in these processes by p53 has been established. For example, the gene *XPC* that is involved in nucleotide excision repair is regulated by p53 through a p53 response element in its promoter. Thrombospondin, an inhibitor of angiogenesis, is also transcriptionally regulated by p53. This further supports the role of p53 as a transcriptional regulator in different biological responses.

Decision making

As the guardian of the genome, p53 prevents damaged DNA from being passed on to daughter cells either by inhibiting the cell cycle or by inducing apoptosis. Cell cycle inhibition and apoptosis are two independent effects of p53. The molecular factors that determine the biological outcome of whether inhibition of the cell cycle or apoptosis takes place are just being elucidated. One model that has been put forth is that different combinations of transcription factors that act as dimers influence the biological response. Oncogene activation (e.g. Myc) is an upstream inducer of p53 that triggers apoptosis. The mechanism of this stress signal acts via the cyclin–cdk inhibitor p21, the main effector of cell cycle inhibition but also an inhibitor of cell death. The regulation of the *p21* gene is a pivotal point in the p53 decision-making process. Both p53 and a transcription factor called Miz-1 are required for *p21* gene expression. Now enter the oncogene, Myc, which competes with p53 for binding with Miz-1. Myc interacts with Miz-1 and inhibits the transcription of *p21*. Through this mechanism of preventing expression of *p21*, Myc not only overrides the p53-regulated block to cell cycle progression but also blocks the p21-mediated inhibition of apoptosis (Figure 6.8). p53 is not altered and is free to induce the expression of pro-apoptotic targets. Additional events are also required for full activation of apoptosis, since p53 phosphorylation

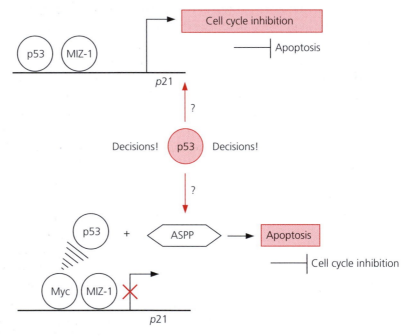

Figure 6.8 Molecular factors in deciding the effects of p53: cell cycle inhibition or apoptosis? The regulation of a gene that codes for a cyclin–cdk inhibitor, the *p21* gene, plays a pivotal role. Top: without competition from Myc, p53 and MIZ-1 bind to the promoter of *p21*, induce transcription, and this results in cell cycle inhibition. Bottom: upon oncogenic activation, Myc competes with the binding of p53. Myc and MIZ-1 bind to the *p21* promoter, inhibit transcription, and block cell cycle inhibition. ASPP binds to p53 and facilitates activation of apoptotic genes to induce apoptosis.

and apoptotic co-factors are required for the induction of some apoptotic genes. Revealing the mechanisms behind other modes of upstream stress inducers of p53, such as oxidative stress, requires further studies.

The apoptosis stimulating proteins of p53 (ASPP) family also plays a role in p53 decision making (Slee and Lu, 2003). These proteins bind to the p53 DNA-binding domain and have been shown specifically to enhance the ability of p53 to activate genes involved in apoptosis and not cell cycle arrest. The selection of apoptotic genes versus growth arrest genes could potentially be accomplished by specific promoter sequences that serve to distinguish the functionally distinct classes of genes. The regulation of ASPP itself requires further study. Mutations in the ASPP binding site of the *p53* gene and epigenetic silencing of the *ASPP* gene have been identified in tumor cells. These tumor cells may have been initiated because they escaped from the apoptotic program normally augmented by ASPP. Other co-activators may also enhance the selectivity of p53 to activate apoptotic genes.

6.5 Mutations in the p53 pathway and cancer

Due to the central role of p53 as a tumor suppressor and guardian of the genome, cell transformation is less likely to occur in cells that maintain a functional p53 pathway. p53 mutant cells are characterized by genomic instability, since mutations are more likely to be maintained in dividing cells, providing an environment that is permissive for tumor initiation. The high frequency of p53 pathway mutations found in tumor cells is most likely to be the result of selective pressure favoring mutant cells that escape tumor suppression. Over 75% of all *p53* mutations are missense mutations and result in single amino acid substitutions. Many mutant p53 molecules are more stable than wild-type p53 protein and can accumulate in cells. More than 90% of the missense mutations are located in the DNA-binding domain (amino acids 102–292) and more than 30% of these affect only six codons and are therefore referred to as 'hotspots' (see Figure 6.4).

In addition to mutation of the *p53* gene, there are other ways to interfere with the p53 pathway. Defects in pathways that lead to the activation of p53 in response to stress, such as mutations in the *chk2* gene, have been identified in cancer cells that do not contain mutations in the *p53* gene. In these cases, the stress signal would not be transmitted to p53 via phosphorylation as in normal cells (see Figure 6.6). Also, over-expression of the MDM2 protein has been demonstrated to alter the regulation of p53, leading to a 'p53-inactivated' phenotype. Inactivation of downstream effectors, such as Bax and FASR, also perturbs the pathway.

Some of these other p53 pathway disruptions may not lead to effects as severe as *p53* mutation, since p53 protein is a central node for receiving and eliciting many stress signals and biological responses, respectively, but may mimic a partial aspect of p53 inactivation and be permissive for tumor formation.

Li–Fraumeni syndrome

Li–Fraumeni syndrome is predominantly characterized by a germline mutation of the *p53* gene and leads to a predisposition to a wide range of cancers. It is an autosomal dominant disease, so an affected individual has a 50% chance of passing the mutation to each offspring. Patients have a 25-fold increased risk of developing cancer before they are 50 years old compared with the general population. The young age at which individuals develop cancer and the frequent occurrence of multiple primary tumors in individuals are characteristic features of the syndrome. The types of cancer seen within families that carry the mutation include sarcomas, breast cancer, leukemia, and brain tumors. Cancer develops at an earlier age over several generations. The protein product of the mutated *p53* gene does not function to protect the genome and an accumulation of mutations goes unchallenged and eventually leads to tumor formation.

More complex than Knudson's two-hit hypothesis

The mechanism of tumor suppressor genes may be more complex than Knudson's two-hit hypothesis suggests. This is particularly clear for *p53*. Loss of heterozygosity is not commonly observed in tumors from cells with only one *p53* allele, suggesting that reduced amounts (haploinsufficiency) of p53 can cause transformation. Mutations may result in varied amounts of tumor suppressor gene expression and therefore tumor suppressor 'dose' may play a role in the cancer outcome. Recent experiments which generated p53 hypomorphs (animals that exhibit reduced levels of p53 expression) using RNA interference (see Section 1.6) support this mechanism (Hemann *et al.*, 2003).

Unlike most other tumor suppressor genes, some *p53* mutations do not lead to loss of function. Some missense mutations form an altered protein that interacts with the product of a normal p53 allele via dimerization to inactivate its function. This type of effect is referred to as dominant negative, whereby the mutated gene product dominates to inactivate the wild-type gene product. In this situation, the autoregulatory loop is affected because p53 fails to induce its inhibitor, MDM2, and as a result p53 mutant protein accumulates. Other mutations can lead to a newly acquired 'gain-of-function' phenotype that can accumulate in and transform cells.

In this instance, mutant *p53* (not wild-type *p53*) can be considered an oncogene having an active role in carcinogenesis.

6.6 Interaction of DNA viral protein products with RB and p53

Viruses are cellular parasites that hijack host cell proteins to maintain their life cycle. Coercing the host cell into S phase is essential for viral propagation. Several DNA viruses have been shown to be carcinogenic to humans. Most notable are papovaviruses, adenoviruses, herpes viruses, and hepatitis B. Interestingly, several of the DNA viruses share a common oncogenic mechanism that involves the interaction of viral proteins with the two important regulators of tumor suppression, RB and p53 (Figure 6.9). The viral proteins adenovirus E1A, papilloma virus E7, and SV40 Large T antigen inactivate RB (Figure 6.9b), adenovirus E1B, and papilloma virus E6 and SV40 Large T antigen, inactivate p53 (Figure 6.9c).

The ability of both E6 and E7 to degrade p53 and RB, respectively, using the ubiquitin-proteasome system, correlates with their oncogenic potential. The biochemical events involved in p53 degradation by E6 are as follows: E6 binds to a ubiquitin-protein ligase (E6-AP) and forms a dimer that subsequently binds to p53. p53 is then ubiquitinated and tagged for recognition by the proteosome for degradation. A similar mechanism is likely for E7-targeted degradation of RB and E1B-targeted degradation of p53.

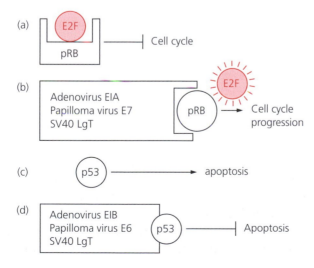

Figure 6.9 Viral protein products interact with RB (pRB) and p53 (parts b and d, respectively) and inhibit their normal function (shown in a and c).

Human papilloma virus (HPV) causes cervical cancer

The *p53* gene is rarely mutated in cervical cancers, suggesting that the causative agent, HPV, may be functionally equivalent to *p53* mutation. A polymorphism in the *p53* gene at amino acid 72 in humans leads to differences in the risk of cervical cancer following exposure to HPV. Patients with two alleles coding for Arg at this position have a seven times higher risk of cervical cancer than those with alleles coding for Pro at this site. The Arg-containing p53 protein is more susceptible to degradation by HPV E6 (probably due to altered protein conformation). As a result of these cells having decreased p53 activity, they are likely to have an increased mutation rate and an increased potential to form tumors.

 Therapeutic strategies

6.7 Targeting of the p53 pathway

The role of p53 as a 'star player' in suppressing tumorigenesis and the high occurrence of mutations in the *p53* gene found in tumors draws attention to the p53 pathway as a promising cancer therapeutic target. As a result, many different strategies that target the p53 pathway have been developed. Several are described below. The variety of p53 pathway aberrations, including both *p53* gene mutations and defective regulation,

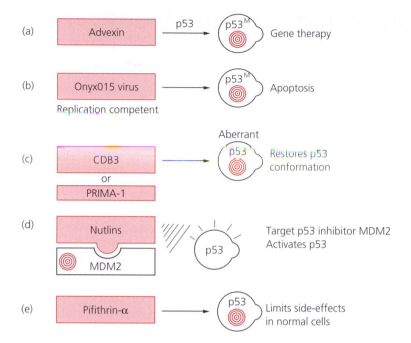

Figure 6.10 Therapeutic strategies that target the p53 pathway. Cell targets are indicated with a (◎) symbol; therapeutic agents (red); p53M, mutant p53; nutlins compete (///) with p53.

suggests that the future success of these therapies will be dependent on knowing the *p53* **genotype** of tumors in patients prior to treatment. We need to know if there are mutations in the *p53* gene itself or in its regulators and, if so, the type of mutations present. You have to know what is wrong before you can fix it. Therapeutics may strive to correct a *p53* mutation or potentiate normal p53 protein function in cases where other alterations in the p53 pathway affect its function. Several different strategies are described below and illustrated in Figure 6.10 (therapeutics are shaded red).

Strategies that aim to correct a *p53* mutation

Gene therapy is one of the most obvious approaches to correct for a *p53* mutation. In fact, many different vectors have been examined in pre-clinical and clinical settings (see Bouchet *et al.*, 2006). Retroviruses have been used in several pre-clinical studies and have shown anti-tumor activity. However, only one Phase I clinical trial using retrovirus-mediated *p53* gene therapy has been published to date (discussed in Bouchet *et al.*, 2006) and expression of *p53* could not be detected, although some clinical responses in lung cancer patients were observed. Unlike retroviruses that integrate into the genome and therefore carry a risk of causing insertional mutagenesis, adenoviruses, which are DNA viruses, do not cause damage to the genome. Frequently used adenoviral vectors can carry large amounts of DNA and can infect a range of cell types via coxsackievirus and adenovirus receptors (CAR) with high efficiencies. Adenoviruses that have been modified to be replication defective have been popular vectors. Advexin® (Introgen Therapeutics; Genedicine®, Shenzhen SiBono GeneTech Co. Ltd) is a replication-defective adenoviral vector that contains the human *p53* gene, driven by a viral promoter (the cytomegalovirus promoter; CMV), within the region of an E1 deletion (Figure 6.10a). Many clinical trials have demonstrated safety and low toxicity. It has been reported recently that Advexin® was used as an adenoviral-mediated *p53* gene therapy to treat one individual with Li–Fraumeni syndrome. Genedicine® obtained a drug license in China and is the world's first commercial gene therapy for cancer.

Replication-competent adenoviruses provide another strategy as the basis of new cancer therapeutics. As mentioned above, wild-type adenovirus can replicate in cells by inactivating p53 and RB (Figure 6.11a). The Onyx 015 virus, a replication-selective adenovirus, was designed to selectively kill cancer cells that contain *p53* mutations (Figure 6.11b). It takes advantage of the fact that interference with the RB and p53 pathways is exploited both by viruses and cancer cells (Ries and Korn, 2002). The Onyx 015 virus contains a deletion of the *E1B* gene and thus it can only replicate within, and subsequently kill, cells that have an inactive p53 pathway (Figure 6.11b). The E1A product of the Onyx 015 virus binds to and inactivates RB and, as a result, induces the G_1–S phase transition of the cell cycle allowing for viral replication and cell destruction. The Onyx

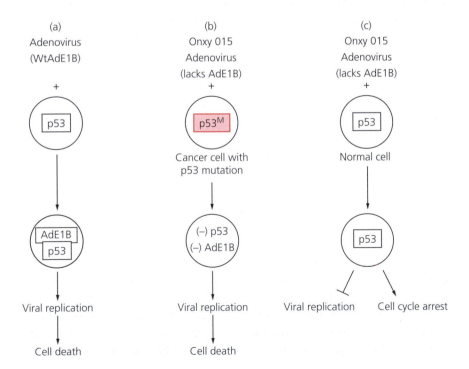

Figure 6.11 The Onyx 015 adenovirus can selectively kill cancer cells with p53 mutations.

015 adenovirus (lacking E1B) triggers a p53 response (growth arrest) in normal cells, resulting in the interference of viral replication (Figure 6.11c). Such selective replication produces a treatment with minimal side-effects. Phase I and II clinical trials have given encouraging results. Intratumoral injection proved safe and specific anti-tumor effects were demonstrated. Phase III trials are ongoing.

Small molecules that can restore wild-type function to products of *p53* gene mutations have been investigated (Bykov *et al.*, 2003). Many missense mutations of *p53* result in aberrant protein conformation and subsequently interfere with the DNA-binding function of the p53 protein. As a result, the p53 inhibitor, MDM2, and target genes essential for apoptosis are not induced. Note that tumors that carry such mutations are more likely to be resistant to conventional chemo- and radiotherapies since these drugs work via the induction of apoptosis. Reactivation of *p53* mutants aims to eliminate tumor cells via the induction of apoptosis. A short (nine residues) synthetic peptide, CDB3, has been shown to stabilize the structure of several *p53* mutants and to restore their transcriptional function (Figure 6.10c.). CDB3 is thought to act as a chaperone protein that aids in the refolding of the mutant p53 protein. Similarly, PRIMA-1 (Figure 6.10c), identified from a chemical library, demonstrates restoration of the wild-type p53 conformation and DNA binding in a number of mutant p53 proteins, including those with mutations in the hotspots (see Figure 6.4). Its specificity for cells expressing mutant p53 is notable. PRIMA-1 has shown low toxicity and mutant p53-dependent anti-tumor effects in human tumor xenografts in animal models.

Strategies that aim to activate endogenous p53

In many tumors wild-type *p53* is expressed but the regulation of the p53 protein is defective and results in an altered p53 pathway. As mentioned above, over-expression of the p53 inhibitor, MDM2, leads to defective regulation and p53 inactivation. Note that cancers caused by viruses do not usually harbor a p53 mutation; instead viral proteins act to inactivate p53 function. An approach on the horizon to activate wild-type p53 protein is the development of inhibitors of the p53–MDM2 interaction (Chene, 2003) (see Pause and Think).

Detailed structural information about the p53–MDM2 complex has been obtained by nuclear magnetic resonance and X-ray crystallography and has revealed that MDM2 has a well-defined binding site for p53. The opposite is not true. Thus, inhibitors are best designed to mimic amino acids of p53. In addition, the binding interface was found to be relatively small, which suggested that it was possible to design small inhibitors that could be taken orally. Following a strategy of high-throughput screening of synthetic chemicals and computer modeling, drugs called nutlins

PAUSE AND THINK

What type of information is required to begin to design inhibitors of the p53–MDM2 interaction?

(Figure 6.10d) were identified and have shown promising results in pre-clinical tests (Vassilev *et al.*, 2004). These results include triggering p53 activation and its biological responses in cancer cells containing wild-type p53. In addition, inhibition of tumor growth by 90% was demonstrated in animal models. Nutlins support the idea that protein–protein interactions are good targets for cancer therapeutic.

Strategies that aim to suppress endogenous p53

It is clear that p53 is important for the disposal of tumor cells. The success of chemo- and radiotherapy is often limited by side-effects in normal tissues. Many of the side-effects of chemo- and radiotherapy are in part mediated by p53. There is normally high expression of p53 in the tissues that are sensitive to these conventional therapies, such as the **hematopoietic** organs and intestinal epithelia, and the DNA damage caused by these agents induces p53 to elicit apoptosis, the mechanism behind the side-effects. Therefore, temporary and reversible suppression of p53 in normal tissue may help alleviate the side-effects of conventional therapies only in patients with tumors that have lost p53 function. A chemical screen has identified pifithrin-α (**p** **fi**fty **thr**ee **in**hibitor) as a potential agent to test this approach (Figure 6.10e). Pifithrin inhibits *p53* gene transcription. Prevention of hair loss and an increase in tolerated dose in irradiated mice show promise in pre-clinical tests.

PAUSE AND THINK

When and where would suppression of p53 be clinically beneficial?

■ **CHAPTER HIGHLIGHTS—REFRESH YOUR MEMORY**

- Tumor suppressor genes act as stop signals for uncontrolled growth or may play a role in DNA repair.

- Knudsons's two-hit hypothesis states that a germline mutation in one tumor suppressor allele predisposes an individual to cancer. Acquiring a second mutation in the second allele later in life triggers carcinogenesis.

- Germline mutations in *BRCA1* and *BRCA2* predispose individuals to breast and ovarian cancer.

- *PTEN* is a tumor suppressor gene that codes for a phosphatase regulating the activity of a potential oncogenic kinase.

- The *Rb* tumor suppressor gene in retinoblastoma follows Knudson's two-hit hypothesis: mutations in both alleles are necessary for tumor initiation.

- The tumor suppressor *p53* has been nicknamed the guardian of the genome because of its central role in maintaining the integrity of the cell's DNA.

- The p53 protein is a transcription factor that regulates genes involved in an antioxidant response, inhibition of the cell cycle, DNA repair, apoptosis, and angiogenesis.

- More than 90% of *p53* missense mutations are located in the DNA-binding domain.

- MDM2 is a main regulator of p53 protein activity.

- The protein product of the *p21* gene, a cdk inhibitor, is key for eliciting the p53 response of cell cycle inhibition.

- Several gene products, including Bax and IGF-BP3, are important for eliciting the apoptotic response of p53.

- The biological response exerted by p53, either inhibition of the cell cycle or apoptosis, is mediated by the regulation of *p21* and by the ASPP family.

- Li–Fraumeni syndrome is a disease that is characterized by an inherited mutation of the *p53* gene. Patients have a predisposition to a variety of cancers.

- Viral proteins from adenovirus, papilloma virus, and SV40 virus inactivate p53 and RB as a common oncogenic mechanism; several utilize the ubiquitin-proteosome system.

- Both the RB pathway and the p53 pathway provide molecular targets for the design of new cancer therapeutics.

ACTIVITY

1. Choose a genetic syndrome that leads to a predisposition to cancer (excluding familial breast cancer and Li–Fraumeni syndrome). Describe in detail the molecular mechanisms involved.

FURTHER READING

Bouchet, B.P., de Fromentel, C.C., Puisieux, A., and Galmarini, C.M. (2006) P53 as a target for anti-cancer drug development. *Crit. Rev. Oncol. Hematol.* **58**: 190–207.

Guimaraes, D.P. and Hainaut, P. (2002) *TP53*: a key gene in human cancer. *Biochimie* **84**: 83–93.

Lane, D.P. and Lain, S. (2002) Therapeutic exploitation of the p53 pathway. *Trends Mol. Med.* **8**: S38–S42.

Levitt, N.C. and Hickson, I.D. (2002) Caretaker tumour suppressor genes that defend genome integrity. *Trends Mol. Med.* **8**: 179–186.

Macleod, K. (2000) Tumor suppressor genes. *Curr. Opin. Genet. Dev.* **10**: 81–93.

Ostman, A., Hellberg, C., and Bohmer, F.D. (2006) Protein-tyrosine phosphatases and cancer. *Nature Rev. Cancer* **6**: 307–320.

Ryan, K.M., Phillips, A.C. and Vousden, K.H. (2001) Regulation and function of the p53 tumour suppressor protein. *Curr. Opin. Cell Biol.* **13**: 332–337.

Scully, R. and Pudget, N. (2002) BRCA1 and BRCA2 in hereditary breast cancer. *Biochimie* **84**: 95–102.

Sherr, C.J. (2004) Principles of tumor suppression. *Cell* **116**: 235–246.

Sulis, M.L. and Parsons, R. (2003) PTEN: from pathology to biology. *Trends Cell Biol.* **13**: 478–483.

Swanton, C. (2004) Cell-cycle targeted therapies. *Lancet Oncol.* **5**: 27–36.

Volgelstein, B., Lane, D., and Levine, A. (2000) Surfing the p53 network. *Nature* **408**: 307–310.

WEB SITES

International Agency for Research on Cancer. Database of p53 mutations
http://www-p53.iarc.fr/index.html

■ **SELECTED SPECIAL TOPICS**

Bykov, V.J.N., Selivanova, G., and Wiman, K.G. (2003) Small molecules that reactivate mutant p53. *Eur. J. Cancer* **39**: 1828–1834.

Chene, P. (2003) Inhibiting the p53-MDM2 interaction: an important target for cancer therapy. *Nature Rev. Cancer* **3**: 102–109.

Hemann, M.T., Fridman, J.S., Zilfou, J.T., Hernando, E., Paddison, P.J., Cordon-Cardo, C., Hannon, G.J., and Lowe, S.W. (2003) An epi-allelic series of p53 hypomorphs created by stable RNAi produces distinct tumor phenotypes. *Nature Genet.* **33**: 396–400.

Ries, S. and Korn, W.M. (2002) ONYX-015: mechanisms of action and clinical potential of a replication-selective adenovirus. *Br. J. Cancer* **86**: 5–11.

Sablina, A.A., Budanov, A.V., Ilyinskaya, G.V., Agapova, L.S., Kravchenko, J.E., and Chumakov, P.M. (2005) The antioxidant function of the p53 tumor suppressor. *Nature Med.* **11**: 1306–1313.

Senderowicz, A.M. (2001) Development of cyclin-dependent kinase modulators as novel therapeutic approaches for hematological malignancies. *Leukemia* **15**: 1–9.

Slee, E.A. and Lu, X. (2003) The ASPP family: deciding between life and death after DNA damage. *Toxicol. Lett.* **139**: 81–87.

Vassilev, L.T., Vu, B.T., Graves, B., Carvajal, D., Podlaski, F., Filipovic, Z., Kong, N., Kammlott, U., Lukacs, C., Klein, C., Fotouhi, N., and Liu, E.A. (2004) activation of the p53 pathway by small-molecule antagonists of MDM2. *Science* **303**: 844–848.

Wang, Z., Shen, D., Parsons, D., Bardelli, A., Sager, J., Szabo, S., Ptak, J., Silliman, N., Peters, B., van der Heijden, M., Parmigiani, G., Yan, H., Wang, T.-L., Riggins, G., Powell, S., Willson, J., Markowitz, S., Kinzler, K., Volgelstein, B., and Velculescu, V. (2004) Mutational analysis of the tyrosine phosphatome in colorectal cancers. *Science* **304**: 1164–1166.

Chapter 7

Apoptosis

Introduction

Apoptosis is a highly regulated process of cell death that not only plays a role in developmental morphogenesis but also controls cell numbers and gets rid of damaged cells. It therefore plays an important role in tumor suppression. As described in Chapter 1, the balance between cell growth, differentiation, and apoptosis affects the net number of cells in the body and aberrant regulation of these processes can give rise to tumors. Apoptosis is a main tumor suppression mechanism within the body because it gets rid of cells that have extensive DNA damage and the potential to lead to cancer. The peeling of your skin after a sunburn is, in fact, due to apoptosis of cells that have had extensive DNA damage after UV exposure. This process is an important defense against skin cancer. Elimination of cells that have damaged DNA helps protect the entire organism from cancer. Defects in apoptosis also influence the effectiveness of those conventional therapies that mainly exert their effect by inducing apoptosis. In this chapter we will describe the molecular mechanisms of apoptosis and examine specific mutations that affect the apoptotic pathway and play a role in carcinogenesis. We will also investigate how mutations in the apoptotic pathway can lead to resistance to chemotherapeutic drugs. Lastly, strategies for the design of new cancer therapeutics that target apoptosis will be presented. Let us begin with a description of apoptosis.

Apoptosis is a type of 'cell suicide' that is intrinsic to the cell. It is an active process requiring the expression of a genetic program that every cell is capable of executing. The apoptotic process is organized, neat, and tidy, leaving behind little evidence of the pre-existing cell. The cell undergoing apoptosis is swept clean during **phagocytosis** by macrophages and neighboring cells that recognize molecular flags (e.g. phosphatidylserine) exhibited by the apoptosing cell. Apoptosis is characterized by cell shrinkage, membrane blebbing and budding, and chromatin condensation and precise fragmentation, all which contribute to the neat disposal of the cell. This sharply contrasts with the 'sloppy' process of **necrosis**, whereby cells swell, cell membranes become leaky, and cells spill out their contents into the surrounding tissue and cause inflammation. Morphological differences between cells undergoing necrosis and apoptosis can be seen in Figure 7.1.

Similar to the central role that kinases have in growth factor signaling pathways, particular **proteases**, called **caspases**, play a central role in apoptosis. Proteolysis, →

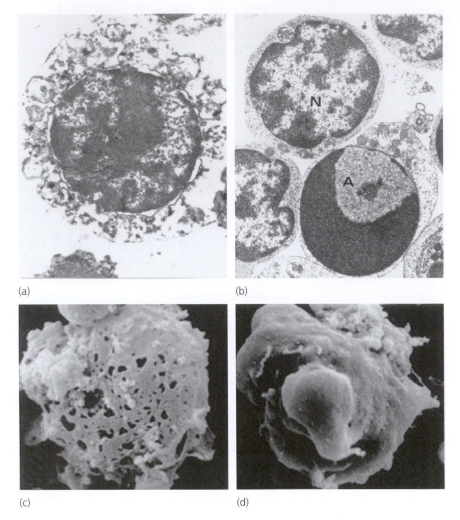

(a)   (b)

(c)   (d)

Figure 7.1 (a) TEM of a necrotic cell: the disruption of the plasma membrane and organelles is observable. A relative preservation of nuclear morphology appears (original magnification ×10,000). (b) TEM of an apoptotic (A) and a normal (N) cell. The characteristic chromatin rearrangement appears in A, strongly different from its normal organization (N). The good preservation of membrane and organelles is also evident (original magnification ×8000). (c) SEM of a necrotic cell. Numerous lesions appear on the cell surface (original magnification ×5000). (d) SEM of an apoptotic cell. Surface blebbing is evident (original magnification ×5000). From Watson, J. (1997) *The Purdue Cytometry CD-ROM*, Vol. 4, guest ed. J. Paul Robinson. Purdue University Cytometry Laboratories, West Lafayette, IN (ISBN 1-890473-03-0).

➔ catalyzed by caspases, helps to break down cellular components for the neat disposal that is characteristic of apoptosis. For example, the shrinkage of the nucleus is aided by caspases that degrade the protein network of lamins that underlie the structure of the nuclear envelope.

7.1 Molecular mechanisms of apoptosis

Cells may be induced to undergo apoptosis by extracellular signals, so-called 'death factors', or by internal physical/chemical insults such as DNA damage or oxidative stress. Subsequently two non-exclusive molecular pathways, the extrinsic and the intrinsic, respectively, may be activated. Caspases are specific proteases that act like molecular scissors to cleave intracellular proteins at aspartate residues (one of the 20 amino acids). Caspases are central to both apoptotic pathways. The term 'caspases' derives from three of the characteristics of the enzymes: they are cysteine-rich **asp**artate prote**ases**. Thirteen mammalian caspases have been identified. They are synthesized as inactive enzymes called procaspases that need to be cleaved at aspartate residues in order to be activated. Although for the most part procaspases are considered inactive, procaspases possess some activity—about 2% of the proteolytic activity of fully activated caspases. This may seem insignificant at the moment but, as we will see below, it is an important feature for some pathways of caspase activation. Moreover, since caspases cleave at aspartate residues and procaspases are themselves activated by cleavage at aspartate residues, caspases participate in a cascade of activation whereby one caspase can activate another caspase in a chain reaction (Figure 7.2). This mechanism, whereby caspases activate procaspases, leads to amplification of an apoptotic signal: only a few initially activated caspase molecules can produce the rapid and complete conversion of a pool of procaspases. Let us examine both the extrinsic and intrinsic apoptotic pathways below.

The extrinsic pathway: mediated by membrane death receptors

The extrinsic pathway for triggering cell death (Figure 7.3) shares some common features with pathways involved in triggering cell growth (see

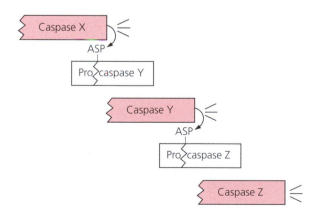

Figure 7.2 A simple caspase cascade.

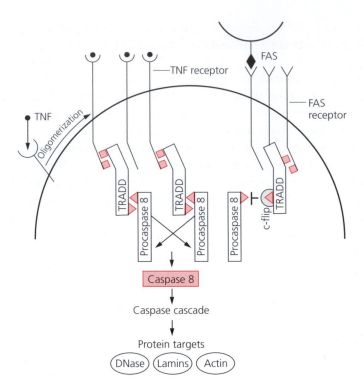

Figure 7.3 The extrinsic pathway of apoptosis. See text for details. The initiator caspase, caspase-8, is shown in red.

Chapter 4). A death factor such as Fas ligand (shown as a filled diamond) or tumor necrosis factor (TNF) (shown as a filled circle) is received by a transmembrane death receptor such as Fas receptor or TNF receptor, respectively. TNF is a soluble factor while Fas ligand is bound to the plasma membrane of neighboring cells. When ligands bind to the death receptors, the receptors undergo a conformational change and oligomerize (several come together) in order to transduce the signal into the cell. The conformational change exposes so-called death domains (red squares) that are located on the receptors' cytoplasmic tail and enable intracellular adaptor proteins such as FADD (Fas-associated death domain protein) and TRADD (TNF receptor-associated death domain protein) to bind via their death domains (see Pause and Think).

The function of adaptor proteins is to transduce the death signal from the receptor to caspases. The adaptors recruit several molecules of procaspase-8 via death effector domains (DEDs; red triangles). Caspase-8 is also known as an initiator caspase since it is the first link between the receptor and the apoptotic proteases and it is key to the extrinsic pathway. Together the death ligands, receptors, adaptors, and initiator caspase are called the death inducing signaling complex (DISC). Molecules of procaspase-8, now in close proximity to each other, become activated by self-cleavage since procaspases have low enzymatic activity, and this initiates a cascade of caspase activation: one activated caspase cleaves and activates other caspases, called executioner caspases (caspase-3, -6, and -7). The cascade ultimately causes the cleavage of specific protein targets and results in apoptosis.

This process can be inhibited by c-Flip (shown in gray in Figure 7.3), an inhibitor of apoptosis. c-Flip can bind to adaptor FADD via a DED and inhibit caspase-8 recruitment and activation.

The breakdown of the cell results from the proteolysis of the target proteins. Target proteins include nuclear lamins allowing for nuclear shrinkage, cytoskeletal proteins such as actin and intermediate filaments for rearranging cell structure, specific kinases for cell signaling, and other enzymes such as caspase-activated DNase for the cleavage of chromatin. The caspase-activated DNase cuts DNA between nucleosomes and generates a DNA ladder (corresponding to multiples of 180 bp—the distance between nucleosomes; Figure 7.4a), that can be detected experimentally and used by scientists as a molecular marker of apoptosis. The TUNEL technique, described in the box below, is another procedure used by scientists to detect apoptosis. Caspases also cleave the tumor suppressor protein, RB (discussed in Chapters 5 and 6), and this cleavage results in the degradation of RB protein. This event is required for apoptosis induced by TNF and points to a role for RB in the inhibition of apoptosis.

PAUSE AND THINK

What do you think is the function of a death domain? A death domain is part of a protein, approximately 70 amino acids, that allows for specific protein–protein interactions to occur and is analogous to the SH2 domain characteristic of growth factor signal transduction pathways.

Self test Close this book and try to redraw Figure 7.3. Check your answer. Correct your work. Close the book once more and try again.

Analysis of apoptosis by the TUNEL technique

Apoptotic cells can be detected by a technique called **t**erminal deoxynucleotidyl transferase-mediated deoxy**u**ridine triphosphate **n**ick **e**nd **l**abeling (TUNEL). As mentioned above, specific fragmentation of DNA at internucleosomal sites is characteristic of apoptosis. The apoptotic endonucleases generate free 3′ OH groups at the ends of the DNA fragments that can be end-labeled using tagged nucleotides. The enzyme terminal deoxynucleotidyl transferase (TdT) catalyzes the addition of labeled deoxynucleotides to the 3′ OH ends of the many DNA fragments within an apoptotic nucleus. The tags most commonly used are biotin or fluorescein. Biotin tags can be detected using diaminobenzidine and a streptavidin–horseradish peroxidase conjugate to generate a color reaction at the site of the DNA ends. Fluorescein can be detected with a fluorescent microscope or by flow cytometry. Alternatively, an alkaline phosphatase-conjugated anti-fluorescein antibody can be used to generate a color reaction. Cells stained by the TUNEL assay using an alkaline phosphatase-conjugated anti-fluorescein antibody are shown in Figure 7.4(b) (see also Plate 4).

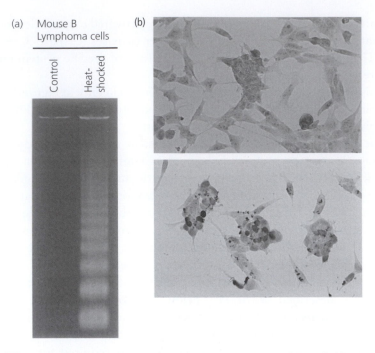

Figure 7.4 Methods for the detection of apoptotic cells. (a) A typical DNA ladder characteristic of cells undergoing apoptosis. Detection by agarose gel electrophoresis and visualized by ethidium bromide staining under UV light. Reprinted from Otsuki, Y, Li, Z., and Shibata, M.A. (2003) Apoptotic detection methods—from morphology to gene. *Progress in Histochemistry and Cytochemistry*, **38**: 275–339, Figure13a. Copyright (2003), with permission from Elsevier. (b) TUNEL staining. The induction of apoptosis in a human neuroblastoma cell line was analyzed by TUNEL staining (described above). Control (top) and induced (bottom) cells. Apoptotic cells (red in Plate 4) are detected using an alkaline phosphatase-conjugated anti-fluorescein antibody. Reprinted from Lui, X.-H., Yu, E.Z., Li, Y.-Y., Rollwagen, F.M., and Kagan, E. (2006) RNA interference targeting Akt promotes apoptosis in hypoxia-exposed human neuroblastoma cells. *Brain Research* **1070**: 24–30, Figure 1. Copyright (2006), with permission from Elsevier. See color plate.

The intrinsic pathway: mediated by the mitochondria

The intrinsic pathway of apoptosis (Figure 7.5) does not depend on external stimuli (e.g. death factors). Stimuli from inside the cell, such as DNA damage and oxidative stress, induce the intrinsic pathway of apoptosis through the Bcl-2 family of proteins that act at the outer mitochondrial membrane. The Bcl-2 family consists of approximately 20 members, all of which contain at least one Bcl-2 homology (BH) domain that mediates protein–protein interactions. Most family members share three or four BH domains. There are two groups within the Bcl-2 family that have opposing functions: one group of Bcl-2 proteins inhibits apoptosis and another group promotes apoptosis (Table 7.1). Within the group of pro-apoptotic molecules is a subset referred to as the BH3-only proteins because they only share

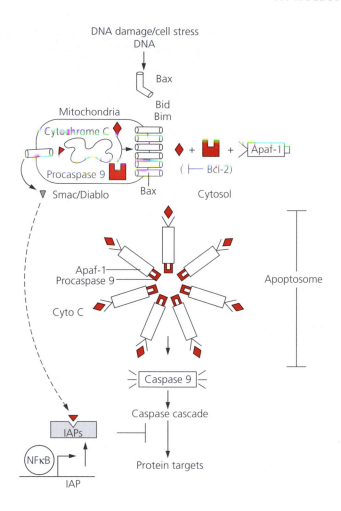

Figure 7.5 The intrinsic pathway of apoptosis, based on current knowledge. See text for details. The initiator caspase, caspase-9, is shown in red.

Table 7.1 Members of the Bcl-2 family

Anti-apoptotic members	Pro-apoptotic members	Pro-apoptotic members—BH3-only members
Bcl-2	Bax	Bad
Bcl-x_L	Bok/Mtd	Bik/Nbk/Blk
Bcl-w	Bcl-x_S	Bid
A1	Bak	Hrk/DP5
Mcl-1	Bcl-G_L	Bim/Bod
Boo		Bmf
		Noxa
		Puma/Bbc3, BNIP3, BNIP3L

one BH domain, BH3. The BH3-only proteins function by either inducing the activity of the pro-apoptotic molecules (BH3-only activators) or by binding and inhibiting the anti-apoptotic Bcl-2 proteins (BH3-only enablers). The Bcl-2 family of proteins is thought to act either by forming channels or blocking channels in the outer mitochondrial membrane to regulate the release of important molecular apoptotic mediators from the mitochondria. The members of this family can associate by protein–protein interactions and it appears that it is the ratio of activity that determines function and hence the outcome. For example, if the activity of the pro-apoptotic factors is high due to low inhibition from anti-apoptotic factors, apoptosis is triggered. The activity of the proteins of the Bcl-2 family can also be regulated by phosphorylation.

The intermembrane space between the two mitochondrial membranes acts as a supply cabinet for apoptotic mediators. The pro-apoptotic Bcl-2 members regulate the release of the apoptotic mediators from this mitochondrial compartment in a process sometimes referred to as **mito**chondrial **o**uter **m**embrane **p**ermeabilization (MOMP). Upon activation by an apoptotic signal, Bax or Bak undergoes a conformational change as it translocates from the cytoplasm to the mitochondria, and inserts into the outer mitochondrial membrane. Oligomerization of six to eight molecules occurs after insertion (six are shown in Figure 7.5) and is induced by the BH3-only proteins Bid and Bim. This new conformation within the mitochondrial membrane increases the permeability of the outer mitochondrial membrane by forming and/or regulating membrane channels and allows the release of apoptotic mediators. A new model has been presented that suggests oligomers of Bax and Bak form polymers within the membrane that lead to generalized membrane disruption (MOMP), and the anti-apoptotic molecules such as Bcl-2 and Bcl-x_L block their action by acting as chain terminators (Reed, 2006).

As shown in Figure 7.5, cytochrome *c*, which also functions in the electron transport chain of aerobic respiration, and procaspase-9 (both shaded in red) are released into the cytoplasm and assemble into a complex called an apoptosome, along with dATP bound to Apaf-1. The binding of cytochrome *c* to cytosolic Apaf-1 triggers the formation of a wheel-like heptameric complex that facilitates the recruitment of procaspase-9 via protein domains, called CARD domains, present on both Apaf-1 and procaspase-9. Recent structural studies suggest that the CARD domains and therefore procaspase-9 molecules reside in a central ring. Further, cytochrome *c* binds to Apaf-1 within clefts formed by a pair of β propellers at the end of the spoke-like helical domain of Apaf-1 with a 1:1 stoichiometry (see Figure 7.5).

Apaf-1 is a protein co-factor that is required for activation of procaspase-9. Caspase-9 is an initiator caspase activated by aggregation that begins another caspase cascade by cleaving and activating downstream caspase-3, -6, and -7. Thus caspase-9 is key to the intrinsic pathway.

HOW DO WE KNOW THAT?

Electron microscopy (see Yu *et al.*, 2005)

Yu *et al.* (2005) used electron cryomicroscopy and single-particle methods to elucidate the structure of the human apoptosome at 12.8 Å resolution. Based on the scientific evidence available at the time, the first edition of this book included a diagram (Figure 7.6) in which the structure of the apoptosome was shown inverted; procaspase-9 was illustrated on the outside of the wheel-like heptameric structure and cytochrome *c* was drawn at the center. This was a model put forth based on stoichiometry. Structural data were not available at the time. The update presented in Figure 7.5 illustrates the progress made in understanding of the apoptosome.

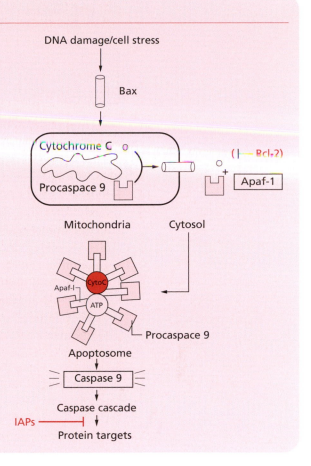

Figure 7.6 The intrinsic pathway of apoptosis as understood in 2005.

Other factors, such as inhibitors of apoptosis proteins (IAPs; eight mammalian IAPs have been identified) and Smac (**s**econd **m**itochondria-derived **ac**tivator)/DIABLO (both shown in gray, Figure 7.5) play a role in modulating the process. The X-chromosome linked member, XIAP, is one member of the IAP family that directly binds to and inhibits the activity of caspase-3 and caspase-7, after they have been processed, by binding to their active site. XIAP also inhibits caspase-9, but does so by binding to monomeric caspase-9 and locking the active site in an aberrant conformation. A transcription factor called NFκB, a major player in inflammation (see Chapter 10), is a potent inhibitor of apoptosis. It induces the transcription of IAPs.

Smac/DIABLO, another regulator released from the mitochondria, eliminates inhibition by IAPs. Smac/DIABLO competes with activated caspase-9 for binding to XIAP. Both caspase-9 and Smac contain a similar tetrapeptide domain that binds to XIAP. Thus, opposing effects on caspase activity are regulated by conserved IAP-binding motifs in caspase-9 and Smac.

Cross-talk between extrinsic and intrinsic pathways

Note that there is cross-talk between the extrinsic and intrinsic pathways and the two converge at the activation of downstream caspases. For example, caspase-8, a key regulator of the extrinsic pathway, can proteolytically cleave and activate Bid, a pro-apoptotic Bcl-2 family member (Figure 7.7). Bid can then stimulate the intrinsic pathway of apoptosis by directly activating Bax and Bak, facilitating the release of cytochrome c from the mitochondria, and inducing the subsequent activation of downstream caspases. In addition, Bid links the intrinsic pathway with the regulation of cell cycle progression in response to DNA damage. Recall from Chapter 2 that ATM kinase is activated upon DNA damage. Recent data demonstrate that phosphorylation of Bid by ATM kinase is required for cell cycle arrest in response to DNA damage (Figure 7.7; Zinkel *et al.*, 2005; Kamer *et al.*, 2005).

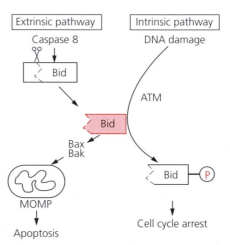

Figure 7.7 Bid links the intrinsic and extrinsic pathways of apoptosis.

→ Dr Korsmeyer was a Professor at Harvard Medical School and Director of the Program in Molecular Oncology at the Dana-Farber Cancer Institute. He received his BS degree in biology and a MD degree from the University of Illinois. He carried out a residency in medicine at the University of California, San Francisco and a post-doctoral tenure under Thomas Waldmann and Philip Leder at the National Cancer Institute.

He was a member of the National Academy of Sciences and the Institute of Medicine. Several awards for distinguished achievement in cancer research are among his honors. Importantly he was an excellent mentor of young scientists who are continuing his work today.

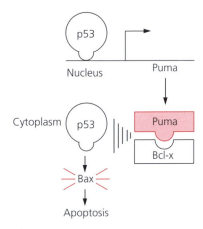

Figure 7.8 Transcription-dependent and transcription-independent functions of p53 linked to PUMA.

p53 and apoptosis

As we saw in Chapter 6, the tumor suppressor protein p53 accomplishes its role as the guardian of the genome, in part, by inducing apoptosis in response to DNA damage and cellular stress. It does this by both transcription-dependent and transcription-independent means. As a transcription factor, p53 induces the expression of genes that code for death receptors and pro-apoptotic members of the Bcl-2 family (see Table 6.2). Examples include *Fas* receptor, *Bax*, and *Bak*. These genes contain a consensus p53-binding site in their promoter regions. p53 can also repress the expression of anti-apoptotic factors, such as Bcl-2 and Bcl-x and IAPs. Recent evidence demonstrates a member of the Bcl-2 family called PUMA (**p**53 **u**pregulated **m**odulator of **a**poptosis), a target of p53, is essential for apoptosis induced by p53. Apoptosis induced by DNA-damaging drugs, irradiation, oncogenic activation, and cell stress was blocked in *PUMA* gene **knock-out mice**. p53 can exert transcription-independent regulation of apoptosis. This has been demonstrated by the induction of apoptosis with p53 mutants incapable of regulating transcription; these p53 mutants included one that lacked the DNA-binding domain, disabling interaction with p53 target genes, one without a nuclear localization signal preventing p53 from reaching the target genes in the nucleus, and one mutated in the p53 transactivation domain preventing the transcriptional activation function. It was also demonstrated that UV-induced apoptosis could be triggered by wild-type p53 strictly from the cytoplasm in cells that were treated with wheatgerm agglutinin, a nuclear import inhibitor. The mechanism of p53 transcription-independent apoptosis involves p53 activation of Bax in the cytoplasm and subsequent release of cytochrome c and caspase activation (Chipuk *et al.*, 2004). Evidence also supports the role of p53 in releasing pro-apoptotic proteins (e.g. Bid) from sequestration by anti-apoptotic proteins (e.g. Bcl-x_L), altering the net functional balance of the Bcl-2 family of proteins. The protein PUMA has provided a link between the transcriptional and cytoplasmic functions of p53 (Chipuk *et al.*, 2005). Data suggest that p53 activates transcription of *PUMA*; PUMA protein then acts as an enabler to release p53 from Bcl-x_L in the cytoplasm so that p53 can directly activate Bax (Figure 7.8). In summary, p53 functions in both the nucleus and the cytoplasm by transcription-dependent and transcription-independent means and these functions are linked by PUMA.

HOW DO WE KNOW THAT?

Immunoprecipitation (see Chipuk *et al.*, 2005)

Ultraviolet treatment of cells results in DNA damage and induction of apoptosis. One question investigated by Chipuk *et al.* (2005) was whether there are any regulators of the Bcl-x_L–p53 complex. They analyzed the extracts of cells that were treated with UV by a technique called immunoprecipitation. Here an antibody against Bcl-x_L was used to isolate proteins complexed to Bcl-x_L and these proteins were analyzed by SDS-polyacrylamide gel electrophoresis and visualized by silver staining and also by western blot. Both p53 and PUMA were identified (look carefully at the data in Figures 1 and S1A in Chipuk *et al.*, 2005).

Another experiment was designed to investigate the kinetics of the formation of the p53–Bcl-x_L complex after treatment with UV. Bcl-x_L was immunoprecipitated at specific time points after UV treatment and analyzed. The data show that the amount of p53 complexed with Bcl-x_L decreased over time after UV treatment and this correlated with the induction of apoptosis (see Figure S2C in Chipuk *et al.*, 2005). What do the asterisks above the fifth band in the row labeled p53 represent? Read the methods and see how they determined the time of induction of apoptosis.

7.2 Apoptosis and cancer

Evasion of apoptosis is one of the six hallmarks of cancer (Figure 1.1). Tumor cells produce many signals, such as those in response to DNA damage and oncogene activation, that normally induce apoptosis. Through tumor suppression pathways, most cells that acquire carcinogenic characteristics are eliminated by apoptosis. However, tumor cells that acquire mutations that allow them to escape from the apoptotic response survive and proliferate. The avoidance of apoptosis permits further accumulation of mutations. This draws our attention to a difference that develops

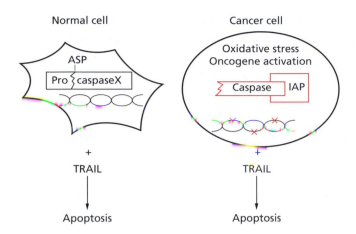

Figure 7.9 Differences in caspase activation and response to TRAIL in normal cells versus cancer cells.

between tumor cells and normal cells (Figure 7.9): since tumor cells receive many apoptosis-inducing signals (such as oxidative stress and oncogene activation) compared with normal cells, tumor cells are 'closer' to triggering an apoptotic response compared with normal cells. However, the apoptotic pathway is often defective in tumor cells. This has stimulated the concept that repair of the apoptotic pathway in tumor cells by targeting p53 may be a valuable strategy for new cancer therapeutics (see Chapter 6).

Evidence suggests that there is a fundamental difference in the state of caspase activation between cancer cells and normal cells due to the stresses characteristic of cancer cells mentioned above: cancer cells contain activated caspases that are inhibited by upregulated IAPs but normal cells contain inactive procaspases that require proteolytic cleavage (Figure 7.9). Therefore, cancer cells are 'closer' to triggering an apoptotic response compared with a normal cell. In support of this, processed caspase-3 has been identified in tumor cells. Tumor cells share this characteristic with the normal *Drosophilia* apoptotic process, whereby activated caspases are inhibited by IAPs in normal cells and induction of apoptosis requires release from IAP inhibition. In summary: apoptotic signals stimulate pro-caspase processing in normal cells, while apoptotic signals stimulate the cessation of IAP inhibition of processed caspases in cancer cells.

TRAIL receptors

A subfamily of TNF receptors, called TRAIL receptors (TRAILR1 and ◎ TRAILR2; also know as death receptor 4 and 5—DR4, DR5), has been found to elicit a differential sensitivity to apoptosis between normal cells and cancer cells. Its ligand, TRAIL (TNF-related apoptosis-inducing ligand), induces apoptosis in many cancer cells (regardless of the *p53* gene profile) but not in most normal cells (Figure 7.9). This subfamily signals apoptosis in a similar manner to TNF receptors recruiting adaptors (e.g. FADD) and an initiator caspase, caspase-8, to the membrane (see Figure 7.3). Since TRAIL and its receptors are expressed in most organs, it is hypothesized that the addition or loss of regulatory molecules determines whether apoptosis will be induced in particular cell types.

The differences identified between normal and tumor cells create an opportunity for designing drugs that target the apoptotic pathways and suggest that attempts to restore apoptotic activity will not affect normal cells. Such drugs are likely to have few side-effects. Before discussing apoptotic therapies, we will first examine a sample of mutations in the apoptosis pathways that have been identified in cancers.

Mutations that affect the extrinsic pathway

Mutations in death receptor genes, such as those encoding the Fas receptor and TRAIL receptor, occur in some cancers. Fas ligand and receptor are induced by UV light. Signaling through Fas receptors induces the development of sunburn in response to UV and is an important defense against skin cancers (Guzman *et al.*, 2003). Somatic mutations in Fas receptors have been reported in melanomas and squamous cell carcinomas.

Suppression of caspase gene expression in the development of particular cancers, such as small-cell lung carcinoma and neuroblastomas, has also been demonstrated. Remember that caspase-8 is the first caspase activated by the death receptors (Figure 7.3) and it maintains a top position in the initiation of the caspase cascade. Loss of caspase-8 expression observed in cancers is due to both epigenetic and mutational alterations; hypermethylation of the caspase-8 promoter, deletions, and missense mutations have been identified. Caspase-8 deficiency is particularly characteristic of neuroblastomas and small-cell lung cancer. Methylation of the caspase gene promoter was found to be the mechanism of loss of expression in a majority of cell lines examined. Also, a deletion of Leu62 was identified in human vulval squamous carcinoma cells and this mutation blocks the interaction of caspase-8 with the adaptor FADD, thus abolishing its link with the death signal and receptor.

Mutations that affect regulators of the intrinsic pathway

Alterations of the intrinsic pathway of apoptosis are much more common than alterations in the extrinsic pathway during carcinogenesis. Mutations that bypass the transduction of apoptotic signals that are triggered by DNA damage, a dominant characteristic of cancer cells, are favored by natural selection. A major contribution to intrinsic pathway alterations occurs through mutations that affect the p53 pathway. Mutations in the *p53* gene itself are the most frequently found mutations in cancer cells, and current estimations may be underestimated since many earlier studies restricted their analysis to exons 5–9 only, rather than the full length of the gene. The *p53* mutations provide the cancer cells with a survival advantage by disrupting apoptosis. Abnormal methylation and loss of heterozygosity for *p73*, a *p53* family member capable of inducing apoptosis, is frequent in lymphomas. Also, the *p73* gene undergoes alternative splicing to generate several RNAs, including amino-terminally deleted variants which can act as inhibitors of *p53*. These variants are over-expressed in many cancers. In addition, mutations in genes involved in the upstream regulation of *p53* (e.g. *ATM* and *Chk2*; see Chapter 6, Figure 6.6) and also in the downstream targets of p53 have also been identified in human tumors. Mutations in molecular components that affect MDM2, the major regulator of p53 activity, are common in tumors that maintain wild-type p53 alleles.

Bcl-2, the first member of the Bcl-2 family of proteins to be discovered, was initially identified from a chromosomal translocation, t(14;18) in B-cell lymphomas, hence the name *bcl*. In t(14;18), the *Bcl-2* gene is translocated to a position juxtaposed to the immunoglobulin heavy chain enhancer. As a consequence of its relocation next to a strong promoter, oncogenic activation of the *Bcl-2* gene occurs. Over-expression of the anti-apoptotic protein Bcl-2 leads to insufficient apoptotic turnover and accumulation of B-cells. This translocation is not only found in most cases of follicular B-cell lymphomas but also in other types of cancer such as gastric, lung, and prostate. Aberrant expression of most of the genes in the Bcl-2 family is linked to carcinogenesis. All anti-apoptotic members of the Bcl-2 family may function as oncogenes, and pro-apoptotic members act as tumor suppressor genes. Mutations in genes that code for pro-apoptotic proteins, such as deletions in the *bak* and *bid* genes, are characteristic of some tumors. *Bax* is mutated in over 50% of a specific class of colon tumors. Remember that p53 regulates many genes of the Bcl-2 family. Thus, many mutations in *p53* that are common in tumors also affect the transcriptional regulation of its target genes, including those of the Bcl-2 family.

Molecules involved in events downstream of the release of mitochondrial apoptotic factors also play a role in tumorigenesis. The gene encoding Apaf-1, the co-activator of caspase-9 upon its release from the mitochondria, is mutated and transcriptionally repressed in metastatic melanoma. Note that epigenetic inactivation, in addition to mutation, plays a role in the inactivation of the apoptotic pathway.

The induction of inhibitors of apoptosis also plays a role in carcinogenesis. XIAP is induced in many types of cancer including leukemias, lung cancer, and prostate cancer. Since XIAP acts to suppress caspase-9, -3, and -7, it affects downstream caspases that are common to both the extrinsic and intrinsic pathways.

Alternative death pathways

The observation that many apoptotic stimuli do not require caspases has led to studies of alternative death pathways. In addition to necrosis, autophagy and mitotic catastrophe are other non-apoptotic mechanisms of cell death. Autophagy (meaning 'eating oneself') acts as a recycling system for the cell whereby proteins and components of damaged organelles that require degradation are targeted to the lysosomes. Cells can recycle the resulting products of degradation. This process is important under starvation conditions and for ridding the cell of defective organelles. Excessive autophagy triggers non-apoptotic cell death. Targeted proteins and organelles are surrounded by a double membraned structure called an autophagosome. The contents of the autophagosome are degraded upon fusion of these vesicles with lysosomes. Mitotic catastrophe, another type of cell death, is caused by aberrant mitosis. Defects in genes (e.g. *BECN1*) required for these processes can contribute to tumorigenesis (see Activity).

The details of the molecular events involved in caspase-independent cell death are not known fully. However, it is known that they also utilize proteases and facilitate permeabilization of the mitochondrial outer membrane. Alternative proteases such as calpains, cathepsins, and serine proteases cleave target proteins to bring about morphological changes characteristic of programmed cell death. Calpains, like caspases, are found as inactive zymogens in the cytoplasm. Cathepsins become activated in lysosomes before being translocated into the cytoplasm and/or nucleus. Apoptosis-inducing factor (AIF) is one molecular player released from the mitochondrial intermembrane space that induces caspase-independent DNA degradation.

The abnormal expression of molecules involved in alternative death pathways is observed in tumor cells. For example, mutations in genes that encode the tumor suppressor proteins, Bin1 and promyelocytic leukemia (PML) protein, which induce alternative death pathways are found in human cancers. Bin activates a caspase-independent pathway that is blocked by a serine protease inhibitor. As more is learned about the molecular players of alternative death pathways, new potential drug targets will be uncovered. In fact, several drugs in clinical trials (e.g. EB1089/seocalcitol, a vitamin D analog) induce calpain-dependent and caspase-independent cell death.

7.3 Apoptosis and chemotherapy

Disruption of the apoptotic pathway has important effects on the clinical outcome of chemotherapy. In order for chemotherapy to be successful, cells must be capable of undergoing apoptosis. Chemotherapeutic agents act primarily by inducing DNA damage. This damage consequently triggers the intrinsic apoptotic pathway. Some types of chemotherapy induce particular cells of the immune system to produce TNF, thus triggering the extrinsic pathway. Drugs with varying structures indirectly elicit the same morphological changes typical of apoptosis. However, remember that one of the hallmarks of cancer cells is that they evade apoptosis. Many tumors have defective apoptotic pathways and are inherently resistant to chemotherapies, regardless of whether or not they have been previously exposed to the drugs. This type of resistance contrasts the classical acquired mechanisms that are associated with drug accumulation and drug stability such as the use of the P-glycoprotein pump (Chapter 2). Since resistance to chemotherapy is a major clinical problem, elucidating the role of apoptosis in drug responses is important for future therapeutic strategies.

Drug resistance can arise through mutations in genes that code for molecular regulators of apoptosis. These mutations serve to uncouple drug-induced damage from the activation of apoptosis. As mentioned above, mutations in the p53 pathway are common in cancer cells and greatly contribute to the inherent drug resistance observed for many cancers. Cells engineered to have a *p53* knock-out are resistant to drug-induced apoptosis. Yet, some 'gain-of-function' *p53* mutations may confer resistance to specific chemotherapies. One p53 mutant induces the expression of the *dUTPase* gene and results in resistance to 5-fluorouracil. Therefore both 'loss-of-function' and some 'gain-of-function' mutations can give rise to resistance. On the other hand one mutant p53 sensitizes some cells to taxanes.

The upregulation of the anti-apoptotic members of the Bcl-2 family and the downregulation of the pro-apoptotic members of the Bcl-2 family in tumors are associated with an increased resistance to chemotherapies. For example, loss of Bax, a pro-apoptotic protein, increases drug resistance in human colorectal cancer cells to the antimetabolite 5-fluorouracil and non-steroidal anti-inflammatory drugs (NSAIDs) used as chemopreventative agents (Zhang *et al.*, 2000). Over-expression of Bcl-2 in metastatic tumors may contribute to the fact that they are notoriously chemoresistant.

Overall, these observations point to an important clinical implication: the genotype of a tumor, especially with respect to the *p53* and *Bcl-2* gene families, is an important factor that influences the effectiveness of therapy.

There is another important implication of treating cells that have non-functional apoptotic pathways with chemotherapy. The lack of an apoptotic effect in response to extensive DNA damage caused by these genotoxic drugs provides an opportunity for the accumulation of mutations. Consequently the risk of carcinogenesis increases. Indeed therapy-related leukemia, whereby a new cancer arises after the administration of chemotherapy, is a clinical problem. Therapy-related leukemias have relatively short latency times. Specific cytogenetic aberrations are associated with different chemotherapeutic agents; chromosomal deletions of chromosome 5 and/or chromosome 7 are characteristic of alkylating drugs. (For a recent case study see Griesinger *et al.*, 2004.)

 Therapeutic strategies

7.4 Apoptotic drugs

The ability to trigger apoptosis in tumor cells is an important strategic design for cancer therapeutics. This is supported by the fact that many successful conventional chemotherapies work by triggering apoptosis, albeit indirectly. Using the knowledge of the molecular players in the apoptotic pathways enables us to design direct apoptotic inducers. Alternatively, endogenous inhibitors can be blocked. This approach by-passes the need for a drug to be mutagenic and avoids therapy-related leukemias. In addition, the induction of apoptotic factors in normal cells should have little effect on these cells since they are not poised to trigger apoptosis to the same degree as tumor cells (see Pause and Think).

Below is a description of strategies targeted against caspases, the Bcl-2 family, and TRAIL.

Direct and indirect activation of caspases

Selective activation of caspases is the most obvious apoptotic target. However, because they comprise a large family of over 12 members and are in every cell type, selectivity has been a problem thus far. Yet screening for small molecule caspase activators is in progress (e.g. Merck Frosst, http://www.merckfrosst.ca/). Procaspase-3, the pro-enzyme of a key effector caspase, is inhibited by an intramolecular interaction facilitated by three aspartate residues, called the 'safety-catch'. Screens are being pursued for small molecules that are able to interfere with this intramolecular inhibitory conformation of procaspase-3. Time is needed to see whether caspases are successful cancer therapeutic targets.

However, the activation of caspases by indirect methods is promising. Since endogenous caspase inhibitor XIAP is over-expressed in many cancers it is a good molecular target for new cancer therapeutics. A synthetic chemical screen aimed at inhibiting XIAP activity identified a class of polyphenylureas that directly relieves the inhibition of caspase-3 and caspase-7 but not caspase-9 (Schimmer *et al.*, 2004). This is feasible because one domain of XIAP directly blocks the active site of caspase-3 and caspase-7 while another distinct domain inhibits caspase-9. The small-molecule inhibitors bind to the XIAP domain known to block the active site of caspase-3 and caspase-7, the downstream caspases. Furthermore, these compounds induced apoptosis in a range of tumor cell lines and showed anti-tumor activity in animal tumor models. Little toxicity was observed for normal cells. This was the first demonstration that relief of caspase inhibition can induce tumor cell apoptosis. Interestingly, other XIAP inhibitors (e.g. Smac peptides) were less successful due to their selective relief of caspase-9 inhibition only, thereby leaving the downstream caspases 3 and 7 available for inhibition.

Regulation of the Bcl-2 family of proteins

The Bcl-2 family is another target for the design of apoptotic drugs. Three main strategies have been used and these are illustrated in Figure 7.10:

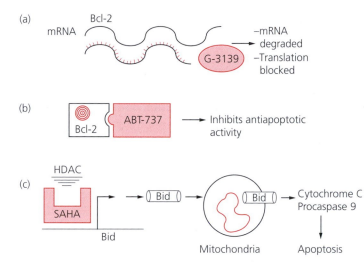

Figure 7.10 Drug strategies that target the Bcl-2 family of proteins. Therapeutic agents are shown in red.

(a) antisense RNA, (b) small molecules to inhibit protein function and protein–protein interactions of anti-apoptotic molecules, and (c) drugs that induce the activity of pro-apoptotic molecules. Since Bcl-2 is over-expressed in a broad range of tumors, inhibition of its expression by antisense is one strategy that has been employed to create a new cancer drug. G-3139 (Genasense) is an 18-mer modified antisense oligonucleotide that is complementary to the first six codons downstream of the translational start site on the Bcl-2 mRNA. Upon hybridization, translation is inhibited and the mRNA is degraded. This alters the balance of pro- and anti-apoptotic factors in favor of apoptosis. Anti-tumor effects have been demonstrated in early clinical trials but it failed to meet the primary survival endpoint in phase III and was denied approval by the US Food and Drug Administration (Banerjee, 2001; Frantz, 2004).

Structural studies of Bcl-2 have revealed that a hydrophobic groove forms the binding site for the BH3 region of pro-apoptotic Bcl-2 family members. Small-molecule inhibitors that bind to Bcl-2/Bcl-x_L and interfere with protein–protein interactions with pro-apoptotic molecules in order to induce apoptosis have been identified (e.g. ABT-737, Abbott Laboratories; antimycin A). ABT-737 binds to the same binding site of Bcl-2 as the pro-apoptotic member Bad. This approach is in pre-clinical and early Phase I trials.

Suberoylanilide hydroxamic acid (SAHA) works by an opposing mechanism; instead of inhibiting an anti-apoptotic factor, it promotes the activity of a pro-apoptotic factor. SAHA is a HDAC inhibitor and therefore acts to induce the expression of epigenetically suppressed genes. SAHA induces the expression of the pro-apoptotic protein, Bid, which translocates into the mitochondria and results in the release of apoptotic factors such as cytochrome *c*. SAHA (vorinostat) has received approval for treatment of Non-Hodgkin's lymphoma.

Targeting TRAIL and its receptor

The differential activity of TRAIL and its receptor in normal cells versus cancer cells suggests that they are good molecular targets for apoptotic therapies. Approximately 80% of cancer cell lines are sensitive to TRAIL ligand and can be induced to undergo apoptosis. In addition, apoptosis induced via a death receptor is thought to be independent of p53 and so the many cancers with inactivated p53 mutations may still be vulnerable to such an approach (see Pause and Think).

The administration of recombinant human TRAIL ligand has exhibited promising anti-tumor activity in animal models and Phase I trials have been initiated for the treatment of solid tumors (Genentech/Amgen). Caution is being exercised because of the hepatic toxicity known to result from related Fas and TNF-α ligand administration and also because of one study that reported a TRAIL-induced apoptotic response in human hepatocytes in culture even though toxicity was not observed in mice and non-human primates. The variability of the effects among different species reminds us that animal studies have limitations for predicting the toxicity of cancer therapies in humans. Also, the critical eye will notice upon reading of the literature that different structural forms of recombinant TRAIL were used in different studies due to variation in the preparation of the recombinant protein and thus may be a source of the different toxicities. TRAIL without extraneous amino acid residues showed no toxicity in non-human primates (see references within Fesik, 2005). Further along is the testing of a TRAIL receptor agonistic monoclonal antibody that recognizes the receptor's extracellular domain. Patients have been enrolled in Phase I and Phase II trials to evaluate drug pharmacology and toxicity (see references within Bremer *et al.*, 2006).

PAUSE AND THINK

What strategy would you use to induce apoptosis through activation of the TRAIL receptor?

■ CHAPTER HIGHLIGHTS—REFRESH YOUR MEMORY

- Apoptosis is an important tumor suppression mechanism.

- Caspases, aspartate proteases, are the main molecular players during apoptosis.

- Apoptosis can be triggered by extracellular death signals or internal stimuli that act via an extrinsic and intrinsic pathway, respectively.

- TNF/TNFR and FAS/FASR signaling are paradigms of the extrinsic pathway.

- The mitochondria stores apoptotic molecules involved in the intrinsic pathway.

- The Bcl-2 family regulates the permeability of the outer mitochondrial membrane.

- p53 induces apoptosis by both transcription-dependent and transcription-independent means.

- Evasion of apoptosis is a hallmark of cancer cells.

- A tumor cell is 'closer' to eliciting an apoptotic response than a normal cell if the apoptotic pathway were to be functional.

- Caspase activity is regulated differently in normal cells and tumor cells: normal cells require procaspase processing while tumor cells require release of processed caspases from IAPs.

- Alterations in the p53 and Bcl-2 related pathways play a major role during carcinogenesis.

- Chemotherapies act indirectly via DNA damage to induce apoptosis.

- Tumors with defective apoptotic pathways are resistant to chemotherapies.

- Mutations in apoptotic proteins enable cancer cells to both survive and become drug resistant.

- Treatment with chemotherapies can cause therapy-related leukemia.

- Apoptotic drugs aim to trigger apoptosis directly and do not require genotoxic activity.

■ ACTIVITY

1. It has been reported that the transcription factor NFκB blocks apoptosis in several cell types. After consulting the scientific literature (Hint: begin with: Li, X. and Stark, G.R. (2002) NFκB-dependent signaling pathways. *Exp. Hematol.* **30**: 285–296) draw a pathway diagram illustrating the molecular components involved in the inhibition of apoptosis by NFκB. Have mutations in this pathway been identified in cancer cells?

2. Beclin-1 is involved in the induction of autophagy in response to starvation. Studies of the gene encoding Beclin, *BECN1*, have demonstrated that impaired autophagy is linked to tumorigenesis. Critically discuss the experimental evidence that supports this link beginning with the following leads: Liang, X.H. *et al.* (1999) *Nature* **402**: 672; Qu, X. *et al.* (2003) *J. Clin. Invest.* **112**: 1809; Yue, Z. *et al.* (2003). *Proc. Natl. Acad. Sci. USA* **100**: 15077.

■ FURTHER READING

Adrian, C., Brumatti, G., and Martin, S.J. (2006) Apoptosomes: protease activation platforms to die from. *Trends Biochem. Sci.* **31**: 243–247.

Bremer, E., van Dam, G., Kroesen, B.J., de Leij, L., and Helfrich, W. (2006) Targeted induction of apoptosis for cancer therapy: current progress and prospects. *Trends Mol. Med.* **12**: 382–393.

Danial, N.N. and Korsmeyer, S.J. (2004) Cell death: critical control points. *Cell* **116**: 205–219.

Er, E., Oliver, L., Cartron, P.-F., Juin, P., Manon, S., and Vallette, F.M. (2006) Mitochondria as the target of the pro-apoptotic protein Bax. *Biochim. Biophys. Acta–Bioenerget.* **1757**: 1301–1311.

Fesik, S.W. (2005) Promoting apoptosis as a strategy for cancer drug discovery. *Nature Rev. Cancer* **5**: 876–885.

Hickman, J.A. (2002) Apoptosis and tumourigenesis. *Curr. Opin. Genet. Dev.* **12**: 67–72.

Hengartner, M.O. (2000) The biochemistry of apoptosis. *Nature* **407**: 770–776.

Hu, W. and Kavanagh, J.J. (2003) Anticancer therapy targeting the apoptotic pathway. *Lancet Oncol.* **4**: 721–729.

Johnstone, R.W., Ruefli, A.A., and Lowe, S.W. (2002) Apoptosis: a link between cancer genetics and chemotherapy. *Cell* **108**: 153–164.

Kirkin, V., Joos, S., and Zornig, M. (2004) The role of Bcl-2 family members in tumorigenesis. *Biochim. Biophys. Acta* **164**: 229–249.

Los, M., Burek, J.C., Stroh, C., Benedyk, K., Hug, H., and Mackiewicz, A. (2003) Anticancer drugs of tomorrow: apoptotic pathways as targets for drug design. *Drug Discov. Today* **8**: 67–77.

Makin, G. and Dive, C. (2001) Apoptosis and cancer chemotherapy. *Trends Cell Biol.* **11**: S22–S26.

Mathiasen, I.S. and Jaattela, M. (2002) Triggering caspase-independent cell death to combat cancer. *Trends Mol. Med.* **8**: 212–220.

Okada, H. and Mak, T.W. (2004) Pathways of apoptotic and non-apoptotic death in tumor cells. *Nature Rev. Cancer* **4**: 592–603.

Reed, J.C. (2006) Proapoptotic multidomain Bcl-2/Bax-family proteins: mechanisms, physiological roles, and therapeutic opportunities. *Cell Death Differentiation* **13**: 1378–1386.

Shiozaki, E.N. and Shi, Y. (2004) Caspases, IAPs and Smac/DIABLO: mechanisms from structural biology. *Trends Biochem. Sci.* **39**: 486–494.

Vousden, K.H. and Lu, X. (2002) Live or let die: the cell's response to p53. *Nature Rev. Cancer* **2**: 594–604.

Zhivotovsky, B. and Orrenius, S. (2003) Defects in the apoptotic machinery of cancer cells: role in drug resistance. *Semin. Cancer. Biol.* **13**: 125–134.

■ **WEB SITES**

Screens for caspase activators: Merck Frosst www.merckfrosst.ca

■ SELECTED SPECIAL TOPICS

Banerjee, D. (2001) Genasense (Genta Inc.). *Curr. Opin. Invest. Drugs* **2**: 574–580.

Chipuk, J.E., Kuwana, T., Bouchier-Hayes, L., Droin, N.M., Newmeyer, D.D., Schuler, M., and Green, D.R. (2004) Direct activation of Bax by p53 mediates mitochondrial membrane permeabilization and apoptosis. *Science* **303**: 1010–1014.

Chipuk, J.E., Bouchier-Hayes, L., Kuwana, T., Newmeyer, D.D., and Green, D.R. (2005) PUMA couples the nuclear and cytoplasmic proapoptotic function of p53. *Science* **309**: 1732–1735 (supporting online material: http://www.sciencemag.org/cgi/content/full/309/5741/1732/DC1).

Frantz, S. (2004) Lessons learnt from Genasense's failure. *Nature Rev. Drug Discov.* **3**: 542–542.

Griesinger, F., Metz, M., Trumper, L., Schulz, T., and Haase, D. (2004) Secondary leukemia after cure for locally advanced NSCLC: alkylating type second leukemia after induction therapy with docetaxel and carboplatin for NSCLC IIIB. *Lung Cancer* **44**: 261–265.

Guzman, E., Langowski, J.L., and Owen-Schaub, L. (2003) Mad dogs, Englishman and apoptosis: the role of cell death in UV-induced skin cancer. *Apoptosis* **8**: 315–325.

Kamer, I., Sarig, R., Zaltsman, Y., Niv, H., Oberkovitz, G., Regev, L., Halmovich, G., Lerenthal, Y., Marcellus, R.C., and Gross, A. (2005) Proaptotic BID is an ATM effector in the DNA-damage response. *Cell* **122**: 593–603.

Schimmer, A.D., Welsh, K., Pinilla, C., Wang, Z., Krajewska, M., Bonneau, M.-J., Pedersen, I.M., Kitada, S., Scott, F.L., Bailly-Maitre, B., Glinsky, G., Scudiero, D., Sausville, E., Salvesen, G., Nefzi, A., Ostresh, J.M., Houghten, R.A., and Reed, J.C. (2004) Small-molecule antagonists of apoptosis suppressor XIAP exhibit broad anti-tumor activity. *Cancer Cell* **5**: 25–35.

Yu, X., Achehan, D., Menetret, J.-F., Booth, C.R., Ludtke, S.J., Riedl, S., Shi, Y., Wang, X., and Akey, C.W. (2005) A structure of the Human Apoptosome at 12.8 Å resolution provides insights into this cell death platform. *Structure* **13**: 1725–1735.

Zhang, L., Yu, J., Park, B.H., Kinzler, K.W., and Vogelstein, B. (2000) Role of BAX in the apoptotic response to anticancer agents. *Science* **290**: 989–992.

Zhivotovsky, B. and Orrenius, S. (2003) Defects in the apoptotic machinery of cancer cells: role in drug resistance. *Semin. Cancer Biol.* **13**: 125–134.

Zinkel, S.S., Hurov, K.E., Ong, C., Abtahi, F.M., Gross, A., and Korsmeyer, S.J. (2005) A role for proapoptotic BID in the DNA-damage response. *Cell* **122**: 579–591.

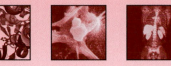

Chapter 8

Stem cells and differentiation

Introduction

As described in Chapter 1, the balance between cell growth, differentiation, and apoptosis affects the net number of cells in the body and aberrant regulation of these processes can give rise to tumors. In this chapter we will describe the characteristics of cells at different degrees of differentiation and discuss the relationship of these characteristics to those of cancer cells. We will also investigate the molecular mechanisms that underlie the regulation of differentiation and examine specific mutations in differentiation pathways that can lead to cancer. Lastly, new cancer therapeutics designed to target different aspects of differentiation pathways are presented. Let us begin with an overview of the process of differentiation during development and in the adult.

We seldom reflect upon our own **ontogeny**, or individual development. The processes involved in the development of a complete person from a formless fertilized egg are almost magical. Hundreds of specialized cell types must form from the fertilized egg and its unspecialized progeny cells called **embryonic stem cells**, that reside in the inner cell mass. The process whereby cells become specialized to perform a particular function is called **differentiation** and relies on the regulation of a particular subset of genes that define a certain cell type. All cells in the body (except red blood cells) contain a full complement of genes of the human genome but it is the *expression* of a subset of genes that makes one cell type different from another: for example a brain cell expresses different genes from a liver cell. Lineage-specific transcription factors responsible for turning on cell type-specific genes are important in this process. During our development, different cell types are organized into varying tissues by pattern formation; although the same cell types are present in an arm and a leg, the morphology, or form of the structures, differs. Regulated gene expression is also important for patterning during development.

In addition to embryonic stem cells, there are also stem cells in the adult that are involved in the regeneration of tissues during the lifetime of the individual. In fact, stem cells are believed to be present in all tissues. Some stem cells are continually active to replace cells as they mature and die off. For example, adult **hematopoietic** stem cells, stem cells that give rise to the blood, self-renew and differentiate to sustain the different types of blood cells over the lifetime of the individual. Other stem cells remain dormant until a physiological signal is received. Hair follicle stem cells respond to a wound. Breast stem cells strongly respond to pregnancy hormones and to a lesser extent to hormones within the female monthly cycle. It has recently been demonstrated that hematopoietic stem cells show differentiation plasticity—that is they can give rise to non-hematopoietic cells (see Pause and Think).

But perhaps this should not be too surprising. Recent cloning experiments have demonstrated that a nucleus from a differentiated cell can be reprogrammed to direct the development of another individual. The cloning of Dolly the sheep from a mammary cell nucleus is a notable demonstration that the pattern of gene expression of a differentiated cell is not permanently fixed.

The process of differentiation is fueled by a source of stem cells in both the embryo and the adult. Stem cells self-renew while at the same time giving rise to cells that are more committed to differentiate along a particular cell lineage. Differentiated cells are associated with withdrawal from the cell cycle. A block in differentiation results in a higher net number of cells and therefore is an important feature for tumor formation in some cancers. Also, despite all the cells from a particular tumor being of clonal origin (see Section 1.2), the tumor contains a mix of cells that have different genetic and physical characteristics. Restated in genetics terminology, a tumor is a mass of genotypically and phenotypically heterogeneous cells despite all the cells being of clonal origin. This heterogeneity may reflect aberrant differentiation and development in addition to accumulation of different mutations. Indeed, the differentiation status of a tumor may be indicative of a patient's **prognosis**. The most malignant tumors often show the smallest number of differentiation markers. Although tumors may exhibit features of differentiation (e.g. teeth in teratomas), the normal pattern formation of cells that underlies the morphology of a normal organ is abandoned. We will examine two features of differentiation pathways that have implications for carcinogenesis: first, the characteristics of stem cells, which are the precursors of differentiated cells, and secondly, the role of lineage-specific transcription factors that act as master switches for sets of genes during the differentiation process.

8.1 Stem cells and cancer

Two defining features of stem cells are their ability to self-renew and their ability to give rise to differentiated cell types of one or more cell lineages. Upon cell division, one daughter cell maintains the characteristics of a stem cell, including the ability to self-renew, and the other daughter cell shows characteristics of commitment towards differentiation (Figure 8.1). The feature of self-renewal is shared with tumor cells. This common feature has led to two proposals for the relevance of stem cell biology to carcinogenesis. The first proposal is that self-renewal provides increased opportunities for carcinogenic changes to occur. The second proposal suggests that altered regulation of self-renewal directly underlies carcinogenesis. We will explore each of these below, where we will find that the concepts from both proposals will intertwine. Note that research into this topic is relatively in its infancy and these proposals require further investigation and substantiation.

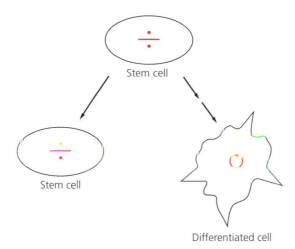

Figure 8.1 Features of stem cells. Stem cells have the ability to self-renew and can also give rise to daughter cells that show a commitment towards differentiation.

Self-renewal provides an extended window of time for mutation

Stem cells are long-lived targets for chance mutations compared with many differentiated cells that die within days or months. The accumulation of mutations necessary for carcinogenesis is more likely to occur in stem cells that self-renew over the lifetime of an individual rather than in mature cells that exit the cell cycle and/or undergo apoptosis after a brief period. This concept supports the proposal the tumors are likely to arise from stem cells. Because restricted progenitor cells self-renew for shorter periods of time they are less likely than stem cells to become oncogenic. Let us look at the process of skin carcinogenesis. Skin is a tissue with a clearly defined hierarchical organization of differentiation. The differentiation pathway begins in the basal layers and leads to the formation of the dead, cornified outer layer of the skin. Epithelial cells of the skin have a turnover rate of 60 days in humans. However, malignant transformation involving the accumulation of specific mutations takes 18 months or more, so the 60-day lifespan of a differentiating cell is not long enough to allow a sufficient number of mutations to accumulate. Self-renewal is a quality of stem cells that allows for the accumulation of transforming mutations, since an individual mutation may be passed on to daughter cells which are themselves susceptible to additional mutations and can pass on accumulated mutations to future progeny cells. This rationale suggests that the accumulation of mutations required for the initiation of skin cancer is likely to occur in the normal stem cell or early progenitor cell compartment.

Deregulation of self-renewal

Stem cells must maintain a balance between self-renewal and differentiation. One proposal for the relevance of stem cell biology to carcinogenesis is that the loss of this balance by stem cells can lead to unregulated self-renewal, a hallmark of cancer. Therefore, tumor cells may arise from stem cells. Alternatively, differentiated cells may acquire a mutation that reactivates a self-renewal program. Perhaps in a manner similar to that in which viruses 'hijack' the cell's machinery for replication, tumor cells 'hijack' the machinery of self-renewal for oncogenesis. Both of these proposals, that cancer can initiate either in a stem cell that has lost regulation of self-renewal or in a differentiated cell that has obtained the ability to self-renew, are supported by the identification of cancer stem cells. These are rare cells within a tumor that have the ability to self-renew and to give rise to phenotypically diverse cancer cells. Some evidence suggests that they drive tumorigenesis.

It has been shown in several types of cancer that tumors are maintained in a growing cancerous state by only a small fraction of particular tumor cells. These cells have surface proteins called markers, which are characteristic of the stem cell normally present in the tissue. For example, it has been established that only about one in a million acute myeloid leukemia cells can develop into new leukemias when transferred *in vivo* and that these cells expressed the same markers ($CD34^+$, $CD38^-$) as normal hematopoietic stem cells. Also, brain cancer stem cells display normal neural stem cell markers. Interestingly, the proportion of brain cancer stem cells identified in a variety of brain cancers correlates with the course of the disease, or prognosis. Fast-growing tumors such as glioblastomas had more brain cancer stem cells than slow-growing tumors like astrocytomas. Evidence for the existence of breast cancer stem cells was obtained by testing whether human breast cancer cells could give rise to new tumors when grown in immunocompromised mice (Al-Hajj, 2003). A minority subpopulation of breast cancer stem cells was isolated based on the expression of cell surface markers ($CD44^+$, $CD24^{-/low}$) and these cells showed a 10- to 50-fold increase in ability to form tumors in animals compared with the bulk of breast tumor cells. Furthermore, these cells were not only able to demonstrate the ability to self-renew but were also able to give rise to cells with different characteristics or phenotypes that made up the bulk of the tumor. These observations support the concept these cells are breast cancer stem cells. Colon cancer stem cells and pancreatic cancer stem cells have recently joined the list (O'Brien *et al.*, 2006; Ricci-Vitiani *et al.*, 2006; Chenwei *et al.*, 2007). Colon cancer stem cells, along with prostate and brain cancer stem cells, over-express the cell surface antigen CD133. Pancreatic cancer stem cells and breast cancer stem cells both express CD44.

Mammary stem cells react to physiological cues, such as hormones, to provide a source of proliferation and differentiation during pregnancy for the creation of a milk-generating breast. A major factor that protects women from breast cancer is an early first full-term pregnancy (Chapter 11).

It is suggested that the depletion of stem cells as a result of the burst of differentiation that occurs during pregnancy is the reason why pregnancy is protective against breast cancer. There may be fewer breast stem cells that have the potential of becoming breast cancer stem cells over time in women who have had children in early adulthood.

In summary, a small minority of cancer stem cells may drive tumorigenesis in some cancers, similar to the small number of adult stem cells that drive the growth of normal tissues.

Molecular mechanisms of self-renewal

Let us examine the molecular mechanisms of self-renewal. The molecular mechanisms that regulate self-renewal of stem cells are just beginning to be understood. There is some evidence that the Wnt signaling pathway, which is important for regulating pattern formation during development, may be involved in the self-renewal process of stem cells during development in the adult, and also in cancer. When the Wnt-regulated transcription factor Tcf (see below) is deleted in mice by gene knock-out procedures, the resulting phenotype is a lack of stem cells in the intestines. In addition, hematopoietic stem cells respond to Wnt signaling *in vivo* and require Wnt signaling for self-renewal (Reya *et al.*, 2003). Data from DNA arrays show that the gene expression pattern in response to Wnt signaling is similar between colon stem cells and colon cancer cells, but differs in differentiated colon cells, suggesting that Wnt signaling plays a role in stem (cancer) cell self-renewal. The Hedgehog signaling pathway too, which is also important for regulating pattern formation in the embryo, has been implicated in the process of stem cell self-renewal. Both the Wnt and Hedgehog signaling pathways will be discussed below.

The Wnt signaling pathway

Wnt proteins (of which there are more than 19 members) are secreted intercellular signaling molecules that act as a ligand to trigger a specific signal transduction pathway (Figure 8.2). It is easiest to examine the cell in the absence of Wnt ligand first (Figure 8.2a). In this state, several proteins associate together in the cytoplasm to form a degradation complex. The degradation complex consists of axin, adenomatous polyposis coli (APC) protein, glycogen synthase kinase (GSK3β), and casein kinase I (CKI). Axin and APC form a structural scaffold for GSK3β and CKI which are serine/threonine kinases. An important transcriptional co-activator, called β-catenin (Figure 8.2a, red triangular shape), is modified by this complex via sequential phosphorylation by CKI and GSK3β and subsequent ubiquitination. These modifications act as molecular flags that target β-catenin for degradation by the proteosome. Since β-catenin is not available

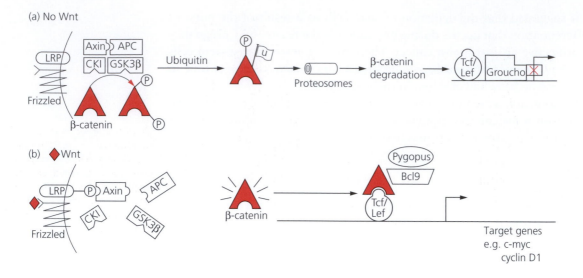

Figure 8.2 The Wnt signaling pathway. See text for details. (P) and (u) mark events of phosphorylation and ubiquitination.

to associate with the Tcf/LEF (**T**-cell factor/lymphoid enhancing factor) family of transcription factors in unstimulated cells, target genes under the regulation of β-catenin–Tcf are repressed. In the absence of β-catenin, Tcf associates with the transcriptional repressor Groucho.

Upon binding of Wnt ligand to its seven-pass transmembrane receptor, Frizzled, and co-receptor LRP (low-density lipoprotein receptor related protein), the cytoplasmic tail of LRP is phosphorylated and axin is recruited to the phosphorylated co-receptor LRP. This disrupts the assembly of the degradation complex (Figure 8.2b). In addition, an inhibitor of GSK3β, dishevelled protein, is activated via phosphorylation (not shown). These events allow β-catenin to escape degradation and move into the nucleus where it can act as a co-activator of the Tcf/LEF family of transcription factors to regulate specific target genes (e.g. c-myc, cyclin D, and adhesion molecules from the EPH family). Activation of target genes also depends on nuclear proteins Bcl9 (also known as legless) and Pygopus (see Pause and Think).

Self test Close this book and try to redraw Figure 8.2. Check your answer. Correct your work. Close the book once more and try again.

Wnt signaling and cancer

Wnt1 was one of the first proto-oncogenes discovered. Viral integration induced oncogene activation and subsequent cancer of the mammary gland. Mutations that constitutively activate the Wnt signaling pathway have been identified in several types of cancer, including intestinal cancers.

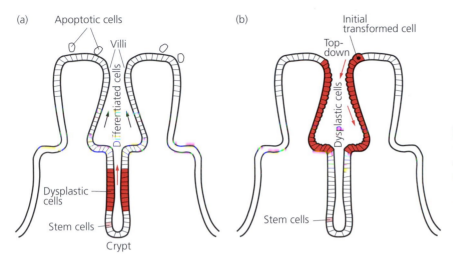

Figure 8.3 Models for the origin of colon cancer. (a) Bottom-up model: stem cells and progenitor cells become unregulated in the crypts of intestinal villi. (b) Top-down model: colorectal tumors may initiate at the top of the villi and spread into crypts. Dysplastic cells are shown in red.

The small intestine/colon is a well-studied model system for examining the link between stem cells, the Wnt pathway, and cancer. Intestinal tissue is highly regenerative; stem cells and epithelial progenitors, also called transit-amplifying cells, that reside in the crypts give rise to more differentiated cells that migrate up along the villi (see Plate 5a and Figure 8.3a). The stem cells renew over the lifespan of the individual, while progenitor cells have a limited self-renewal capacity (about four divisions). Upon reaching the top of the villi, fully differentiated cells undergo apoptosis. The intestinal epithelium is renewed within a few days. Normally, Wnt signaling is required to maintain the stem cells and progenitors of the crypt. Colorectal cancer seems to follow a sequence of progression from benign polyps or adenoma (see Plate 5b) to carcinoma *in situ*, and finally invasive carcinoma. The sequence is paralleled by the accumulation of mutations.

Adenoma cells maintain the properties of progenitor cells, allowing time for the accumulation of mutations. However, the location of the initial event is not known and two models have been proposed. The bottom-up model suggests that the renewal properties of stem cells and progenitor cells become unregulated and initiate tumorigenesis in the crypts (Figure 8.3a). Alternatively, the top-down model was proposed and is supported by a report that found that *APC* mutations associated with colorectal cancers were only present in **dysplastic** cells found at the top of the crypts in pre-cancerous lesions (adenomas), and not in the stem cells at the base of the crypt (Shih *et al.*, 2001; Figure 8.3b, dysplastic cells shown in red). Microscopic examination of pre-cancerous lesions revealed an abrupt transition between the dysplastic compartment at the top of the crypts and the normal epithelium at the bottom of the crypts.

Mutations that result in the constitutive activation of the Wnt pathway are responsible for 90% of colorectal cancer. This translates in human

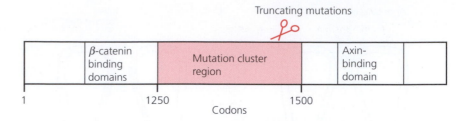

Figure 8.4 The mutation cluster region of *APC*.

terms to 50,000 lives per year in the USA alone. Most of the mutations inactivate the function of APC or activate β-catenin, but rarely alter the ligand Wnt. Colorectal cancer can be classified into two forms: familial forms and sporadic forms. Patients with the inherited cancer predisposition syndrome, familial adenomatous polyposis coli (FAP), carry a germline mutation in the *APC* gene and develop high numbers of polyps in the colon (polyposis) in early adulthood. As a result of having many polyps, these patients have an increased risk of colorectal cancer. The *APC* gene acts as a true tumor suppressor gene in that both copies of the *APC* gene are inactivated in colorectal tumors. Most mutations occur in the coding sequences for the central region of the APC protein (codons 1250–1500), referred to as the mutation cluster region, in both germline and somatic cases (Figure 8.4) (see Pause and Think).

Mutations in the Wnt signaling cascade also promote other types of cancers. Activating mutations of β-catenin that affect the regulatory sequences essential for its targeted degradation can lead to skin tumors. Mutations in the axin gene are found in hepatocellular carcinoma. Many of the axin gene mutations lead to protein truncations that delete the axin–β-catenin binding sites. Therefore, these observations suggest that some transforming mutations may function to reactivate the self-renewal pathway. The cells carrying these mutations can be thought of as *de novo* stem cells, that is cells that have acquired stem cell characteristics as a result of mutation, and were not produced from self-renewal of other stem cells.

PAUSE AND THINK

What is the ultimate molecular consequence of having inactivating mutations in *APC*? Constitutive activation of Tcf transcriptional activators.

◎ The Hedgehog signaling pathway

The Hedgehog (Hh) signaling pathway also plays important roles in embryonic development, tissue self-renewal, and carcinogenesis. It is essential for pattern formation in many tissues including the neural tube, skin, and gut. Similar to Wnt proteins, Hh proteins (three members: Sonic, Desert, and Indian) are secreted intercellular signaling molecules that act as a ligand to trigger a specific signal transduction pathway (Figure 8.5). Two transmembrane proteins, Patched and Smoothened (related to Frizzled described above), are responsible for signal transduction by Hh. In the absence of Hh (Figure 8.5a), Patch inhibits Smoothened and thus

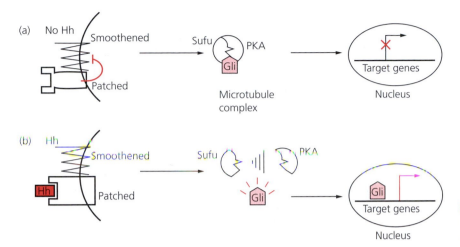

Figure 8.5 The Hedgehog signaling pathway. See text for details.

suppresses the pathway. Upon binding of Hh to Patched (Figure 8.5b), inhibition of Smoothened is relieved. The signal is transduced into the cell and causes a large protein complex to dissociate and release the zinc finger transcription factor Gli (shown in red) so that it can be translocated to the nucleus and regulate the expression of its target genes. The signaling events downstream of Smoothened are not well defined in mammals but the **su**ppressor of **fu**sed (Sufu) and protein kinase A (PKA) have been identified as negative regulators that reside in the protein complex.

Self test Close this book and try to redraw Figure 8.5. Check your answer. Correct your work. Close the book once more and try again.

A LEADER IN THE FIELD . . . of differentiation: Cliff Tabin

Cliff Tabin once told me that he never really wanted a science career that required only working at the bench; he preferred to formulate hypotheses about molecular developmental biology and to teach. He is now renowned worldwide for his discovery of the protein Sonic Hedgehog, and the many functional studies of this protein that have followed.

Drosophila larvae that carry mutations in a specific gene have a phenotype characterized by bristles. Hence, the name given to the protein product of that gene was hedgehog. The vertebrate homolog was named Sonic Hedgehog by the Tabin laboratory after the character from a British comic book. Coincidently their scientific paper describing the cloning of the vertebrate gene came out in the same year as the US release of the Sega Sonic Hedgehog video game. Scientists do have fun at play.

Cliff carried out his PhD in Robert Weinberg's laboratory at MIT, Boston. His postdoctoral tenure was carried out at the Department of Biochemistry at Harvard University and the Department of Molecular Biology at Massachusetts General Hospital. Cliff is currently a Professor of Genetics at the Harvard Medical School in Boston.

Hedgehog signaling and cancer

Patched is defined as a tumor suppressor gene; patients with Gorlin's syndrome carry a germline mutation in one copy of Patched and have a predisposition to develop skin, cerebellar, and muscle tumors (basal cell carcinoma (BCC), medulloblastomas, and rhabdomyosarcomas, respectively). Inactivating mutations in Patched and activating mutations of Smoothened were identified in sporadic (opposed to familial) human BCC tumors and Gli-1 expression was found in nearly all BCCs. In fact, all sporadic BCCs possess an activated Hh signaling pathway.

It has been suggested that since BCC are tumors that include hair follicle differentiation, they may originate from a source of stem cells that reside in a structure of the hair follicle, called the hair follicle bulge, which has acquired an aberrant Hh signaling pathway. These cancer stem cells could self-renew and give rise to the differentiated hair follicle cells observed in BCC tumors. Similarly, it has been proposed that medulloblastoma, the most common childhood malignant brain tumor, arises from neuron precursors that possess an inappropriately activated Hh pathway. Activation of this pathway by mutation is observed in 30% of sporadic medulloblastomas. Molecular evidence of an activated Hh pathway was also reported for gliomas. Gli was originally identified as an amplified gene in cultured glioma cells. Unlike Wnt, where mutations involved in carcinogenesis rarely affect this ligand, Hh is over-expressed in upper gastrointestinal tumors. Taken together, it is apparent that the Hh signal pathway is relevant for several types of human cancer.

> **PAUSE AND THINK**
>
> Does Smoothened act as a tumor suppressor gene or an oncogene? It is an oncogene since activating mutations have been isolated.

Additional properties of stem cells and tumor cells

Cancer stem cells, in addition to being able to self-renew, also have the ability to give rise to more differentiated cell types with limited proliferative capacity. Teratocarcinoma is an obvious example whereby the tumor contains undifferentiated stem cells and non-proliferative differentiated cells such as bone and cartilage. Although the degree of differentiation for other cancers is less obvious, cancer stem cells from other cancers have been shown to generate more cells with different phenotypes. The cell heterogeneity present in a tumor may be derived from cancer stem cells that can not only self-renew but can simultaneously give rise to more differentiated cells. A striking demonstration has suggested that tumor cells can be reprogrammed to become normal and totipotent during experimental manipulation (like fully differentiated cells during cloning experiments). When placed in early mouse embryos, teratocarcinoma cells can mimic stem cells and can contribute to normal development. In addition, the degree of differentiation of a cell may also affect the outcome of oncogene activation. The use of selective gene promoters to drive the expression of a Ras oncogene in different cell populations with different degrees of differentiation (e.g. stem cells or committed progeny cells) resulted in tumors with different malignant potential (i.e. malignant carcinomas versus benign papillomas). Although additional studies are needed, this suggests that the activation of an oncogene may be carcinogenic in some states of differentiation and not in others within a particular cell lineage.

Another feature of stem cells that is shared with tumor cells is the ability to migrate to other tissues of the body. In contrast, most differentiated cells remain localized to a specific tissue. Transplantation of stem cells has demonstrated the migratory nature of stem cells. For example, bone marrow cells migrate to several non-hematopoietic tissues such as the brain, liver, and lung. Metastasis of tumor cells from a primary site to secondary sites is a characteristic that makes cancer lethal (details are discussed in Chapter 9).

It has been proposed that the origin of the transformed cell determines the potential for metastasis: tumors arising from a stem cell are more likely to metastasize than tumors arising from more differentiated cells which are less likely to spread. The inherent ability of a stem cell to migrate may cause these cells to be aggressively metastatic, if transformed. The myeloid leukemias support this view: transformed stem cells are likely to be malignant while transformed committed progenitor cells are likely to be benign.

Moreover, telomerase activity (discussed in Chapter 3), which is necessary for tumor proliferation and progression and is present in 90% of human cancers, is present in normal stem cells and proliferative cells. This supports the hypothesis that cancer cells are derived from normal stem cells.

Summary

This discussion leads to the question of the nature of the cell that initiates carcinogenesis. It may be hypothesized that tumors arise from stem cells within a tissue or alternatively from more differentiated cells that acquire the stem cell quality of self-renewal. There is supporting evidence for both. Alternatively, a continuum of target cells relative to different states of differentiation may exist: stem cells, progenitor cells, and terminally differentiated cells may all be targets for transformation. Further, the stage of differentiation of the target cell may affect the malignant potential and severity of the cancer.

8.2 Differentiation and the regulation of transcription

We have thus far discussed one of the two defining properties of stem cells, that is their ability to self-renew. Next, let's examine the ability of stem cells to generate differentiated progeny. The process of differentiation is

---

PAUSE AND THINK

Do you think that the proportion of cancer stem cells in different tumors can help explain differences in the ability of the tumor to spread or metastasize? Yes, the success of metastasis may be based on the number of cancer stem cells in the primary tumor; non-tumorigenic cancer cells may not have the ability to form new tumors at distant sites.

dependent upon the expression of a specific subset of genes that defines a particular type of cell. Regulation of gene expression can include both inhibitory and inductive mechanisms. The polycomb group of protein repressors and hematopoietic lineage-specific transcription factors are two examples of important regulatory mechanisms involved in a stem cell's ability to form differentiated progeny.

Polycomb proteins silence gene expression in stem cells and cancer

The **polycomb group** (PcG) of proteins repress the transcription of specific sets of genes by epigenetic modifications (see Chapter 3). As p53 has been nicknamed the 'guardian of the genome', the polycomb group proteins have been nicknamed the 'guardians of stemness'. This is because the target genes that they repress include a large number of developmental regulators that promote differentiation (Figure 8.6). Transcription factors such as the homeobox proteins of the Dlx and Pax family and the Fox, Sox family that are crucial during development are among the hundreds of target genes identified by mapping of PcG proteins to human DNA. Thus, polycomb group proteins are implicated in stem cell maintenance. In addition, they also repress key tumor suppressor pathways. This can be seen by repression of the genetic locus *INK4a/CDKN2A* that encodes the cdk inhibitor INK4a (p16), and ARF (p14), an inducer of p53, and suggests that the polycomb group proteins have oncogenic potential.

The mechanism of epigenetic regulation involves the formation of two **PcG repressive complexes**, PRC 2 and PRC1. PRC2 consists of proteins EED, EZH1, EZH2, and SUZ12. This complex contains histone methyltransferase activity and targets lysine 27 (and lysine 9) of histone H3. The trimethylated histone H3 may serve as an anchor for PRC1. It is proposed that repression involves direct inhibition of the transcriptional machinery, recruitment of methyltransferases, and chromatin compaction.

Figure 8.6 Polycomb group proteins repress the expression of many developmental regulators (only a sample is shown). The role of PcG proteins in stem cell maintenance and in repressing tumor suppressor genes suggests that they may have oncogenic potential.

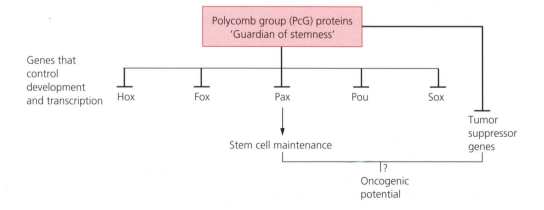

Upon differentiation, there is de-repression of PcG target genes. Although the mechanism for the de-repression is unknown, some evidence suggests that PcGs are removed from the promoter regions of their target genes and/or a specific histone lysine demethylase is involved in reversing the epigenetic modifications initiated by the PcG proteins.

PcG proteins and cancer

The ability of polycomb group proteins to suppress the differentiation of stem cells implicates them in oncogenesis since abnormal regulation of differentiation can lead to cancer. In acute myeloid leukemia, most leukemic cells have a limited capacity for proliferation but are replenished by rare leukemic stem cells (see Section 8.1). Therefore, the ability of stem cells to self-renew is important in the maintenance of this disease. A PcG protein repressor, Bmi-1, has been demonstrated to be essential for the control of self-renewal in hematopoietic stem cells and in leukemic stem cells (Lessard and Sauvageau, 2003). *In vitro*, leukemic stem cells that lack Bmi-1 show growth arrest in the G_1 phase of the cell cycle and begin to differentiate. *In vivo*, mice with a *Bmi-1* gene knock-out show a progressive depletion of all blood cells indicating the essential role of Bmi-1 in hematopoietic stem cells. In addition, in mouse models using leukemic stem cells lacking Bmi-1, smaller numbers of leukemic cells are detected in the peripheral blood compared with controls, indicating that these cancer stem cells have proliferative defects. This is an example of how a common gene can regulate self-renewal in both normal and cancer stem cells. Bmi-1 normally exerts its effects partially by repressing the expression of two cdk inhibitors p16 and p14 via chromatin remodeling. The role of *Bmi-1* as a human oncogene is supported by the identification of *Bmi-1* gene amplification in some lymphomas. Several other PcG proteins are linked to oncogenesis: SUZ12 is over-expressed in breast and colon cancers and EZH2 is over-expressed in lymphoma and breast and prostate tumors. This evidence supports the theory that cells with stem cell properties drive tumor formation and progression. PcG proteins may contribute to carcinogenesis by both the silencing of tumor-suppressing pathways and by inducing and maintaining the stem cell state (Figure 8.6).

Role of lineage-specific transcription factors in blocked differentiation

The induction of lineage-specific gene transcription is dependent on lineage-specific transcription factors. Acute myeloid leukemia serves as an important paradigm for examining how disruption of the function of a transcription factor can interfere with differentiation and lead to cancer.

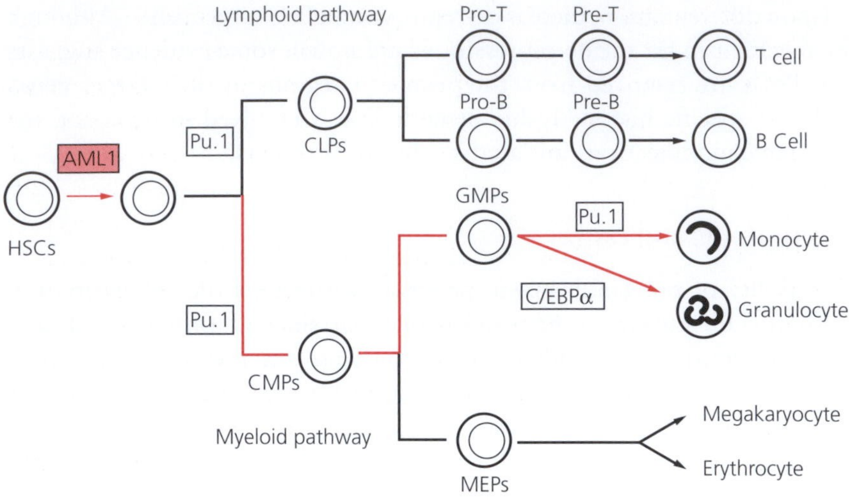

Figure 8.7 Hematopoietic lineages: disruption in the granulocyte or monocyte lineage (shown in red) leads to AML. From Tenen, D.G. (2003) Disruption of differentiation in human cancer: AML shows the way. *Nature Rev. Cancer*, 3: 89–101. Copyright 2003, with permission from D.G. Tenen.

Acute myeloid leukemia (AML) is a disease characterized by a block in the differentiation of the granulocyte or monocyte lineage (Figure 8.7). There are several subtypes of acute myeloid leukemia. The classification system of this disease is still evolving but should eventually reflect molecular features at the point of the differentiation block. The lineage is organized as a hierarchy that begins with pluripotent hematopoietic stem cells (HSCs). These cells self-renew and form progenitor cells. The progenitor cells differentiate into several types of precursor cells including myeloid precursor cells. Myeloid precursor cells are common to both the monocyte and granulocyte lineages. Several transcription factors have been identified to be important in the development of hematopoietic lineages. One factor, AML1, is involved in almost all lineages. Others are lineage-specific factors (differentiation factors), such as PU.1 and CCAAT/enhancer-binding protein α (C/EBPα). Lineage-specific transcription factors activate a particular set of lineage-specific genes and/or inhibit the cell cycle for terminally differentiated cells. PU.1 is involved in the differentiation of the common myeloid progenitor (CMP) cell and, later on, in the differentiation of monocytes/macrophages. Most myeloid-specific genes have PU.1 sites in their promoters. C/EBPα, a zinc finger transcription factor, functions in the differentiation of granulocytes.

Many mutations that are typically found in acute myeloid leukemia affect specific transcription factors; both chromosomal translocations (e.g. t(8;21)) and coding region mutations are common. The gene for the AML1 transcription factor is disrupted in the t(8;21) translocation and this translocation leads to acute myeloid leukemia. The chromosomal translocation t(8;21) is identified in both hematopoietic stem cells and more differentiated cells in patients, thus providing additional evidence that the transforming mutations of acute myeloid leukemia occur in hematopoietic stem cells.

Mutations in lineage-specific transcription factors are found in patients with acute myeloid leukemia subtypes that are consistent with their role in normal hematopoiesis. PU.1 mutations are found in the earliest stage (M0: very immature leukemia) and in monocytic leukemias reflecting PU.1's early role in myeloid precursor cells and in the development of monocytes/macrophages. Approximately 10% of patients with acute myeloid leukemia carry a mutation in c/EBPα, and most of these cases are associated with the granulocytic subtype reflecting the role of c/EBPα in granulocyte differentiation. Thus, mutation of transcription factors involved in differentiation is an important mechanism behind oncogenesis.

Acute promyelocytic leukemia, a subtype of acute myeloid leukemia, is most often characterized by the chromosomal translocation t(15;17), that results in the fusion of the *PML* gene with the retinoic acid receptor alpha (RARα) gene to create a hybrid protein, PML–RAR, with altered functions. As described in Chapter 3, RARs (α, β, and γ) are members of the steroid hormone receptor superfamily and act as ligand-dependent transcription factors that are important effectors of the essential role of retinoic acid in cell differentiation. The wild-type receptors bind to the retinoic acid response element in target genes as RAR–RXR heterodimers. In the absence of retinoic acid (RA), the receptors associate with HDAC–co-repressor complexes that silence target genes by histone deacetylation and subsequent chromatin compaction (Figure 8.8a). Upon binding of

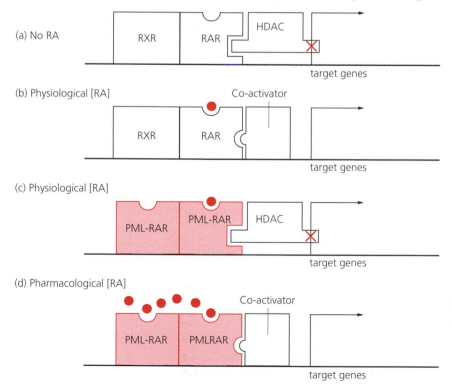

(a) No RA

(b) Physiological [RA]

(c) Physiological [RA]

(d) Pharmacological [RA]

Figure 8.8 The activity of the RAR and the PML–RAR fusion protein in varying conditions of retinoic acid concentration. Expression of target genes leads to differentiation.

RA, the receptor undergoes a change in shape that causes the receptor to dissociate from the HDAC–co-repressor complex and allows the receptor to interact with co-activators in order to transcriptionally induce its target genes and promote differentiation (Figure 8.8b). Co-activators recruit HATs and also mediate interactions with the basal transcriptional machinery. The oncogenic fusion protein (shown in red) maintains both the DNA-binding domain and the ligand-binding domain of the RARα receptor. It has a higher affinity for HDAC and does not dissociate in the presence of physiological concentrations of RA (Figure 8.8c). In addition, the ability of the fusion protein to form homodimers is essential for the development of the disease, suggesting that they act in a dominant negative manner by blocking wild-type RAR–RXR heterodimers or by recruiting novel co-repressors. The normal role of the PML protein may also be disrupted in the fusion protein. PML protein is normally found in nuclear organelles called nuclear bodies and, as a co-activator of p53, acts as a pro-apoptotic protein. Thus, although altered gene expression of retinoic acid target genes is most likely the predominant mechanism of the oncogenic effect of PML–RAR, additional possibilities exist, such as affecting PML function exist (Salomoni and Pandolfi, 2002).

 ## Therapeutic strategies

The concept of cancer stem cells has important implications for the design and testing of new cancer drugs. First, since cancer stem cells support the growth and migration of the tumor, drugs need to target this small subset of cells within the tumor. Many existing conventional drugs give hopeful initial responses that are followed by disappointing latter reoccurrences. Drugs targeted at cancer stem cells may prevent reoccurrence and actually cure metastatic cancer.

PAUSE AND THINK

Consider the possible side-effects of drugs that target cancer stem cells. Such drugs may destroy normal stem cells. Depending on the tissue, this may or may not be acceptable. For example, the loss of breast stem cells may be acceptable for most patients since breast cancer usually strikes after child-bearing years and the breast is not a vital organ. On the other hand, destruction of skin stem cells would result in serious problems since the skin would be unable to self-renew.

The best scenario would be to find a drug that would target cancer stem cells without affecting normal stem cells of the same tissue. In fact, there is evidence that suggests this may be possible (Yilmaz *et al.*, 2006). It has been demonstrated in mice that deletion of PTEN (a tumor suppressor phosphatase protein) resulted in leukemia-initiating cells that could transfer disease upon transplantation to irradiated mice but also caused initial proliferation and later depletion of normal hematopoietic stem cells. Thus a distinction was made between the cancer stem cells and normal stem cells of the hematopoietic system: PTEN deletion promotes the generation of leukemia-initiating cells but the depletion of normal stem cells. A drug that is able to reverse the downstream effects of PTEN deletion would lead to a depletion of leukemia-initiating cells and prevent the depletion of normal stem cells.

The efficacy of such new drugs should be determined by their effect on the cancer stem cell population and not on overall tumor regression. Drugs may be successful at killing all of the cells of a tumor except cancer stem cells, so that measuring tumor regression would not reflect the fact that the most dangerous tumor cell types remained unaffected. Differences in drug resistance between cancer stem cells and other tumor cells is a possible explanation for such a scenario. Stem cells express high levels of ATP-binding cassette (ABC) transporters (e.g. P-glycoprotein), members of the multi-drug-resistance gene family (see Chapter 2). The ability of the ABC transporters in stem cells to inhibit the accumulation of the fluorescent dyes Hoechst 33342 and rhodamine 123 provides a means of helping to sort stem cells. The population of tumor cells that do not accumulate these dyes are referred to as 'side-population' cells. Stem cells are predominantly found in this population. This is a property that protects these long-living cells from foreign toxins and is not usually maintained upon differentiation. A side-population of cells with high efflux capacity has also been identified in tumor cells. This suggest that cancer stem cells have inherent drug resistance and is an alternative mechanism to the acquired drug resistance discussed in Chapter 2. Therefore, therapeutic strategies involving the administration of ABC inhibitors along with chemotherapies are being investigated.

Below are examples of drug strategies that target self-renewal or differentiation pathways.

8.3 Inhibitors of the Wnt pathway

The importance of the Wnt pathway in several cancers, particularly colorectal cancer, suggests that the molecular components of this pathway are good targets for new therapeutics (see Pause and Think).

Disruption of the protein–protein interaction between β-catenin and the Tcf transcription factors (Figure 8.9) is one strategy that has been

PAUSE AND THINK

What molecules would you target in this pathway?

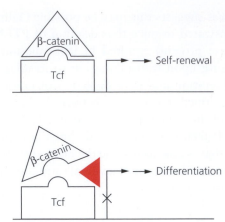

Figure 8.9 Drug strategy to inhibit the β-catenin–Tcf interaction.

investigated (Lepourcelet *et al.*, 2004). This interaction occurs downstream of the APC degradation complex and is the endpoint effect of Wnt signaling. Drugs acting at this stage would counter both inactivating mutations in APC, axin, and GSK3β, and activating mutations in β-catenin that cause inappropriate formation of β-catenin–Tcf complexes. The observation that Tcf inhibition induces the differentiation of colorectal cancer cells into epithelial villi is evidence that supports this approach. From a high-throughput screen Lepourcelet *et al.* (2004) identified three natural compounds that acted as inhibitors of the β-catenin–Tcf interaction. Also, these compounds that share a core chemical structure inhibited the expression of two Tcf target genes and inhibited proliferation of colorectal cancer cells. Although in its early stages, this strategy holds promise for the development of new cancer therapeutics. Since these drugs target a molecular pathway that is important in self-renewal, they have a greater chance of tumor eradication rather than just tumor regression.

8.4 Inhibitors of the Hh pathway

Inhibitors of the Hh signaling pathway are being investigated as cancer therapeutics (Figure 8.10). One example is cyclopamine, a steroidal alkaloid that is found in high levels in wild corn lilies. (Its name comes from the cyclopic effects – formation of a single eye – observed from its action as a teratogen. Pregnant sheep that ingested high quantities of wild corn lilies gave birth to cyclopic lambs. There are obvious implications for treating woman of child-bearing age with this teratogen.) Cyclopamine suppresses the Hh pathway by inhibiting the activity of the transmembrane protein, Smoothened. As a result of the inhibition of Smoothened, transcription of target genes is repressed. In medulloblastoma cell lines

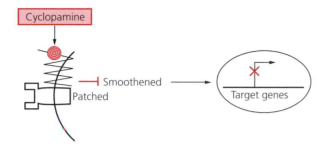

Figure 8.10 Inhibition of the Hedgehog pathway by cyclopamine. Inhibition of Smoothened represses the expression of target genes.

(see 'How do we know that?' below), cyclopamine treatment blocked the growth of medulloblastoma cells and affected the regulation of genes involved in differentiation (Berman *et al.*, 2002). Expression of a neuronal stem cell marker, neurofilament nestin, was decreased while expression of a marker of neuronal differentiation, Neuro D, was increased.

A small molecule inhibitor of Smoothened, HhAntag-691, has shown promise in a transgenic mouse model (Romer *et al.*, 2004). Treatment resulted in the reduction of expression of several genes associated with the Shh pathway, a decrease in tumor growth, and an increase in apoptosis.

HOW DO WE KNOW THAT?

Pre-clinical testing of anti-tumor activity

Examine the method of investigation used in the Berman *et al.* (2002) study and in the Romer *et al.* (2004) study discussed above and compare the two.

In the studies by both Berman *et al.* (2002) and Romer *et al.* (2004), a transgenic mouse model that mimicked the molecular defect of human tumors and the anatomical location of the tumors was created. The mice were **heterozygous** for the *Ptc1* gene and null for the *p53* gene. These mice have a 100% incidence of developing medulloblastoma. In Berman's study, growth inhibition by cyclopamine was examined in **allografts** of these tumors and cell lines originating from the allografts. Allografts involve the transplantation of tissue from one individual to another. In this case, tumor cells from the medulloblastomas were taken from the transgenic mice and transplanted subcutaneously in nude mice. In Romer's study, the effect on tumor growth by a small-molecule inhibitor, HhAntag-691 (a benzimidazole derivative), that can enter the brain, was examined *in vivo*.

PAUSE AND THINK

The choice of experimental model for developing an anticancer drug is vital for predicting the outcome in patients. Which do you suppose produces the strongest evidence for proceeding to clinical trials?

Ex vivo analysis (xenografts, allografts) remove the tumor from its normal environment and cell culture lines may not truly represent the disease in humans. Romer's study examines the effects of a drug on a tumor located in its normal anatomical location.

Genetech is involved in the development of small-molecule antagonists and Hedgehog-blocking antibodies as means of inhibiting the Hh pathway for new cancer treatments.

8.5 Leukemia and differentiation therapies

Differentiation therapy aims to promote the maturation and differentiation of cells such that a malignant phenotype changes into a benign phenotype. The mechanisms may include the induction of growth arrest and apoptosis via gene regulation. The use of differentiation therapy for the treatment of acute promyelocytic leukemia (APL), a subtype of AML, has been one of the great success stories of the last few decades. Retinoid treatment, using all-trans retinoic acid (ATRA) has transformed a deadly leukemia into one of the most treatable forms of cancer. Retinoid therapy along with chemotherapy results in complete remission with 80% survival at 5 years. Note that treatment with retinoic acid alone causes retinoic acid syndrome in 10–15% of patients but administration with chemotherapy reduces this side-effect. The high concentration of retinoids administered 'push' RA binding to the ligand-binding domain of the RARα–PML fusion protein (Figure 8.8d). This results in a conformational change that induces the exchange of the HDAC–co-repressor complex for a co-activating complex. Consequently, the target genes of RARα are expressed and the block of differentiation is overcome. The gene encoding the differentiation specific transcription factor C/EBP is one of the targets of retinoid treatment. Another strategy for developing a new therapy may be to inhibit homodimerization of the fusion proteins, an idea that is supported by the work of Kwok *et al.* (2006).

■ CHAPTER HIGHLIGHTS—REFRESH YOUR MEMORY

- Stem cells provide a source of cells for differentiation.

- Stem cells are characterized by their ability to self-renew and to form more differentiated progeny, simultaneously.

- Self-renewal is a characteristic that is shared with tumor cells.

- Stem cells are more likely to accumulate mutations compared with other cells.

- Cancer stem cells are rare cells within tumors that self-renew and drive tumorigenesis.

- Evidence suggests that the Wnt signaling pathway is involved in self-renewal.

- The transcriptional co-activator, β-catenin, is stabilized in the presence of Wnt.

- Mutations that inappropriately activate the Wnt signaling pathway promote carcinogenesis, particularly colon cancer.

- A germline mutation in the *APC* gene causes familial adenomatous polyposis coli.

- The Hedgehog (Hh) signaling pathway is also implicated in self-renewal.

- Hh signaling exerts its effects via the Gli zinc finger transcription factors.

- Inappropriate activation of the Hh pathway is linked to many cancers.

- A germline mutation in the *Patched* gene causes Gorlin's syndrome.

- Both stem cells and malignant tumor cells migrate to other tissues in the body.

- The degree of differentiation of the transformed founder cell may determine metastatic potential.

- Cancer may originate from stem cells or may involve reactivation of the self-renewal process.

- The polycomb group of proteins are nicknamed the 'guardians of stemness'.

- Polycomb group proteins act as epigenetic gene silencers and maintain the stem cell state.

- AML is an important paradigm for the role of differentiation in cancer.

- Lineage-specific transcription factors are commonly mutated in AML.

- Drugs that target the self-renewal pathways of cancer stem cells are more likely to achieve a cure.

- Interference with both the Wnt and Hh signaling pathways is a recent therapeutic strategy that is being explored.

- Retinoid therapy is successful as a differentiation therapy for APL.

■ ACTIVITY

1. The tumor suppressor gene *PTEN* has recently been found to be an important regulator of proliferation of neural stem cells. Critically analyze the evidence that supports this and discuss its relevance to specific cancers. (Hint: start with *Nature Med.* **8**: 16 (2002).)

■ FURTHER READING

Altucci, L. and Gronemeyer, H. (2001) The promise of retinoids to fight against cancer. *Nature Rev. Cancer* **1**: 181–193.

Dean, M., Fojo, T., and Bates, S. (2005) Tumour stem cells and drug resistance. *Nature Rev. Cancer* **5**: 275–284.

Giles, R.H., van Es, J.H., and Clevers, H. (2003) Caught up in a Wnt storm: Wnt signaling in cancer. *Biochem. Biophys. Acta* **1653**: 1–24.

Gregorieff, A. and Clevers, H. (2005) Wnt signaling in the intestinal epithelium: from endoderm to cancer. *Genes Dev.* **19**: 877–890.

Lee, T., Jenner, R., Boyer, L., Guenther, M., Levine, S., Kumar, R., Chevalier, B., Johnstone, S., Cole, M., and Isono, K. (2006) Control of developmental regulators by polycomb in human embryonic stem cells. *Cell* **125**: 301–313.

Owens, D.M. and Watt, F.M. (2003) Contribution of stem cells and differentiated cells to epidermal tumors. *Nature Rev. Cancer* **3**: 444–451.

Pardal, R., Clarke, M.F., and Morrison, S.J. (2003) Applying the principles of stem-cell biology to cancer. *Nature Rev. Cancer* **3**: 895–902.

Perez-Losada, J. and Balmain, A. (2002) Stem-cell hierarchy in skin cancer. *Nature Rev. Cancer* **3**: 434–443.

Polakis, P. (2000) Wnt signaling and cancer. *Genes Dev.* **11**: 1837–1851.

Radtke, F. and Clevers, H. (2005) Self-renewal and cancer of the gut: two sides of a coin. *Science* **307**: 1904–1909.

Reya, T. and Clevers, H. (2005) Wnt signaling in stem cells and cancer. *Nature* **434**: 843–850.

Reya, T., Morrison, S.J., Clarke, M.F., and Weissman, I.L. (2001) Stem cells, cancer, and cancer stem cells. *Nature* **414**: 105–111.

Ruiz, I. Altaba, A., Sanchez, P., and Dahmane, N. (2002) Gli and Hedgehog in cancer: tumours, embryos and stem cells. *Nature Rev. Cancer* **2**: 361–372.

Smalley, M. and Ashworth, A. (2003) Stem cells and breast cancer: a field in transit. *Nature Rev. Cancer* **3**: 832–844.

Sparmann, A. and van Lohuizen, M. (2006) Polycomb silencers control cell fate, development and cancer. *Nature Rev. Cancer* **6**: 846–856.

Tenen, D.G. (2003) Disruption of differentiation in human cancer: AML shows the way. *Nature Rev. Cancer* **3**: 89–101.

Vescovi, A.L., Galli, R., and Reynolds, B.A. (2006) Brain tumor stem cells. *Nature Rev. Cancer* **6**: 425–436.

■ WEB SITES

Wnt homepage http://www.stanford.edu/~rnusse/wntwindow.html

■ SELECTED SPECIAL TOPICS

Al-Hajj, M., Wicha, M.S., Benito-Hernandez, A., Morrison, S.J., and Clarke, M.F. (2003) Prospective identification of tumorigenic breast cancer cells. *Proc. Natl. Acad. Sci. USA* **100**: 3983–3988.

Berman, D.M., Karhadkar, S.S., Hallahan, A.R., Pritchard, J.I., Eberhart, C.G., Watkins, D.N., Chen, J.K., Cooper, M.K., Taipale, J., Olson, J.M., and Beachy, P.A. (2002) Medulloblastoma growth inhibition by hedgehog pathway blockade. *Science* **297**: 1559–1561.

Chenwei, L., Heidt, D.G., Dalerba, P., Burant, C.F., Zhang, L., Adsay, V., Wicha, M., Clarke, M.F., and Simeone, D.M. (2007) Identification of pancreatic cancer stem cells. *Cancer Res.* **67**: 1030–1037.

Kwok, C., Zeisig, B.B., and So, C.W. (2006) Forced homo-oligomerization of RARalpha leads to transformation of primary hematopoietic cells. *Cancer Cell* **9**: 73–74.

Lepourcelet, M., Chen, Y.-N.P., France, D.S., Wang, H., Crews, P., Petersen, F., Bruseo, C., Wood, A.W., and Shivdasani, R.A. (2004) Small-molecule antagonists of the oncogenic Tcf/beta-catenin protein complex. *Cancer Cell* **5**: 91–102.

Lessard, J. and Sauvageau, G. (2003) Bmi-1 determines the proliferative capacity of normal and leukemic stem cells. *Nature* **423**: 255–260.

O'Brien, C.A., Pollett, A., Gallinger, S., and Dick, J.E. (2006) Identification of a human colon cancer cell capable of initiating tumour growth in immunodeficient mice. *Nature* **445**: 106–110.

Reya, T., Duncan, A.W., Ailles, L., Domen, J., Scherer, D.C., Willert, K., Hintz, L., Nusse, R., and Weissman, I.L. (2003) A role for Wnt signaling in self-renewal of haematopoietic stem cells. *Nature* **423**: 409–414.

Ricci-Vitiani, L., Lombardi, D.G., Pilozzi, E., Biffoni, M., Todaro, M., Peschle, C., and De Maria, R. (2006) Identification and expansion of human colon-cancer-initiating cells. *Nature* **445**: 111–115.

Romer, J.T., Kimura, H., Magdaleno, S., Sasai, K., Fuller, C., Baines, H., Connelly, M., Stewart, C.F., Gould, S., Rubin, L.L., and Curran, T. (2004) Suppression of the Shh pathway using a small molecule inhibitor eliminates medulloblastoma in *Ptc1*$^{+/-}$ *p53*$^{-/-}$ mice. *Cancer Cell* **6**: 229–240.

Salomoni, P. and Pandolfi, P.P. (2002) The role of PML in tumor suppression. *Cell* **108**: 165–170.

Shih, I.-M., Wang, T.-L., Traverso, G., Romans, K., Hamilton, S.R., Ben-Sasson, S., Kinzler, K.W., and Vogelstein, B. (2001) Top-down morphogenesis of colorectal tumors. *Proc. Natl. Acad. Sci. USA* **98**: 2640–2645.

Yilmaz, O.H., Valdez, R., Theisen, B.K., Guo, W., Ferguson, D.O., Wu, H., and Morrison, S.J. (2006) *Pten* dependence distinguishes haematopoietic stem cells from leukaemia-initiating cells. *Nature* **441**: 475–482.

Chapter 9

Metastasis

Introduction

Most cells of the body normally remain resident within a particular tissue or organ (though hematopoietic stem cells are a notable exception). Liver cells remain in the liver and cannot be found in the lung and vice versa. Organs have well-demarcated boundaries defined by surrounding **basement membranes**. Basement membranes are acellular structures made up of a fabric of extracellular matrix (ECM) proteins: predominantly laminins, type IV collagen, and proteoglycans. Cancer is distinctly characterized by the spreading of tumor cells throughout the body. The process by which tumor cells migrate from a primary site to other parts of the body is called **metastasis**. Metastasis is the fundamental difference between a benign and malignant growth and represents the major clinical problem of cancer. A primary tumor can be surgically removed relatively easily, whereas once hundreds or more metastases have been established throughout the body they are practically impossible to remove. Sadly, over 50% of solid tumors have metastasized at the time of diagnosis

The spread of cells throughout the body results in physical obstruction, competition with normal cells for nutrients and oxygen, and invasion and interference with organ function. Interestingly, specific cancers metastasize to particular sites. Many of the preferences observed for the spread of specific cancers to specific metastatic locations can be explained by the directionality of blood flow. Since the bloodstream is the predominant means of long-distance transport, organs in close proximity 'en route' are likely to be main sites of metastasis for a particular primary tumor. However, about one-third of the locations of frequent metastases is puzzling in this regard. For example, breast cancer metastasizes to bone more frequently than anatomy would suggest. One explanation of this observation was described over 100 years ago in the 'seed and soil' theory proposed by Paget. It described cancer cells as 'seeds' requiring a match with optimal environments or 'soils' to succeed. The ability of cancer cells to metastasize is dependent on the interactions of their cell surface molecules with the microenvironment, including neighboring cells and the extracellular matrix. Recent molecular observations suggest that receptors lining the capillaries in the organs to which cancer spreads influence the destination of metastasized cells, and these findings support the 'seed and soil' theory. This theory is also supported by the concept of the establishment of a **pre-metastatic niche**, a site of future metastasis that is altered in preparation for the arrival of tumor cells. Further studies are needed to discover the factors needed for a tumor cell to be successful in metastasis. Although cancers are largely successful in metastasizing in the long run, on the cellular level, only 1 in 10,000 metastasizing cells survives transport.

9.1 Steps of metastasis

There are several major steps involved in metastasis: migration, **intravasation**, transport, **extravasation**, and metastatic colonization (Figure 9.1). The first step (migration) and the last step (metastatic colonization) have been demonstrated to be rate limiting and their rate dictates the overall metastatic ability of the cancer. As we examine each of the major steps below, try to evaluate the molecular components as possible therapeutic targets and think about strategies that may be used to develop new drugs. Examples of therapeutic strategies will be described at the end of the chapter.

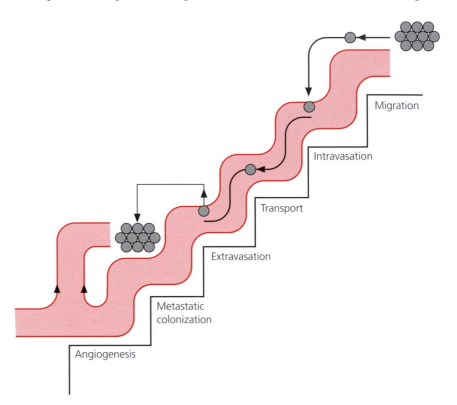

Figure 9.1 Steps of metastasis.

9.2 Tools of cell migration: cell adhesion molecules, integrins, and proteases

Cell adhesion molecules

In order for cells to migrate away from the primary tumor (top right, Figure 9.1), cells must break free from the normal molecular constraints that link adjacent cells to each other. Cell adhesion molecules (CAMs)

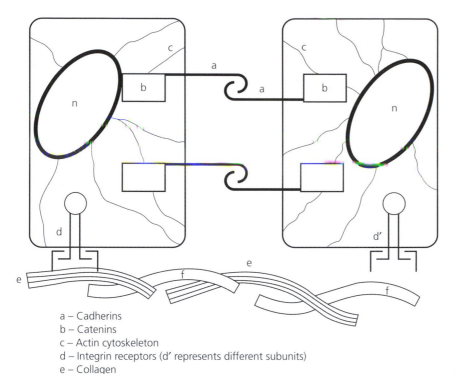

a – Cadherins
b – Catenins
c – Actin cytoskeleton
d – Integrin receptors (d' represents different subunits)
e – Collagen
f – Fibronectin
n – Nucleus

Figure 9.2 Cell adhesion molecules and associated components.

and cadherins are two families of proteins that mediate homotypic (same cell type) and heterotypic (different cell types) recognition. They 'hook' cells into place extracellularly (Figure 9.2). Cadherins (Figure 9.2a) are calcium-dependent transmembrane glycoproteins that interact, via catenins (Figure 9.2b), with the cytoskeleton (Figure 9.2c).

Catenins also bind to transcription factors and induce gene expression in the nucleus. Thus intercellular interactions are networked to mediators of intracellular functions. Several lines of evidence suggest that these molecules are important during metastasis. Cells treated with antibodies that block the function of cadherins became invasive in collagen gels, indicating an increased metastatic potential. Furthermore, **transfection** of the *E-cadherin* gene into metastatic epithelial cells can render them non-invasive. Mutations in the extracellular domain and methylation in the promoter region of the *E-cadherin* gene, the gene encoding the predominant cell adhesion molecule in epithelial cells, have been identified in gastric and prostate carcinomas. It has been suggested that E-cadherin acts as a tumor suppressor that normally functions to secure cell–cell adhesion and suppresses metastasis of tumor cells to distant sites.

PAUSE AND THINK

Do you think the cytoskeleton is important for cell migration? Why?

Integrins

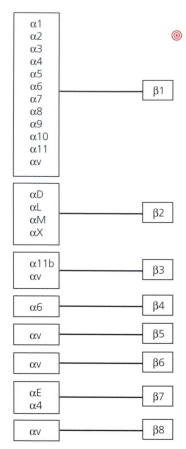

◎ Cells must also break free from the normal molecular constraints with the ECM. Integrin receptors (Figure 9.2d) are a family of more than 24 heterodimers made up of a range of α and β subunits (Figure 9.3) that mediate cell–ECM interactions and intracellular signal transduction. The recognition of the different components of the ECM, e.g. collagen (Figure 9.2e), fibronectin (Figure 9.2f), or laminin, depends on the α and β subunit composition. Many ligands for integrin receptors contain an Arg–Gly–Asp sequence that is involved in binding. Upon ligand binding, the integrins cluster in the membrane and affect the cytoskeleton through interaction with actin-binding proteins and specific kinases, such as focal adhesion kinase (FAK). In contrast to most transmembrane receptors, the cytoplasmic tail of integrins does not exhibit any catalytic activity (e.g. kinase activity) itself. Data suggest that FAK mediates cell motility through recruitment of Src and activation of the RAS pathway (discussed in Chapter 4). In addition to this typical outside of the cell to inside of the cell signaling, integrins also mediate 'inside–outside' signaling. Intracellular signals mediated at the cytoplasmic domain of integrins induce a conformational change in the extracellular domain and thus regulate the affinity of the integrins for their ECM ligands. Integrins also have a role in anoikis, apoptosis triggered in response to lack of ECM ligand binding. Integrins without suitable ECM ligands recruit caspase-8 to the membrane and trigger apoptosis. Thus, integrin-dependent cell anchorage is crucial for survival of the cell.

Altered integrin receptor expression in tumor cells can enable the mobility of metastasizing cells by modifying membrane distribution and/or allowing adherence to different ECMs. Regulation by the cancer cell must result in precise intermediate strengths of adhesion to produce the maximum rate of cell migration, allowing cells to advance their leading edge and to release their lagging edge. The role of integrins in motility is obvious in melanoma cells in which their invasive front edge shows a strong pattern of expression of integrin αvβ3 that is absent in pre-neoplastic melanomas. At the moment, the complexity of ligand-binding affinity and variable ligand concentrations available to the various receptors makes it difficult to predict the outcome of altered integrin expression with respect to migration; sometimes integrins are downregulated and in some contexts they are induced. An altered expression of a specific integrin heterodimer may be permissive for invasion. For example, an increase of α6β4, a laminin-binding integrin, promotes invasion through the basement membrane and the laminin matrix often secreted by epithelial tumors. Further still, altered integrin expression may facilitate invading cells to overcome anoikis.

Figure 9.3 The integrin family: α and β subunit heterodimers.

Proteases

Invasion of tumor cells into the surrounding tissue requires the action of specific proteases that degrade a path through the ECM and stroma. ◉ Serine proteases and matrix metalloproteases (MMPs) are two families that are important. Although some tumor cells can synthesize MMPs, more often tumor cells induce surrounding stromal cells to produce MMPs. One appropriately named protein, called extracellular matrix metalloprotease inducer (EMMPRIN), is upregulated on the membrane of tumor cells and induces production of MMP in adjacent stromal cells. The family of MMPs can not only degrade all structural components of the ECM, but also other proteins residing on the outside of cells (e.g. endothelial cell growth factors), and thus are likely to play an important role in metastasis, including angiogenesis (see Sections 9.6 and 9.7). Normally, these zinc-dependent proteinases are tightly regulated at several levels in addition to gene expression. First, they are synthesized as latent enzymes and require proteolytic cleavage to be activated. Also, endogenous tissue inhibitors (TIMPs) regulate their function. A tip in the balance between MMPs and TIMPs can signal invasion. MMPs are upregulated in almost all tumors and their expression profile can indicate the degree of tumor progression in some cancers.

9.3 Intravasation

Intravasation is the penetration of a cell into a blood or lymphatic vessel. The process requires several steps: the tumor cell must attach to the stromal face of the vessel, degrade the basement membrane (absent in lymphatic vessels), and pass between the endothelial cells (trans-endothelial migration) into the bloodstream. The chick egg provides a model system for the study of intravasation (Figure 9.4). Malignant human cells can be inoculated through a window made in the shell of an egg onto the chorionic epithelium, beneath which lies a rich bed of blood vessels (Figure 9.4, top red arrow). Successful intravasation of the human tumor cells into the bloodstream of the egg is followed by metastasis to distant sites and subsequent formation of secondary tumors. Human cells from these secondary tumors can be detected by DNA amplification (polymerase chain reaction, PCR) in samples taken opposite the inoculation site. Repetitive DNA sequences (approximately 300 bp long) called Alu sequences are present in the human genome and are not present in the chick genome. Genetically modified human cells created to test the role of a specific molecule in intravasation can be

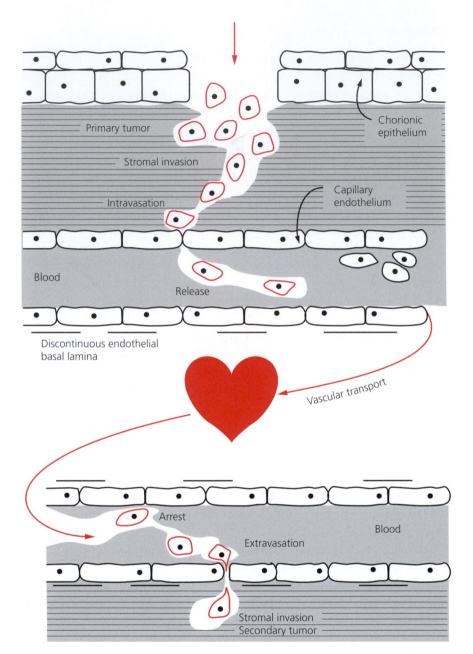

Figure 9.4 Model system for studying intravasation. See text for details. Reprinted from Quigley, J. and Armstrong, P. (1998) Tumor cell intravasation: Alu-cidated: the chick embryo opens the window. *Cell*, **94**: 281–284, Copyright (1998), with permission from Elsevier.

easily tested in this system. For example, cells experimentally altered to express reduced quantities of a particular protease receptor (urokinase receptor) result in reduced levels of Alu PCR product at sites opposite the inoculation site. This implies that this protease receptor normally plays a role in intravasation.

9.4 Transport

Transport through the bloodstream is one-way. Tumor cells travel singly or as clumps with platelets, called emboli, in the direction of blood flow. Specific cancers have favored sites of metastasis and this is partly due to the concept of the **first-pass organ**. The first-pass organ is the first organ *en route* via the bloodstream that lies downstream from the primary tumor site. The lung is the first pass organ for cells of the breast via the superior vena cava that also receives drainage from the lymphatic vessels. Thus, the lung is a common site of metastasis from breast cancer. The liver is the first pass organ for cells via the hepatic portal vein and is particularly vulnerable due to sinusoids, areas where blood is in direct contact with hepatocytes.

9.5 Extravasation

Extravasation is the escape of a tumor cell from a blood or lymphatic vessel. The steps involved are the same for intravasation but in reverse: the tumor cell must attach to the endothelial side of the blood vessel, pass through the endothelial cells and basement membrane, and migrate into the surrounding stroma.

Members of the selectin family of adhesion molecules, particularly E-selectin, are specifically expressed on endothelial cells and are important for the attachment of cancer cells to the endothelium. They are calcium-dependent transmembrane receptors that mediate interactions with cancer cells by binding to various glycoprotein ligands presented on adhering cells. Endothelial selectins are differentially expressed on the vasculature of different organs and may support the 'seed and soil' theory discussed above. E-selectin expression in liver sinusoidal cells is triggered by Lewis lung carcinoma cells and may explain the preference of these cells to metastasize to the liver. Signaling between the selectins and their ligands appears to be bidirectional, in that signal transduction in both participating cells has been demonstrated. That is, signaling initiates from both the selectin cytoplasmic tails and from their activated ligands. For example, cross-linking of E-selectin induces tyrosine phosphorylation in *endothelial cells* and also modifies endothelial cell shape. In contrast, stress-activated protein kinase-2 (SAPK2/p38), an isoform of MAPK, is induced in *cancer cells* upon binding of E-selectin (on endothelial cells) and is necessary for transendothelial migration (Laferriere *et al.*, 2002). This suggests that binding to E-selectin on the endothelium by cancer cells not only mediates adhesion to the endothelium but also triggers a signal transduction cascade that is important for transendothelial migration by the cancer cells.

9.6 Metastatic colonization

The words in the term 'metastatic colonization' have been precisely chosen to describe the last stage of metastasis. Let us examine the 'familiar' concept of colonization. The British established distant colonies in the New World, the growth of which was dependent on the surrounding waterways and harbors. As the settlers moved west, some of the new environmental conditions were unfavorable for growth. Other locations encouraged the development of a new means of water access and resulted in a flourishing settlement. Metastatic colonization is the establishment of a progressively growing tumor at a distant site, involving angiogenesis as an essential process to provide nutrients and oxygen. It is important to contrast this process with the situation of metastasized tumor cells that do not expand and remain dormant for years as micrometastases. Micrometastases maintain an overall balance between proliferation and apoptosis, and due to the lack of angiogenesis, do not demonstrate progressive growth. Metastatic colonization identifies the last step of metastasis that can be targeted to halt the complete clinical cancer phenotype.

A new class of genes, called metastasis-suppressor genes, have been identified by their low expression in metastatic cells compared with non-metastatic tumor cells. Thus loss of function (analogous to the mechanism of tumor suppressor genes) increases the metastatic propensity of a cancer cell. Since the discovery of the first, *NM23*, seven additional genes have been identified to date, of which the protein products of some affect metastatic colonization. *MKK4* is one example. It is hypothesized that MKK4 protein induces apoptosis in response to the stress of a new microenvironment and thus suppresses metastatic colonization. The mechanism of action of metastasis suppressor proteins includes regulation of common signal-transduction pathways (e.g. MAPK) and gap–junction communication, though these are only beginning to be elucidated.

The concept of a pre-metastatic niche, a site of future metastasis that is altered in preparation for the arrival of tumor cells supports the 'seed and soil' theory. An examination of the migration of tagged bone marrow cells in mice after the inoculation of specific mouse tumor cells provides some evidence for the establishment of a pre-metastatic niche. Investigators observed that the location of clusters of tagged bone marrow cells was dependent on where the specific tumor cells would normally metastasize. Similar results were obtained when human cancer cells were tested. As discussed in Oppenheimer (2006) and Kaplan *et al.* (2006), these data suggest that cancer cells secrete factors that facilitate changes to the local microenvironment of a future colonization site before tumor cells arrive. Bone marrow cells respond to these factors by migrating to the pre-metastatic niche and are involved in preparing a favorable environment for the cancer cells to colonize (for more on migrating bone marrow cells and cancer see also Section 10.2).

As alluded to above, metastatic colonization cannot be successful without the formation of new blood vessels. **Angiogenesis** is the process of forming new blood vessels from pre-existing ones by the growth and migration of endothelial cells in a process called 'sprouting'. Although this process is common during embryogenesis it rarely occurs in the adult, being reserved for wound healing and the female reproductive cycle. With respect to cancer, angiogenesis is essential for metastasized tumors since all cells must be within 100–200 µm of a blood vessel (the diffusion limit of oxygen) in order to receive essential oxygen and nutrients. Sprouting of pre-existing vessels requires major reorganization involving destabilization of the mature vessel, proliferation and migration of endothelial cells, and maturation. It is regulated by the interaction of soluble mediators and their cognate receptors. Malignant cells in culture and host stromal cells induced by a tumor *in vivo* have been shown to be sources of these soluble mediators. The neovasculature that is formed in cancer is unlike that formed in wound healing. It is leaky and tortuous and provides direct entry, allowing cells easy access to the circulation. The neovasculature is also different at the molecular level from resting endothelium. For example, the integrins $\alpha v \beta 3$ and $\alpha v \beta 5$ are upregulated in angiogenic vessels compared with mature vessels. The proliferating endothelial cells of the sprouting vessel need to interact with components of the ECM that it is invading. The pro-angiogenic factors VEGF and bFGF induce the expression of these integrins. Molecular differences are not limited to the endothelium since the supporting pericytes and ECM show specific angiogenic markers (e.g. NG2 and oncofetal fibronectin, respectively). Therefore, all components of angiogenic vasculature are molecularly distinct from normal vessels.

A LEADER IN THE FIELD . . . of angiogenesis: In memory of Judah Folkman

Judah's pioneering discoveries into the mechanism of angiogenesis opened up a new field of cancer research and supported his ground-breaking idea that tumors are dependent on angiogenesis. His laboratory identified the first angiogenic inhibitor and he is currently carrying out clinical trials of anti-angiogenic therapies. He is also investigating the observation that some tumors remain dormant, sometimes indefinitely, due to the production by the tumor of an angiogenic inhibitor, but can become angiogenic when production of the inhibitor decreases.

Judah received his BA from Ohio State University and his MD from Harvard Medical School. He has made advancements in a range of fields, including the development of the first atrioventricular implantable pacemaker and implantable polymers for controlled release of contraceptive. He is currently the Director of Surgical Research and Professor of Cell Biology at Harvard Medical School, Children's Hospital in Boston.

9.7 The angiogenic switch

Figure 9.5 The angiogenic switch. Adapted from Madhusudan and Harris (2002).

The regulation of angiogenesis is dependent upon the dynamic balance of angiogenic inducers and inhibitors. Increasing the activity of the inducers or decreasing the activity of the inhibitors tips the balance of the 'angiogenic switch' to the 'on' position, and vice versa (Figure 9.5). We will focus on only a few of these.

Anti-angiogenic factors

Proteolytic fragments
Angiostatin
Endostatin
Serpin antithrombin
Canstatin
PEX
Prolactin (16 kD)
Restin
Tumstatin
Arresten
Vasostatin
Kringle 1-5
Fibronectin fragments
Cytokines and chemokines
Interleukin-1,-4,-10,-12 and -18
Interferon-α,-β,-γ
EMAP II
gro-β
IP-10
Monokine induced by interferon-γ
Platelet factor 4
Soluble receptors
Soluble FGFR-1
Soluble VEGFR-1
Collagenase inhibitor
TIMP-1,-2,-3 and -4
Vitamins
1,25-(OH) vitamin D_3
Retionic acid
Tumour suppresor genes
p16
p53
Other inhibitors
Angiopoietin
Angiotensin
Angiotensin-2-receptor
Caveolin
Meth-1,-2
2-Methoxy oestradiol
Osteopondin cleavage product
Pigment epithelium derived factor
Prostatic specific antigen
Protamine
Thrombospondin-1,-2
Transforming growth factor-β1
Troponin 1

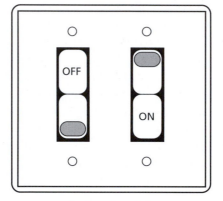

Angiogenic switch

Pro-angiogenic factors

Growth factors
VEGF
FGF (acidic and basic)
Hepatocyte-derived growth factor
Platelet-derived growth factor
EGF
Granulocyte colony-stimulating factor
Tumor necrosis factor α
Cytokines
Interleukin-1,-6 and -8
Enzymes
Cathepsin
Gelatinase A,B
Stromelysin
Small adhesion molecule
$α_v,β_3$ integrin
Metal ions
Copper
Others
Angiostatin-2
Angiopoietin-1
Angiotropin
Angiogenin
Adrenomedullin
Erythropoeitin
Endothelin
Hypoxia
Midkine
Nitric oxide synthase
Prostaglandin E
Pleiotropin
Platelet activating factor
Plasminogen activator inhibitor
Thymidine phosphorylase
Thrombopoietin
Urokinase tissue plasminogen

Angiogenic inducers

Growth factors, both non-specific and endothelial-specific, dominate the list of angiogenic inducers. Although the non-specific growth factors (e.g. FGF) affect many cell types, they are still important for angiogenesis. Three families of vascular-endothelium-specific growth factors and their transmembrane receptors have been identified: vascular endothelial growth factors (VEGFs) and VEGF receptors (VEGFRs), angiopoietins and Tie receptors, and ephrins and ephrin receptors. All of these receptors are tyrosine kinase receptors.

VEGF is the star player involved in the initiation of angiogenesis, while angiopoietins and ephrins are important for subsequent maturation. The VEGF family currently consists of five family members (VEGFA–E) which transmit their signal via three VEGF receptor tyrosine kinases (VEGFR-1, VEGFR-2, and VEGFR-3). VEGFA is secreted by a range of tumor cells. The tumor microenvironment also affects the surrounding stromal cells, and induction of the VEGF promoter in surrounding non-transformed cells has been demonstrated suggesting a collaboration between host and transformed cells. Also, reserves of VEGF are found in the ECM and are released by MMPs. Not only does VEGF induce endothelial cell proliferation but it can also induce permeability and leakage. This feature may be important for the initiation of angiogenesis since it has been suggested that the existing mature vessels must be destabilized before sprouting begins. VEGFR-2 mediates the endothelial effects of VEGF, while VEGFR-1 is inhibitory and VEGFR-3 is vital for lymphatic vessels. Although many of the details of the signal transduction pathway of VEGFs have yet to be elucidated, the VEGFA signal transduction pathway (Figure 9.6) appears to be very similar to the signal transduction pathways for EGFs (compare with Figure 4.2): dimerization, autophosphorylation, creation of high-affinity binding sites for proteins with SH2 domains(e.g. VEGFR-associated protein (VRAP), Sck, and phospholipase Cγ), and subsequent activation of the RAS, Raf, MAP kinase cascade. VEGF-responsive genes include the EGFR ligand, epiregulin, *COX2* and matrix-metalloproteinases *MMP1* and *MMP2*. In addition, a PI3K-dependent pathway is triggered. This activates AKT and leads to a block in apoptosis and, via nitric oxide production, to increased vascular permeability. Several other important intracellular molecules, such as Src, are also implicated.

PAUSE AND THINK

Could VEGFRs, Tie receptors, and ephrin receptors be additional targets for kinase inhibitor therapeutics?

Angiogenic inhibitors

Angiogenic inhibitors normally found in the body (endogenous inhibitors) maintain the angiogenic switch in the 'off' position by inhibiting endothelial cell migration and proliferation. Some angiogenic inhibitors are stored

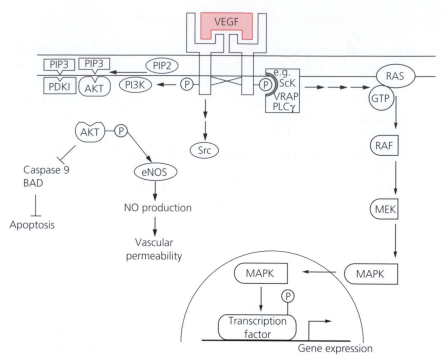

Figure 9.6 The VEGFA signal transduction pathway. One molecule of VEGFA binds to two VEGFR2 receptors facilitating dimerization and autophosphorylation. Proteins containing SH2 domains (shaded in gray) bind to the phosphorylated receptor and trigger activation of the RAS–Raf–MAP kinase cascade. In addition, PI3K is activated. AKT leads to inhibition of apoptosis. AKT also stimulates endothelial nitric oxide synthase and stimulates vascular permeability via nitric oxide (NO) production. Src is one of several other molecules that are activated by VEGFR2.

as cryptic parts within larger proteins that are not themselves inhibitors (Figure 9.7). Plasminogen can be cleaved by proteinases, including several MMPs, to release the angiogenic inhibitor, angiostatin. Angiostatin binds to its endothelial cell surface receptor, annexin II, to exert its inhibitory effects. Endostatin is a fragment of collagen XVIII and can be proteolytically released by elastase and cathepsin. It blocks MAPK activation in endothelial cells and also MMPs.

It has been observed that sometimes, when a tumor is removed by surgery or irradiation, dormant metastases are often activated and growth and angiogenesis are initiated. This phenomenon has been termed 'concomitant resistance'. Evidence suggests that the production of angiogenic inhibitors, such as angiostatin and endostatin, by certain tumors prevents the growth of remote micrometastases via the blood. When the primary tumor is removed so are these inhibitors, and the angiogenic switch is activated for the micrometastases. Also, surgery is known to cause induction

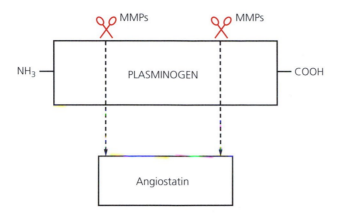

Figure 9.7 Cryptic angiogenic inhibitors.

of angiogenic growth factors and thus may exacerbate malignant disease through this mechanism (Ian Judson, personal communication).

The angiogenic switch is regulated in two ways during tumorigenesis. First, as a tumor grows it creates conditions of hypoxia (low oxygen concentration), and this induces angiogenesis via the hypoxia-inducible factor-1α (HIF-1α). One target of HIF-1α that is important for angiogenesis is the *VEGF* gene. HIF is actually a heterodimeric transcription factor comprising one HIF-1α and one HIF-1β subunit. The activity of HIF is regulated by oxygen concentration, not at the level of mRNA expression as both subunit mRNAs are constitutively expressed, but rather at the protein level of HIF-1α (Figure 9.8). Under normoxic conditions (20% oxygen) HIF-1α is rapidly degraded. The von Hippel–Lindau (VHL) tumor suppressor protein is an important regulator of HIF-1α degradation (Kim and Kaelin, 2003). The first step in targeting HIF-1α for degradation under normoxic conditions is modification (hydroxylation) by the enzyme prolyl 4-hydroxylase (shown in red in Figure 9.8). This enzyme directly binds and links molecular oxygen to specific proline residues on HIF-1α, and thus acts as a direct oxygen sensor in this pathway. VHL binds to hydroxylated HIF-1α and activates a complex of proteins responsible for the addition of ubiquitin (indicated by a 'U' in a red diamond, Figure 9.8) that target HIF-1α for proteosomal degradation. In the absence of HIF-1α, HIF-1α target genes cannot be transcriptionally activated and angiogenesis does not occur.

Under hypoxic conditions the enzyme prolyl 4-hydroxylase is inactivated, HIF-1α is not hydroxylated, and VHL cannot bind and target HIF-1α for proteosomal degradation. HIF-1α is rapidly stabilized and transported to the nucleus. The heterodimeric HIF transcription factor can then activate its target genes. As mentioned above, the most notable target is the *VEGF* gene that contains a hypoxia response element (HRE) in its promoter region.

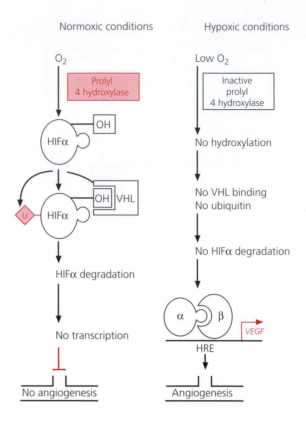

Normoxic conditions   Hypoxic conditions

Figure 9.8 The induction of angiogenesis by hypoxia.

Secondly, oncogenic proteins and loss of tumor suppressors contribute to the modification of the angiogenic switch. In contrast to the well-known direct contribution of oncogenes and tumor suppressors to proliferation, apoptosis, and differentiation, indirect roles in angiogenesis are now recognized. Approximately 30 oncoproteins have been shown to tip the balance towards angiogenesis (Table 9.1). Aberrant production of growth factor, in addition to acting in an autocrine manner to stimulate proliferation of tumor cells, can also act in a paracrine manner to stimulate

Table 9.1 Oncogenes and altered tumor suppressor genes that are pro-angiogenic. From Kerbel, R. and Folkman, J. (2002) Clinical translation of angiogenesis inhibitors. *Nature Rev. Cancer* **2**: 727–739, Copyright (2002), with permission

Oncogene	Mechanism of pro-angiogenic activity
Bcl-2	VEGF upregulation
EGFR	VEGF, bFGF, IL-8 upregulation
Fos	VEGF upregulation
Her2	VEGF upregulation
Jun	VEGF upregulation, thrombospondin downregulation
KRAS, HRAS	VEGF upregulation, thrombospondin downregulation
Myb	Thrombospondin downregulation
Myc	Angiogenic properties in epidermis
Src	VEGF upregulation, thrombospondin downregulation
Wnt	Increased VEGF
PTEN	Increased VEGF
p53	VEGF upregulation, thrombospondin downregulation
VHL	Increased VEGF
Rb	Decreased thrombospondin

the growth of endothelial cells. 'Star' oncogenic proteins including receptor tyrosine kinases (e.g. EGFR), intracellular tyrosine kinases (e.g. Src), intracellular transducers (e.g. Ras), and transcription factors (e.g. Fos), have been shown to upregulate the 'star' angiogenic inducer, VEGF. Some of these oncogenic proteins simultaneously downregulate angiogenic inhibitors (e.g. thrombospondin).

As one may have predicted, the multi-functional roles of the tumor suppressor p53 include the regulation of angiogenesis. As a transcription factor, p53 normally binds to and activates the promoter of the thrombospondin-1 gene. Mutations in the *p53* gene, commonly associated with the cancer phenotype, result in a decrease of the angiogenic inhibitor so that the angiogenic switch favors angiogenesis.

9.8 Parallels between early development and metastasis

In contrast to the adult, the early embryo requires cell invasiveness and motility during early development and pattern formation. For example, gastrulation and the formation of the neural tube require coordinated cell movement and detachment and invasivenss from/into adjacent tissue. In fact, the process called the **epithelial–mesenchymal transition (EMT)**, which involves the conversion of a sheet of closely connected epithelial cells into highly mobile mesenchymal or neural crest cells, is common during embryogenesis. These qualities are also characteristic of metastatic cells. A molecular link between EMT and metastasis has recently been reported. In a comparison of tumors derived from cell lines with varying capabilities for metastasis, gene expression profiling revealed the transcription factor, Twist, as one of the most differentially expressed genes. Inhibition of Twist resulted in the loss of several steps of metastasis, including intravasation. Twist expression has been documented for several human tumors (e.g. metastatic melanoma). Twist can also induce the EMT and developmental mutations of Twist result in the failure of neural tube closure. Therefore, Twist is not only an inducer of the EMT during development but is also a key regulator of metastasis. It is possible that EMT pathways may provide new targets for diagnostics, prognostics, and therapeutics.

9.9 Other means of tumor neovascularization

Recent evidence has suggested that, in addition to angiogenesis, vasculogenic mimicry and vasculogenesis contribute to the formation of tumor vessels (Figure 9.9a–c). Vasculogenic mimicry describes the process whereby

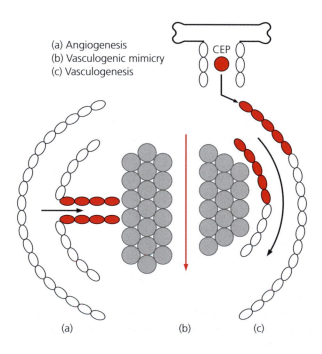

(a) Angiogenesis
(b) Vasculogenic mimicry
(c) Vasculogenesis

CEP

(a)   (b)   (c)

Figure 9.9 Tumor neovascularization.

tumor cells (e.g. melanoma cells; shown as gray circles in Figure 9.9) act as endothelial cells and form vascular-like structures (Figure 9.9b, red arrow). Vasculogenesis involves the differentiation and proliferation of endothelial cells from endothelial progenitor cells. Studies have demonstrated that up to 40% of tumor endothelial cells originated from circulating endothelial progenitor cells (CEPs; shown as a red circle) derived from the bone marrow. Angiogenic factors from the tumor, such as VEGF, are involved in the recruitment of these cells that express VEGFR-2. After reaching the tumor, CEPs differentiate and contribute to the tumor neovasculature (Figure 9.9c, red ovals). It seems likely that different cancers may differ in their requirement for CEP contributions to the new tumor vasculature. It is known that they are necessary for lymphomas and colon cancer.

 Therapeutic strategies

Perhaps one could envisage a therapy targeted at each of the major steps of metastasis. However, since the first and last steps are rate-limiting, these have been the targets most often tried. Protease and integrin inhibitors have been obvious molecular targets to block migration. Therapies aimed at the tumor vasculature have been designed either to halt the angiogenic process (anti-angiogenic drugs) or to destroy the tumor vasculature which has already been formed (vascular targeting). Some examples of the therapies that have been developed are discussed below.

9.10 Metalloproteinase inhibitors (MPIs)

There was a rapid response by pharmaceutical companies to develop metalloproteinase inhibitors because of the evidence of the role of MMPs in metastasis. These molecules appear to function in several steps of metastasis, including migration and metastatic colonization. The initial wave of clinical trials proved to be disappointing although informative for future trials. The development of drugs exceeded the rate at which basic research was able to uncover the details of the MMP family. First, about 24 different family members have been identified. The knowledge of temporal and spatial expression patterns, functional roles, and roles in different cancers of the individual family members, lagged behind the development of small-molecule inhibitors and natural product drugs. The trials were hindered by unexpected side-effects (musculoskeletal pain) and poor design. There was difficulty in measuring efficacy and the drugs were administered only to patients with advanced disease even though pre-clinical evidence suggested that administration at early stages of disease was crucial. Although no MPIs have received approval as a cancer therapy thus far, modifications have been made and several MPIs are still in clinical trials. These include Marimastat, BMS-275291 (lacks named side-effects), Prinomastat, Metastat, and Neovastat (isolated from shark cartilage).

9.11 Anti-angiogenic therapy and vascular targeting

Anti-angiogenic therapy is designed to prevent the formation of new blood vessels. Rather than target the tumor cells directly, the aim of anti-angiogenic therapy is to interfere with the responsiveness of endothelial cells that is essential to the tumor's survival. Drugs may be designed to prevent the cells from responding to pro-angiogenic signals or may be targeted to block the activity of the inducers (Figure 9.10). Overall, these drugs are cytostatic rather than cytotoxic, and therefore may need long-term continuous administration. Anti-angiogenic therapies, together with vascular targeting (discussed below), differ from the therapies discussed previously, and the differences have several implications. First, since angiogenesis only occurs on occasion in the adult, drugs that inhibit

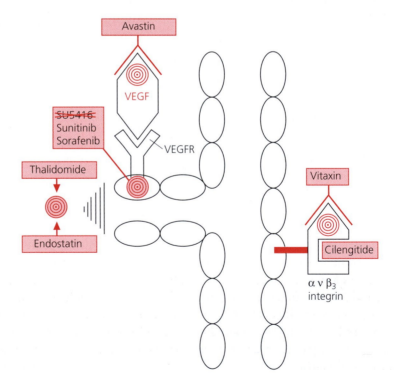

Figure 9.10 Anti-angiogenic therapies and their molecular targets. Endothelial cells are shown as black ovals. Therapeutic agents are shown in red and cellular targets are indicated by a (◎) symbol. Clinical development of SU5416, the first VEGFR tyrosine kinase inhibitor to enter clinical trials, has been stopped (shown by a red cross).

Table 9.2 Angiogenesis inhibitors in clinical trials

Drug	Company	Mechanism	Phase of trial
Drugs that block activators of angiogenesis and their receptors			
SU5416	Sugen	Blocks VEGFR signaling	Withdrawn
SU6668	Sugen	Blocks VEGFR, FGFR, PDGFR	Withdrawn
Sorafenib (BAY 43–9006)	Bayer	Blocks VEGFR, PDGFR, FLT3, KIT, and Raf	Approved
Sunitinib (SU-11248)	Pfizer	VEGFR, PDGFR, FLT3, KIT	Approved
Avastin	Genetech	Monoclonal Ab to VEGF	Approved
IMC-1C11	Imclone System	Monoclonal Ab to VEGF	I
Angiozyme	Ribozyme Pharm	Inhibition of VEGFR synthesis	I/II
AZD2171	AstraZeneca	VEGFR1/2 tyrosine kinase inhibitor	II
ZD6474, Zactima™ (vandetanib)	AstraZeneca	VEGFR1/2 tyrosine kinase inhibitor	Approved orphan drug/III
VEGF-Trap	Regeneron Pharm	Soluble decoy VEGFR	II/III
Drugs that inhibit endothelial-specific integrin signaling			
Vitaxin II	MedImmune	Inhibitor of $\alpha v \beta 3$ integrin	II
Cilengitide	Merck KGaA	Antagonist of integrins $\alpha v \beta 3$ and $\alpha v \beta 5$	II
Drugs that inhibit endothelial cells			
Thalidomide	Celgene	Unknown	III
Endostatin	EntreMed	Inhibition of endothelial cells	II (approved in China, 2005)
Angiostatin	EntreMed	Inhibition of endothelial cells	I
ABT-510	Abbott Labs	Thrombospondin-1 analog	II
Drugs that block matrix breakdown			
Marimastat	British Biotech	Inhibitor of MMPs	III
Neovastat	Aeterna Zentaris	Inhibitor of MMPs	III
BMS-275291	Bristol Myers Squibb	Inhibitor of MMPs	III
Miscellaneous			
Combretastatin	Oxigene	Binds to tubulin; disrupts the cytoskeleton	I

Ab, antibody.

it are predicted to cause minimal side-effects. More importantly, the target endothelial cells recruited during angiogenesis are genetically stable, unlike the tumor cells that have accumulated mutations, and are therefore less likely to develop drug resistance rapidly. Approximately 80 anti-angiogenic drugs are currently in clinical trials (some are listed in Table 9.2). Examples of several different strategies that have been employed are described below.

One strategy involves targeting angiogenic factors such as VEGF. Avastin (bevacizumab), a recombinant human monoclonal antibody that recognizes all VEGF isoforms, has been tested in clinical trials (for example see Yang *et al.*, 2003) and approved for treatment of colorectal cancer. Interestingly, the drug failed to show a response (life extension) in an early breast cancer trial. Why was there a different response observed in the two different cancers? The answer lies in the angiogenic switch: colon tumors are more dependent on VEGF for the induction of angiogenesis while this is true only for early stages of breast cancer. Advanced breast cancer utilizes a broader arsenal of angiogenic inducers, and thus inhibition of just one activator does not have an effect.

Small-molecule tyrosine kinase inhibitors have been used to target the VEGFR. Semaxanib (SU5416) was the first VEGFR inhibitor to enter Phase III clinical trials. Its mechanism of action is that it inhibits receptor autophosphorylation. Although semaxanib demonstrated promising results in patients with Kaposi's sarcoma, significant toxicity and poor responses in patients with colorectal cancer led to the withdrawal of the drug. Its further development was also discontinued due to unfavorable pharmacology, namely a particularly short half-life of only several hours. As a result of the short half-life of the drug, effective doses were unable to be maintained even after bi-weekly intravenous administration. Similarly, the drug SU6668, which has a similar mode of action to semaxanib and is orally active, was also withdrawn. However, this strategy has proved successful by the approval of two multi-targeted tyrosine kinase inhibitors, sunitinib and sorafenib, for the treatment of advanced renal cell carcinoma in 2006. Sunitinib targets VEGF receptors as well as PDGFR, KIT, and FLT3. Sorafenib targets VEGF receptors, PDGFR, KIT, FLT3, and Raf kinase (as mentioned in Chapter 4) (see Pause and Think).

Administration of recombinant human endogenous inhibitors is another anti-angiogenic treatment strategy that held much promise but which thus far has not delivered the expected results. Endostatin, which was only discovered in 1996, was the first to enter clinical trials. Although it was demonstrated to be non-toxic, no clinical response was observed. This negative result may, again, be due to suboptimal design of the clinical trial rather than inefficacy of the drug, since patients with advanced solid tumors were selected despite pre-clinical success with early stage cancer models. The company (EntreMed Inc., Rockville, MD) has announced that it will halt production of endostatin due to financial difficulties.

Antagonists to integrins αvβ3 and αvβ5 would block endothelial integrin–ECM interactions and specifically induce apoptosis of angiogenic vessels with little effect on mature vessels. Two integrin inhibitors have entered clinical trials: Vitaxin is a humanized monoclonal antibody

PAUSE AND THINK

Do you remember another example where a small molecule inhibitor was used to target a tyrosine kinase receptor? Hint, see Chapter 4.

against αvβ3 and cilengitide is a synthetic cyclic peptide antagonist that mimics the Arg–Gly–Asp 'ligand' sequence and inhibits integrins αvβ3, and αvβ5 (Gutheil *et al.*, 2000; Tucker, 2002).

Thalidomide, a drug cursed in the past as being teratogenic, is one of the most effective drugs for treating patients with multiple myeloma. It has been shown to inhibit angiogenesis induced by bFGF or VEGF, and reduced plasma levels of these proteins correlate with the efficacy of thalidomide treatment. However, the anti-angiogenic activity of thalido- mide is linked to its teratogenicity and thus patient education regarding pregnancy is crucial.

Anti-angiogenic effects may be 'side-effects' of other cancer therapies. Cancer therapies targeted at oncogene products often affect angiogenesis. Herceptin (the antibody directed against ErbB2, see Chapter 4) has been shown to be anti-angiogenic by inhibiting the production of angiogenic inducers (e.g. TGF-α and angiopoietin-1) by tumor cells and upregulating angiogenic inhibitors (e.g. thrombospondin). Chronic frequent adminis- tration of conventional chemotherapy at doses of one-tenth to one-third of the MTD, known as metronomic scheduling, has also resulted in anti- angiogenic effects.

Vascular targeting

Vasculature targeting is a therapeutic approach designed to destroy the existing neovasculature in order to starve the tumor of oxygen and nutrients and lead to tumor regression. This approach is possible due to the identification of molecular differences between tumor and normal vasculature. Clinical trials in both the UK and USA have begun to test combretastatin compounds, first isolated from the African bushwillow, *Combretum caffrum*, which are selectively toxic to neovasculature (Griggs *et al.*, 2001). Combretastatin compounds bind tubulin and disrupt the cytoskeleton. Their effects have been explained by the hypothesis that immature endothelium may have a more intrinsic need for a tubulin cyto- skeleton to maintain its shape than stable mature vasculature which is firmly supported by a basement membrane. Loss of shape and rounding up of the endothelial cells in new blood vessels block blood flow and/or lead to vascular collapse thereby depriving the tumor of oxygen and nutri- ents (Figure 9.11; compare images before (a) and after (b) treatment with combretastatin A4). As a result, necrosis occurs at the core of the tumor. Unfortunately, a ring of tumor cells at the periphery remain viable (Figure 9.11b) and indicate the need for combination therapy. Other mech- anisms of action responsible for the apoptotic effects of combretastatins are also probable. Anti-vascular effects are seen at doses of one-tenth of the MTD. ZD6126 is another vascular targeting agent in clinical trials

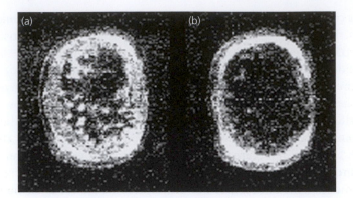

Figure 9.11 Effects of combretastatin on tumor neovasculature. Anti-vascular effects were analyzed by magnetic resonance imaging. The image intensity indicates tumor vasculature. A primary tumor before (a) and after (b) treatment with combretastatin A4. Strong anti-vascular effects are seen in the core of the tumor after treatment but a small viable rim of tumor tissue can be seen at the periphery. Reprinted from Beauregard, D.A. *et al.* (1998) Magnetic resonance imaging and spectroscopy of combretastatin A(4) prodrug induced disruption of tumor profusion and energetic status. *Br. J. Cancer* 77: 1761–1767, Copyright (1998), with permission from Nature Publishing Group.

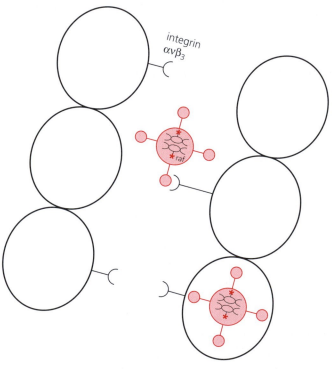

Figure 9.12 Vascular targeting by nanoparticle technology.

that targets the tubulin cytoskeleton. Anti-vascular effects have been seen without cytotoxicity (Blakey *et al.*, 2002). We must be aware for long-term administration that both drugs are selective for all neovasculature and are not only tumor specific.

Nanoparticle technology, gene therapy, and vascular targeting have come together in an exciting report with hints at future applications. Knowledge of several biochemical areas has been combined specifically to target an anti-angiogenic gene to the neovasculature of tumors in mice (Hood *et al.*, 2002) (Figure 9.12). Lipid-based nanoparticles (Figure 9.12, shaded red) were coated with a ligand to a neovasculature-specific receptor, integrin αvβ3. This integrin is not only specific to newly growing vessels but also internalizes viruses and small particles and thus can facilitate gene delivery. A mutant form of the *Raf* gene (Figure 9.12, marked by an asterisk) was coupled to the nanoparticles and was used to inhibit the Raf pathway critical for angiogenesis *in vivo*. Systemic delivery to mice resulted in apoptosis of tumor endothelial cells and concentric rings of apoptotic tumor cells around the targeted vessels. Regression of primary and metastatic tumors was demonstrated. Since viruses were not used for gene delivery, the disadvantages of viral delivery (e.g. risk of further carcinogenesis and an immunogenic response) were bypassed.

9.12 Targeting several steps of metastasis at once

As we have seen in this chapter, there are several steps involved in the metastasis of a cell from a primary tumor to a secondary site. Recently, sets of genes or 'gene signatures' that are associated with primary tumor growth and risk of metastasis have been identified. Four genes of a lung metastasis gene signature (the EGFR ligand *epiregulin*, *COX2*, and *MMP1* and *MMP2*) in human cancer cells were shown to mediate tumor growth, angiogenesis, migration, intravasation, and extravasation in mice (Gupta *et al.*, 2007). The experimental approach involved generating cells that simultaneously targeted four genes for reduced expression by using the technique of short hairpin RNA interference and examining each of the biological parameters mentioned above. More interesting from a therapeutic context, a combination of existing drugs (cetuximab, an anti-EGFR antibody, celecoxib, a COX inhibitor, and GM6001, a MMP inhibitor) was also able to target the protein products of the four genes and demonstrated inhibition of growth and metastasis. These results hold great potential for the future because if we can block metastasis we have a hope of managing the disease.

HOW DO WE KNOW THAT?

In vivo assays to analyze tumor growth and stages of metastasis (see Gupta *et al.*, 2007)

The procedure for the *in vivo* assays is as follows: inject human cancer cells (originally obtained from cells that had metastasized to the lung in a breast cancer patient) into a mouse, allow 24 days for primary tumor growth, treat mice with named drugs, and harvest tissues from mice at specified times.

To assess the effects on primary tumor growth, tumor volume was measured and compared with controls (see Figure 4b of Gupta *et al.*, 2007). Results are attributed to tumor cell apoptosis. How do they know that? You will need to refer to the online supplementary information associated with the article. To assess

the effects of these drugs on intravasation, the presence of human cells in the mouse blood was examined by the detection of human-specific GAPDH expression using real-time PCR (see Figure 4c of Gupta *et al.*, 2007). To assess extravasation and colonization of the lung, cryosections of lung tissue were analyzed by immunohistochemistry using a human-specific fluorescent antibody to detect tumor cells and DAPI (4,6-diamidino-2-phenylindole) stain to detect all nuclei (see Figure 4d of Gupta *et al.*, 2007). The metastatic burden (number and size distribution of metastases) is calculated as the area of fluorescence normalized to the area of DAPI staining (data shown in Figure 4f of Gupta *et al.*, 2007).

■ CHAPTER HIGHLIGHTS—REFRESH YOUR MEMORY

- The major steps involved in metastasis are: migration, intravasation, transport, extravasation, and metastatic colonization.

- Different cancers metastasize to specific locations due to the direction of blood flow and molecules which support the 'seed and soil' hypothesis.

- Integrins are receptors that mediate cell–ECM interactions and, with respect to the exterior and interior of a cell, mediate bidirectional signaling.

- The steps involved in intravasation and extravasation are similar but are the reverse of each other.

- Metastatic colonization is characterized by progressive growth of a tumor at a distant site and requires angiogenesis.

- Micrometastases do not show net growth and may stay dormant for years.

- Loss of function of metastasis-suppressor genes results in an increase in metastatic capability.

- Members of the VEGF family are specific endothelial cell growth factors that are key players in angiogenesis. Their signals are mediated through transmembrane tyrosine kinase receptors.

- Hypoxia inducible factor is a heterodimeric transcription factor that targets genes important for angiogenesis, such as VEGF.

- The angiogenic switch is regulated by the dynamic balance of pro- and anti-angiogenic factors.

- Vasculogenic mimicry and vasculogenesis also contribute to neovascularization of tumors.

- Anti-angiogenic therapy is designed to *prevent the formation of* new blood vessels while vasculature targeting is designed to *destroy* the neovasculature.

■ ACTIVITY

1. Using the web sites on page 210, update Table 9.2. Have certain drugs progressed to advanced clinical trials? Have some been terminated? Have new drugs been added? Can you think of any additional strategies not mentioned? Can you think of any strategies that target HIF-1α?

■ **FURTHER READING**

Bergers, G. and Benjamin, L.E. (2003) Tumorigenesis and the angiogenic switch. *Nature Rev. Cancer* **3**: 401–410.

Carmeliet, P. and Jain, R.K. (2000) Angiogenesis in cancer and other diseases. *Nature* **407**: 249–257.

Chang, C. and Werb, Z. (2001) The many faces of metalloproteases: cell growth, invasion, angiogenesis and metastasis. *Trends Cell Biol.* **11**: S37–S43.

Coussens, L.M., Fingleton, B., and Matrisian, L.M. (2002) Matrix metalloproteinase inhibitors and cancer: trials and tribulations. *Science* **295**: 2387–2392.

Cross, M.J., Dixelius, J., Matsumoto, T., and Claesson-Welsh, L. (2003) VEGF-receptor signal transduction. *Trends Biochem. Sci.* **28**: 488–494.

Folkman, J. (2006) Antiangiogenesis in cancer therapy-endostatin and its mechanism of action. *Exp. Cell Res.* **312**: 594–607.

George, D.J. and Moore, C. (2006) Angiogenesis inhibitors in clinical oncology. *Update Cancer Ther.* **1**: 429–434.

Hood, J.D. and Cheresh, D.A. (2002) Role of integrins in cell invasion and migration. *Nature Rev. Cancer* **2**: 91–100.

Kaplan, R.N., Rafii, S., and Lyden, D. (2006) Preparing the 'Soil': the premetastatic niche. *Cancer Res.* **66**: 11089–11093.

Kerbel, R. and Folkman, J. (2002) Clinical translation of angiogenesis inhibitors. *Nature Rev. Cancer* **2**: 727–739.

Madhusudan, S. and Harris, A.L. (2002) Drug inhibition of angiogenesis. *Curr. Opin. Pharm.* **2**: 403–414.

Malik, A.K. and Gerber, H.-P. (2004) Targeting VEGF ligands and receptors in cancer. *Targets* **2**: 48–57.

McCarty, M.F., Liu, W., Fan, F., Parikh, A., Reimuth, N., Stoeltzing, O., and Ellis, L.M. (2003) Promises and pitfalls of anti-angiogenic therapy in clinical trials. *Trends Mol. Med.* **9**: 53–58.

Matter, A. (2001) Tumour angiogenesis as a therapeutic target. *Drug Discov. Today* **6**: 1005–1020.

Oppenheimer, S.B. (2006) Cellular basis of cancer metastasis: a review of fundamentals and new advances. *Acta Histochem.* **108**: 327–334.

Ruegg, C., Hasmim, M., Lejeune, F., and Alghisi, G.C. (2006) Antiangiogenic peptides and proteins: from experimental tools to clinical drugs. *Biochim. Biophys. Acta* **1765**: 155–177.

Ruoslahti, E. (2002) Specialization of tumour vasculature. *Nature Rev. Cancer* **2**: 83–90.

Steeg, P.S. (2003) Metastasis suppressors alter the signal transduction of cancer cells. *Nature Rev. Cancer.* **3**: 55–63.

Taraboletti, G. and Margosio, B. (2001) Antiangiogenic and antivascular therapy for cancer. *Curr. Opin. Pharm.* **1**: 378–384.

Yang, J., Mani, S.A., and Weinberg, R.A. (2006) Exploring a new twist on tumor metastasis. *Cancer Res.* **66**: 4549–4552.

■ **WEB SITES**

The Angiogenesis Foundation http://www.angio.org/
Clinical trials http://www.cancer.gov/clinicaltrials

■ **SELECTED SPECIAL TOPICS**

Blakey, D.C., Ashton, S.E., Westwood, F.R., Walker, M., and Ryan, A.J. (2002) ZD6126: A novel small molecule vascular targeting agent. *Int. J. Radiat. Oncol. Biol. Phys.* **54**: 1497–1502.

Griggs, J., Metcalfe, J.C., and Hesketh, R. (2001) Targeting tumor vasculature: the development of combretastatin A. *Lancet Oncol.* **2**: 82–87.

Gupta, G.P., Nguyen, D.X., Chiang, A.C., Bos, P.D., Kim, J.Y., Nadal, C., Gomis, R.R., Monova-Todorova, K., and Massague, J. (2007) Mediators of vascular remodeling co-opted for sequential steps in lung metastasis. *Nature* **446**: 765–770.

Gutheil, J.C., Campbell, T.N., Pierce, P.R., Watkins, J.D., Huse, W.D., Bodkin, D.J., and Cheresh, D.A. (2000) Targeted antiangiogenic therapy for cancer using Vitaxin: a humanized monoclonal antibody to the integrin $\alpha v\beta 3$. *Clin. Cancer. Res.* **6**: 3056–3061.

Hood, J.D., Bednarski, M., Frausto, R., Guccione, S., Reisfeld, R.A., Xiang, R., and Cheresh, D.A. (2002) Tumor regression by targeted gene delivery to the neovasculature. *Science* **296**: 2404–2407.

Kim, W. and Kaelin Jr, W.G. (2003) The von-Hippel-Lindau tumor repressor protein: new insights into oxygen sensing and cancer. *Curr. Opin. Genet. Dev.* **13**: 55–60.

Laferriere, J. Houle, F., and Huot, J. (2002) Regulation of the metastatic process by E-selectin and stress-activated protein kinase-2/p38. *Ann. NY Acad. Sci.* **973**: 562–572.

Tucker, G.C. (2002) Inhibitors of integrins. *Curr. Opin. Pharmacol.* **2**: 394–402.

Yang, J.C., Haworth, L., Sherry, R.M., Hwu, P., Schwartzentruber, D.J., Topalian, S.L., Steinberg, S.M., Chen, H.X., and Rosenberg, S.A. (2003) A randomized trial of bevacizumab, an anti-vascular endothelial growth factor antibody for metastatic renal cancer. *New Engl. J. Med.* **349**: 427–434.

Chapter 10

Infections and inflammation

Introduction

One-sixth of all cancers are caused by infectious agents and inflammation. This may be a surprising fact, and suggests the logical question: 'Can we "catch" cancer?'. The answer to this question is not straightforward. One does not 'catch' cancer in the same way as one 'catches a cold'. Exposure to an infectious agent does not immediately trigger cancer. However, we now know that long-term exposure to specific infectious agents, some causing chronic inflammation, can lead to cancer. In addition, there is evidence that **chronic** inflammation, in the absence of an infectious agent, leads to an increased risk of cancer. This is good news for cancer prevention and treatment, since we have learned a lot about the prevention and treatment of some types of infection related to other diseases and also about prevention and treatment of chronic inflammation. Infection and inflammation may be major preventable causes of human cancer.

Infectious agents involved in carcinogenesis include DNA and RNA viruses and bacteria. DNA viruses contain viral genes that do not have cellular homologs. As we discussed in Chapter 6 (Figure 6.9), they act by producing proteins that interact and inhibit tumor suppressor genes (e.g. *p53* and *Rb*) to promote cell proliferation. RNA viruses, or retroviruses, carry altered forms of cellular genes, called oncogenes, or disrupt normal gene expression via insertional mutagenesis (discussed in Chapter 4). The mouse mammary tumor virus (MMTV), an oncogenic retrovirus, is an important model system that induces breast cancer in mice through insertional mutagenesis. However, conflicting evidence for a role of MMTV-like sequences in human breast cancer has been reported.

Some viral and bacterial infections induce a chronic inflammatory response that contributes to the process of carcinogenesis. Inflammation is a host defense mechanism against infectious agents and injury, as it is a consequence of wound healing. Under normal conditions it is highly regulated and short lived: such acute inflammation typically resolves itself with the help of anti-inflammatory factors. By contrast, recent evidence suggests that it is lingering, chronic inflammation that plays an important role in causing cancer. In addition, cancer has been referred to as a 'wound that never heals'. The body responds to a tumor by creating an inflammatory microenvironment around the tumor. Inflammatory cells, growth factors, and reactive oxygen/nitrogen species characterize the site of the inflammatory response. These factors of inflammation set the stage for cell proliferation, mutagenesis, angiogenesis, and metastasis.

In this chapter we will identify infectious agents that are considered to be carcinogens and discuss several modes of action of these infectious agents. The molecular mechanisms of chronic inflammation (in the presence or absence of an infectious agent) that contribute to carcinogenesis will also be described. Finally, the chapter will conclude with a report on the major therapeutic applications of this knowledge.

10.1 Identifying infectious agents as carcinogens

In order to identify which infectious agents actually *cause* cancer several general criteria are applied. First there must be a consistent association between infection and the cancer that is supported by either epidemiological or molecular evidence. In addition, cell transformation or induction of tumors in animal models by the infectious agent must be demonstrated. In some instances, infectious agents may not reside in the transformed cells but may cause cancer indirectly, through inflammation and chronic tissue injury or paracrine growth stimulation (see below under Kaposi's sarcoma-associated herpesvirus). A list of some of the infectious agents that are known to be carcinogenic is shown in Table 10.1 and discussed below.

Epstein–Barr virus (EBV)

Epstein–Barr virus, a DNA virus, is a good starting point for examining the role of infectious agents as carcinogens. Upon close evaluation it has

Table 10.1 Infectious agents and their role as cancer-causing agents (data from Pagano *et al.*, 2004)

Infectious agent	Type	Presence in tumor	Type of cancer	Causative	Major effector
Human papillomaviruses	DNA virus	100%	Cervical	Yes	E6, E7
Epstein–Barr virus	DNA virus	100%	Nasopharyngeal carcinomas	Yes	
		98% (endemic)	Burkitt's lymphoma	No	LMP1
Kaposi's sarcoma-associated herpesvirus	DNA virus	>95%	Kaposi's sarcoma	Yes	LANA
		100%	Primary effusion lymphoma	Yes	LANA
Human T-cell leukemia virus	RNA virus	100%	T-cell leukemia	Yes	Tax protein
Hepatitis B virus	DNA virus	100%	Hepatocellular carcinoma	Yes	HBV X
Helicobacter pylori	Bacterium	+/–	Gastric cancer	Yes	CagA

been shown to act as a causative factor in B-cell lymphoproliferative diseases and probably nasopharyngeal carcinoma. However, it is thought to be only a contributing factor for a type of cancer called Burkitt's lymphoma (Pagano *et al.*, 2004). Let's look at the evidence. In support of a causative role of EBV in the former two cancers, it has been demonstrated that EBV can transform lymphoid cells in culture and documented that all cases of nasopharyngeal carcinoma are associated with EBV infection, regardless of geographical location. In contrast, Burkitt's lymphoma is not always associated with EBV although Burkitt's lymphoma *is* associated with EBV in geographical regions that are also endemic for malaria (Table 10.1). This suggests that EBV may be an important co-factor along with malaria for the disease. Thus, epidemiological evidence is lacking to support a causative role for EBV in Burkitt's lymphoma. Further studies examining the role of EBV, perhaps in subtypes of Burkitt's lymphoma, are required.

Epstein–Barr virus encodes several viral proteins that affect host gene expression. One of these, oncoprotein LMP1, is able to transform cells in culture. Its multi-functional effects include activation of genes important for promoting cell proliferation (e.g. *EGFR*) and inhibiting apoptosis (e.g. *Bcl-2*). It also activates a nuclear transcription factor called NF-κB. As we will see below, activation of cell growth pathways and anti-apoptotic pathways, as well as activation of the key player, NF-κB, are important molecular themes that run throughout this chapter.

Human papillomavirus (HPV)

Human papillomavirus infection is strongly associated with cervical cancer: virtually 100% of all cervical cancer cells contain HPV (see Plate 6). There is a lag time between HPV infection and cervical cancer of at least 10 years. Genital HPV may be the most common sexually transmitted viral infection, and the risk of infection increases with the number of sexual partners. This DNA virus requires access to the proliferating cells of the cervical epithelium. It uses entry points created by micro-erosion of the overlying cell layers to reach the basal layer of the epithelium, where stem cells and progenitor cells reside. The development of cancer involves expression of viral genes, integration of viral DNA into the host chromosomes, and changes to host cell genes and gene products. The HPV gene products E6 and E7 are major players in carcinogenesis that target tumor suppressor proteins in the host cell. E7 binds to and triggers the degradation of RB, thus preventing the sequestration of E2F. E6 forms a complex with a ubiquitin ligase. The complex binds p53, and p53 degradation is triggered (see Chapter 6). Viral products E6 and E7 are able to transform cultured human cells and induce tumors in mice.

Note that only a subset of the total of 130 types of HPV that have been identified is considered 'high risk' for cervical cancer (see Figure 10.1).

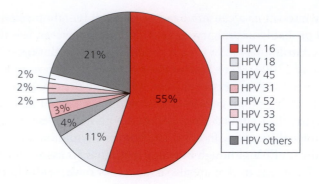

HPV16 and HPV18 account for over 65% of the global distribution of HPV types in cervical cancer. Viral genotype analysis, distinguishing between the different types, was crucial in establishing the link with cervical cancer; if all HPVs were considered as one agent the link would not have been established.

Human T-cell leukemia virus type-1 (HTLV-1)

Almost all cases of adult T-cell leukemia exhibit molecular evidence for the presence of HTLV-1. This is the only virus known to have a causal link to human leukemia. Also, it is the only retrovirus that is linked to human cancer. HTLV-1 infection is prevalent in Japan, the Caribbean, South America, and Central Africa. About 2–5% of infected individuals develop T-cell leukemia/lymphoma.

Transmission of the virus is through intimate contact and includes transmission through breast milk, semen, unscreened blood, and contaminated needles among drug users. In Japan, breast-feeding for more than 6 months has been discouraged; as a result transmission of HTLV-1 to infants has been greatly reduced.

As a retrovirus, HTLV-1 genomic RNA is copied into DNA by reverse transcriptase, before viral proteins are synthesized by the host cell's machinery. The Tax protein of HTLV-1 is a key player in the mechanism of HTLV-1-induced carcinogenesis. It is a molecule that activates host cell genes through the transcription factor NF-κB (see below), and interferes with several tumor suppressor proteins (e.g. p53) to promote cell proliferation and ultimately leukemia.

◎ Hepatitis B virus (HBV) and liver cancer

There is a strong association between hepatitis B virus infection and liver cancer (hepatocellular carcinoma). Hepatitis B, a DNA virus, is a potent carcinogen as demonstrated by the fact that HBV carriers have a 10–25-fold greater risk of developing hepatocellular carcinoma than

> **LIFESTYLE TIP**
>
> Cancer is a rare but possible consequence of contracting a sexually transmitted disease. This may be one reason to consider necessary precautions.

uninfected individuals (see Pagano *et al.*, 2004). Host–viral interactions evoke an immune response that results in liver necrosis, inflammation, and regeneration. These effects are sustained in the 10% of adults who develop chronic infections. It has been proposed that increased proliferation and/or oxidative stress from inflammation may lead to oncogenic mutations. Inflammation caused by Hepatitis B virus is important for the development of hepatocellular carcinoma, in a manner that parallels mechanisms observed in gastric cancer (see below).

The multifunctional viral protein, HBV X, is thought to be important for HBV-induced carcinogenesis and it was shown to induce liver cancer in transgenic mice. It is thought to function by activating proto-oncogenes via various signaling cascades, including many kinase cascades (e.g. the RAS–RAF–MAPK pathway, Chapter 4); interacting with NF-κB (see below); and binding to and inactivating p53.

Note that Hepatitis C virus is also a risk factor for hepatocellular carcinoma but details will not be included here.

Kaposi's sarcoma-associated herpesvirus (KSHV)

Kaposi's sarcoma-associated herpesvirus (KSHV) is a DNA virus. It is strongly linked with a vascular tumor of heterogeneous cell composition usually associated with the skin, called Kaposi's sarcoma (>95%), and primary effusion lymphomas (100%). Although Kaposi's sarcoma is associated frequently with AIDS patients, there are types found in different populations where AIDS is not prevalent. Classic Kaposi's sarcoma is seen in the Mediterranean and eastern Europe while an endemic type is prevalent in parts of Africa where HIV may act as a co-factor.

KSHV is thought to contribute to tumorigenesis through several mechanisms. Firstly, several viral gene products have been shown to transform cells in culture and in transgenic mice. Also, some viral products induce the production of cytokines and growth factors that can influence uninfected neighboring cells. It has been suggested that KSHV tumorigenesis involves a paracrine process whereby uninfected cells are transformed by these induced cytokines and growth factors secreted by the infected cells. This may explain the heterogeneous cell composition of some KSHV-induced tumors. In addition, KSHV produces several viral anti-apoptotic proteins (e.g. vBcl-2) and a viral protein called LANA, that interferes with the function of RB and p53. This mechanism of targeting two crucial tumor suppressor proteins is shared with HPV.

Helicobacter pylori infection and gastric cancer   ◎

Helicobacter pylori is a bacterium capable of inducing chronic inflammation in the stomach and initiating carcinogenesis. It has been identified as a carcinogen for humans by the International Agency for Research on Cancer (IARC)/World Health Organization. However, only less than 1%

of those infected will develop gastric cancer. Gastric carcinogenesis depends on the bacterial strain, host response, and environmental factors. It is a multi-step process where inflammation is considered the initial and required step in the process: *Helicobacter pylori* infection→chronic superficial gastritis→atrophic gastritis→intestinal dysplasia→gastric carcinoma.

Gastric atrophy is characterized by the loss of normal glandular cells and results in a decrease of acid production. These conditions allow additional bacteria to colonize the stomach and trigger an inflammatory response.

Epidemiological studies show that the prevalence of gastric cancer corresponds to the prevalence of particular strains of *H. pylori* in specific geographical locations and that gastric cancer develops in *H. pylori*-infected individuals and not in uninfected individuals. Overall, it is estimated that 60–90% of all gastric cancers are caused by *H. pylori* infection. Experimental evidence includes the induction of gastric cancer in animals by *H. pylori* infection and reduction in gastric cancer risk and the prevention of pre-cancerous lesions by eradication of *H. pylori* infection.

Let's examine the proposed mechanism by which this bacterium can cause cancer. Many high risk strains of *H. pylori* code for a protein called cytotoxin-associated antigen A (CagA). Epidemiological studies show that CagA-positive strains are predominant in regions with a high prevalence of gastric cancer. The bacterial CagA protein is an effector protein that is injected into cells by the bacterial secretion system to elicit cellular effects, such as stimulation of cell growth (Figure 10.2a). CagA is phosphorylated by cellular tyrosine kinases that are members of the Src family of kinases. Phosphorylated CagA interacts with SH2 domain-containing proteins

(a)

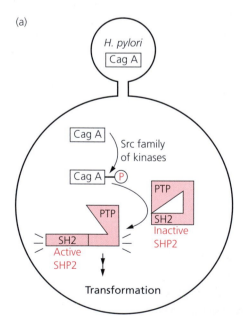

(b)

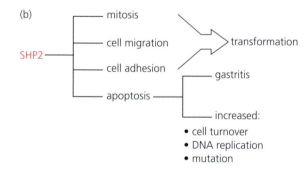

Figure 10.2 Molecular mechanisms involved in *H. pylori* infection that contribute to carcinogenesis. (a) Phosphorylated cytotoxin-associated antigen A (CagA) causes a conformational change and activates an oncogenic protein tyrosine phosphatase (PTP) called SHP-2. (b) Cellular effects of SHP-2 activation that may lead to transformation.

such as SHP-2 (an oncogenic tyrosine phosphatase, see Chapter 4) and Grb2. SHP-2 normally maintains an inactive conformation by a mechanism similarly described for Src (see Figure 4.6): an amino-SH2 domain of SHP-2 blocks substrate access by an intramolecular interaction. Binding of CagA may cause a conformational change that relieves the intramolecular inhibition and leads to the stimulation of SHP-2 phosphatase activity (note the change in shape of SHP-2, shown in red in Figure 10.2a). Thus, CagA binding of SHP-2 mimics a gain-of-function oncogenic mutant form of SHP-2. A signal transduction pathway is initiated that affects cell mitosis, migration, and adhesion (Figure 10.2b). Sustained activation of SHP-2 by CagA leads to apoptosis in cell culture, most likely due to it causing an imbalance of mitogenic signals. Long-term apoptosis of the gastric mucosal cells may be the cause of gastritis and also lead to increased cell turnover. Increased DNA replication increases the risk of mutation and may lead to transformation.

In addition to the effect of bacterial proteins on cell signaling and cell biology, other mechanisms seem to be involved in carcinogenesis due to *H. pylori*. These include effects of chronic inflammation and stem cell recruitment (see page 223). In addition to CagA, *H. pylori* also delivers proteins to cells that induce pro-inflammatory mediators through the NF-κB pathway. *Helicobacter pylori*-induced inflammation stimulates DNA methyltransferases and results in epigenetic changes by hypermethylation. Inflammation may induce oxidative stress and ultimately increase the rate of mutations. *Helicobacter pylori* may also induce oxidative stress by production of superoxide and reduction of the antioxidant vitamin C.

Note that although causality has not yet been proven, associations between other bacterial infections and cancer have been noted. These include *Salmonella typhi* infection and gall bladder cancer, *Streptococcus bovis* and colon cancer, *Bartonella* and vascular tumors, and *Chlamydia pneumoniae* and lung cancer.

> **PAUSE AND THINK**
>
> Try to make a list of the infectious agents discussed above and describe how their major effector molecule(s) exert its (their) effects. Check your answer with Table 10.1.

10.2 Inflammation and cancer

The link between inflammation and cancer is clearly illustrated by the association of chronic inflammation in both Hepatitis B virus and *H. pylori*-induced cancers, as seen above. Furthermore, inflammation plays a causative role, independent of infection. There are a number of chronic inflammatory conditions caused by non-infectious agents that are associated with cancer. It has been proposed that asbestos causes cancer by acting as an inflammatory stimulus in the lungs, predisposing individuals to bronchial carcinoma. Similarly, esophageal reflux causes injury of the esophagus and may induce an inflammatory response that increases the risk of esophageal carcinoma. Rheumatoid arthritis is linked with non-Hodgkin's lymphoma. In an animal model prototype of inflammation-associated cancer, genetically altered mice that develop liver inflammation also subsequently develop cancer (this animal model is used in the study by Pikarsky *et al.* (2004) discussed below in How do we know that?). Let's examine the molecular events of the inflammatory response.

The key cells of a chronic inflammatory response are macrophages. These cells produce tumor necrosis factor-alpha (TNF-α), a cytokine that helps orchestrate the inflammatory response by inducing a range of effector molecules, some of which help perpetuate the inflammatory response. In addition, leukocytes produce reactive oxygen and nitrogen species (ROS and NOS, respectively) to help fight infection, but these products (via the formation of peroxynitrite) also cause DNA mutations. Chronic inflammation is associated with an increased production of ROS and NOS, and therefore the risk of DNA damage is increased. Tissue regeneration and cell renewal induced by Hepatitis B virus and *H. pylori* infections, respectively, involve cell division, during which DNA is most susceptible to DNA damage. Thus the interplay between infection and an immune response can be seen.

Several pro-inflammatory products, such as TNF-α, interleukins, and chemokines, mediate processes known to be critical in carcinogenesis: proliferation, apoptosis, angiogenesis, and metastasis. The expression of the genes that code for these products is regulated by the transcription factor NF-κB. Since NF-κB is induced by carcinogens, including oncogenic viral products, it is an important link between inflammation and cancer and will be discussed in detail below.

Once a tumor has developed, the immune response continues to play a role in tumor progression. Both the tumor cells and non-malignant cells residing in or near the tumor are involved in the process of inflammation-associated malignant progression (Figure 10.3). Chemoattractive molecules, called chemokines, are involved in the recruitment and the infiltration of leucocytes, including tumor-associated macrophages (TAMs), into the tumor. The expression of growth factors, cytokines, and chemokines, by both the TAMs and the tumor cells, impacts on the cells in that location and promotes proliferation and survival. TNF-α produced by TAMs and a variety of tumor cells is a key player in the inflammatory response, as mentioned above, and when unregulated can act as a tumor promoter. TNF-α can affect cell motility and tumor metastasis. The enzyme, inducible nitric oxide (NO) synthase, is one target stimulated by TNF-α. This enzyme is implicated in several stages of carcinogenesis including cell transformation and growth of transformed cells. The cytokine interleukin-6 (IL-6), produced by liver macrophages, has been shown to be important in hepatocarcinogenesis (Naugler *et al.*, 2007). Production of IL-6 requires the activation of transcription factor NF-κB (see below). In addition to

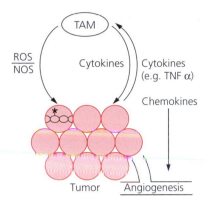

Figure 10.3 Molecular events of the inflammatory response at the site of a tumor. Tumor cells (red) secrete chemokines that recruit leukocytes including tumor-associated macrophages (TAMs). TAMs produce cytokines and reactive oxygen/nitrogen species (ROS/NOS, respectively) which can mutate DNA (shown by the asterisk). Tumor cells also produce cytokines. Chemokines promote angiogenesis.

their role in recruiting leukocytes to the site of inflammation, chemokines play an important role in the angiogenic switch. Chemokines signal via G-protein-coupled receptors, and this results in the transcription of target genes. Pro-inflammatory chemokines promote angiogenesis.

NF-κB is a key player in the inflammatory response

A key mediator of the inflammatory response is the transcription factor NF-κB. It is induced by several cell types, such as macrophages, target cells of inflammation, and cancer cells. Figure 10.4 shows some of the upstream activators of NF-κB in both macrophage and cancer cells (see Aggarwal, 2004; Karin, 2006). NF-κB is activated by specific macrophage products (e.g. TNF-α), *H. pylori* CagA protein, viral proteins (e.g. KSHV), carcinogens (cigarette smoke), stress, and chemotherapeutic agents. In addition to inflammation, NF-κB has other downstream effects that contribute to tumorigenesis, such as the inhibition of apoptosis and the promotion of metastasis and angiogenesis (Figure 10.4). Thus, NF-κB provides a molecular link between inflammation and cancer. Oncogenic activation of the NF-κB gene has also been identified in human tumors, including multiple myeloma, acute lymphocyte leukemia, prostate, and breast cancers.

Let's describe the molecular regulation of the NF-κB pathway (Figure 10.5). NF-κB (shown in red) is a dimeric transcription factor made up of hetero- or homodimers of protein members in the NF-κB family. The five NF-κB family members are grouped into two groups. The first group consists of p65 (RelA), Rel B, and c-Rel. The second group consists of NF-κB 1 (p50), and NF-κB 2 (p52). The first group of proteins

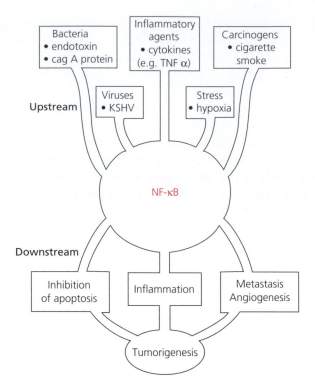

Figure 10.4 Upstream activators and downstream effects of NF-κB.

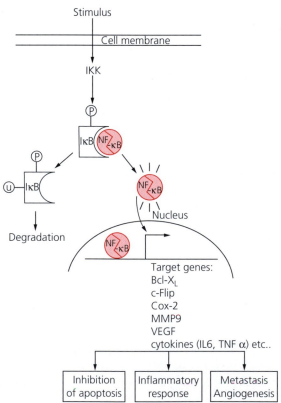

Figure 10.5 Regulation of the NF-κB pathway. See text for details.

are synthesized as mature products, whereas the second group of proteins must be proteolytically processed to produce the mature p50 and p52 proteins. Only the first group contain transactivation domains and therefore proteins of the second group cannot activate transcription on their own. The most predominant NF-κB dimer activated by the classical pathway is p65–p50. (Note: An important finding linking NF-κB to carcinogenesis was the discovery that c-rel is the proto-oncogene of the v-rel oncogene.) Normally, NF-κB is sequestered in the cytoplasm by an inhibitor of NF-κB (IκB). Upon cell activation, the kinase IκB kinase, (IKK) phosphorylates IκB and targets it for degradation via a ubiquitin ligase complex. This causes the release and translocation of NF-κB to the nucleus. Here NF-κB can transcriptionally regulate its target genes at NF-κB DNA response elements (GGGRNNYYCC). NF-κB regulates more than 200 genes to elicit its varied effects.

One of the most important cellular effects of activation of NF-κB is the inhibition of apoptosis via the induction of anti-apoptotic gene expression (e.g. induction of Bcl-X$_L$, cellular inhibitor of apoptosis (c-IAP), cFLIP). In this way NF-κB prevents an important tumor suppressing mechanism and promotes carcinogenesis.

PAUSE AND THINK

Can you remember similar types of molecular mechanisms regulating other transcription factors? Hint: One is an important transcription factor involved in angiogenesis and another is involved in an important developmental program.

HOW DO WE KNOW THAT?

Functional knock-out mice

The role of NF-κB in tumorigenesis was investigated in a mouse model system whereby the mouse strain develops hepatitis and is prone to hepatocellular carcinoma (Pikarsky *et al.*, 2004). Transgenic animals containing a hepatocyte-inducible NF-κB inhibitor, IκB, were examined as a means of creating an equivalent of a NF-κB knockout.

Why and how was this hepatocyte-inducible regulation accomplished?

Since NF-κB is involved in many crucial cellular responses, a total eradication of activity would lead to embryonic lethality. An experimental system that can be turned on and off would allow for normal development and investigation of the role of NF-κB in one tissue-specific context.

The IκB gene was linked to a tetracycline-regulated promoter so that IκB was only expressed in the presence of a tetracycline transactivator. The gene for the transactivator was under the control of a hepatocyte-specific promoter so that it was only expressed in liver cells. In the presence of the tetracycline derivative, doxycycline, the tetracycline-controlled transactivator could not bind to its target DNA sequences (sequences of the tetracycline operon) and transcription of

IκB was blocked. Treatment of mice with the doxycycline suppressed the transgene (in this case, the inhibitor of NF-κB). So doxycycline-treated transgenic mice contained active NF-κB, while untreated mice contained inactive NF-κB due to the expression of its inhibitor (see Pause and Think).

The results showed that when NF-κB is inactive, only a small percentage (10%) of pre-cancerous adenomas progressed to carcinoma compared with controls. Blocking NF-κB activity induced hepatocyte apoptosis as detected by antibody staining for activated caspase-3 and also led to a dramatic decrease in tumor progression as shown by magnetic resonance imaging and histological analysis. In addition, they showed that the inflammatory factor, TNF-α, produced by residing inflammatory cells controlled the activation of NF-κB in the hepatocytes. PCR analysis of cell fractions showed that the source of TNF-α was in the non-hepatocyte fraction of the liver. A block in →

PAUSE AND THINK

See if you can sketch a diagram that shows the transgene (labeling promoter and coding sequences), the transactivator, and the consequences of no treatment versus doxycycline treatment. Check your answer with Figure 10.6.

→ NF-κB activation was demonstrated by using an anti-TNF-α antibody to block TNF-α function. Thus, NF-κB in the liver is controlled through a paracrine manner via TNFα produced by inflammatory cells.

This work supported the findings from another laboratory (Greten *et al.*, 2004) that also used knock-out transgenic mice to ablate (knock out) NF-κB activity. An essential activator of NF-κB, called IKKβ, was ablated in intestinal epithelial cells in a mouse model of colon cancer. These mice showed an 80% reduction in tumor incidence relative to control animals. Tumor size was not affected. Analysis of the colon revealed that apoptosis was not inhibited by NF-κB in these altered mice. Thus, apoptosis acts as an important tumor-suppressing mechanism in the absence of NF-κB activation. Ablation of IKKβ in myeloid cells in this mouse model reduces the expression of cytokines that influence tumor growth and results in a

decrease in tumor size. Thus, inhibition of the NF-κB pathway in these two cell types affects tumorigenesis in two different ways (Table 10.2).

Table 10.2 Summary of NF-κB pathway inhibition experiments

Deletion of IKKβ[a]	Intestinal epithelial cells	Myeloid cells
Tumor incidence	Decrease	
Tumor size	No effect	Decrease
Production of pro-inflammatory cytokines		Decrease

[a]Functionally equivalent to inactive NF-κB.

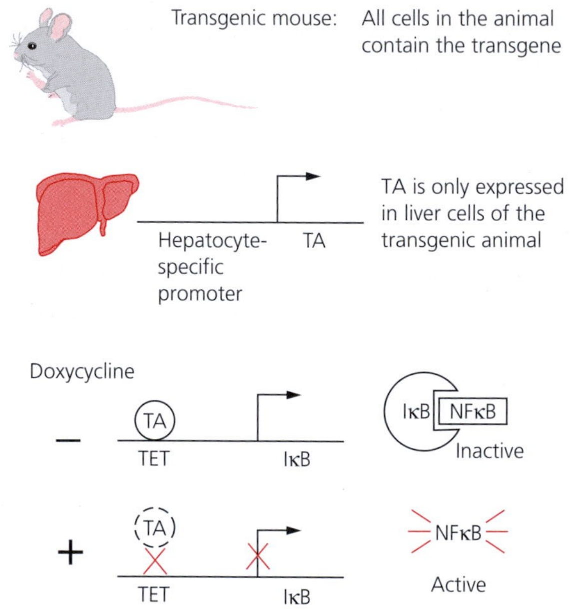

Figure 10.6 Hepatocyte-inducible regulation of a transgene used to experimentally control NF-κB activity. TA, transactivator; IκB, inhibitor of NF-κB; TET, tetracycline-regulated promoter sequence.

Other roles of NF-κB

NF-κB activates the *cyclin D1* gene, and thus plays a role in regulating the cell cycle. In addition, NF-κB activates the expression of pro-inflammatory genes (e.g. the *COX-2* gene and cytokine genes) and metastasis and angiogenic genes (e.g. *MMP9*, chemokine receptors, *VEGF*). COX-2 is an enzyme that is involved in the synthesis of prostaglandin, PGE-2, a potent pro-inflammatory molecule (see below). An NF-κB DNA-binding element has been identified in the *MMP9* gene. Thus NF-κB helps maintain the inflammatory response and promotes metastasis. It is important to note that NF-κB also has anti-tumorigenic effects in certain tissues (e.g. skin) and so complexities of cell context exist and must be kept in mind when considering therapeutic strategies.

Inflammation and tissue injury in gastric cancer recruits bone marrow stem cells

In Chapter 8 we discussed that cancer may arise from cancer stem cells and reviewed the data in support of tissue-specific cancer stem cells. An alternative proposal suggests that the stem cells that contribute to cancer may originate from a different tissue. The environment of tissue injury and inflammation has been linked to the recruitment of bone marrow-derived stem cells. Bone marrow-derived stem cells respond to inflammatory mediators and tissue injury, and because of their demonstrated plasticity may serve as a backup when tissue-specific stem cells are damaged. In a mouse model of gastric cancer induced by chronic infection with *H. pylori*, bone marrow-derived stem cells were shown to be recruited to the stomach and to contribute to gastric cancer (Houghton *et al.*, 2004). Acute inflammation and/or injury did not cause recruitment of these stem cells.

Conclusion

In conclusion, as can be seen from the above, several mechanisms of infection and inflammation are involved in the process of cancer initiation and promotion. We have seen examples of infectious agents that carry oncogenes or produce products that inhibit tumor suppressors. Many infective agents trigger chronic inflammation, and this plays a part in their mechanism of action. However, chronic inflammation, even in the absence of an infectious agent, plays its own role in carcinogenesis. Key cells of the inflammatory response produce factors that influence major processes involved in carcinogenesis and, as reported more recently, trigger the migration of stem cells that may themselves contribute to cancer.

◎ Therapeutic strategies

Cancers caused by infections could be prevented if infections could be eradicated. The impact of this can be fully appreciated by looking at some numbers: there are 405,000 deaths per year worldwide from gastric carcinoma and 35,000 women per year die from cervical cancer in the

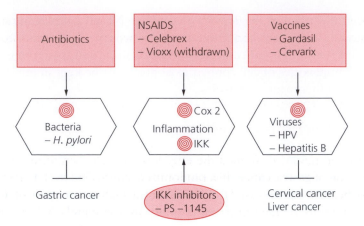

Figure 10.7 Cancer prevention strategies targeted against infection and inflammation.

USA and Europe. Infections are implicated in the occurrence of these diseases. Wouldn't it be extraordinary if we could prevent the suffering and death of these people?

Below is a discussion of several strategies targeted against infection and inflammation for the prevention of cancer (Figure 10.7). Some of these are used today, others have just been approved or are on our doorstep, and one has been tried but is no longer administered due to severe side-effects.

10.3 A national vaccination program against Hepatitis B virus in Taiwan

In Taiwan, in 1982, 15–20% of the population were carriers of Hepatitis B virus. In addition, 20% of all cancer deaths were due to hepatocellular carcinoma, and more than 80% of these cases were due to chronic hepatitis B infection. As a result of this public health problem, a nationwide hepatitis B vaccination program was initiated in 1984. In the first 2 years, infants born to carrier mothers were vaccinated. Two years later, all newborns were vaccinated, and from 1987 pre-school children were vaccinated. Later adolescents and adults were also vaccinated. The incidence of hepatocellular carcinoma in children decreased significantly

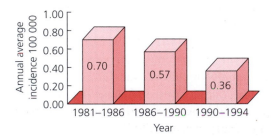

Figure 10.8 Graph showing the effects of HBV vaccination on liver cancer in children.

(Figure 10.8), demonstrating that a majority of cases of hepatocellular carcinomas in children can be prevented by hepatitis B vaccination.

10.4 Eradication of *H. pylori* and the relationship to prevention of gastric cancer

Wong *et al.* (2004) examined the effects of *H. pylori* eradication on the prevention of gastric cancer in a randomized, controlled trial. Participants (1630 healthy carriers of *H. pylori* from a high-risk region of China) were randomly divided into two groups: approximately half received a 2-week course of triple therapy (omeprazole, amoxicillin plus clavulanate potassium, and metronidazole) and half received a placebo. They were followed up for 7.5 years from 1994–2002. The study found that the incidence of gastric cancer was similar between the two groups. However, eradication of *H. pylori* resulted in a significant decrease of the incidence of gastric cancer in the group of *H. pylori* carriers who did not have pre-cancerous lesions. Thus, these results suggest that eradication of *H. pylori* should be considered in all patients without pre-cancerous lesions in high-risk areas.

10.5 Cancer vaccines to prevent cervical cancer

The world's first cervical cancer vaccine called Gardasil® (Merck), was approved in June 2006 by the US Food and Drug Administration (FDA). The hope is that, over time, after implementation of vaccination strategies, the number of women diagnosed with cervical cancer in the world (currently about 470,000 cases per year) will decrease dramatically.

The major capsid protein, L1, from four HPV types (6, 11, 16, 18) was used to form virus-like particles (VLPs) for the production of this quadrivalent vaccine. When the capsid protein is expressed in eukaryotic cells using recombinant DNA techniques, the L1 capsid protein self-assembles into particles that mimic the virus. These particles, along with an adjuvant, are administered as the vaccine. The vaccine has been demonstrated to prevent cervical cancer caused by HPV16 and HPV18 and also pre-cancerous lesions and warts caused by HPV6, -11, -16, and -18, in clinical trials (Villa *et al.*, 2005). Since the ideal time to administer a preventative vaccine is before infection, Gardasil has been approved for administration in adolescent girls/young adults, ages 9–26. Clinical trials are also being carried out to test a HPV16 and HPV18 bivalent vaccine, Cervarix® (sponsored by GlaxoSmithKline), and these too are showing promising results (Harper *et al.*, 2004).

PAUSE AND THINK

Why were these four HPV types chosen for the production of Gardasil? We can see from Figure 10.1 that HPV types 16 and 18 account for approximately 70% of cases of cervical cancer. What is not shown on the graph is that HPV6 and -11 cause approximately 90% of genital warts and give rise to lesions that are clinically indistinguishable from pre-cancerous lesions caused by HPV16 and -18. Abnormal lesions called by HPV6 and -11 lead to false positives and trigger additional investigations. Thus, by eliminating these lesions, abnormal Pap results (see below) will be easier to interpret.

LIFESTYLE TIP

Although we now have an HPV vaccine to help prevent against cervical cancer, screening programs are still important for detecting cervical cancer caused by HPV strains not covered by the vaccine or for previously infected women.

A little lesson about Pap and HPV DNA screening

The most common method of screening for cervical cancer is the Papanicolaou cytology technique or Pap smear test. Cells from the cervix are harvested for microscopic analysis and examined for changes in cell morphology that may represent pre-cancerous cell changes called cervical intra-epithelial neoplasia (CIN) or cancer. Limitations of this technique include poor sample collection and/or slide preparation leading to abnormal cell morphology, and errors of interpretation by the laboratory scientist. However, routine Pap screening in some countries has resulted in a substantial reduction in cervical cancer mortality. Significantly, cervical cancer mortality rates in the UK have decreased over 60% in the last 30 years (http://info.cancerresearchuk.org/cancerstats/types/cervix/mortality/).

The addition of testing for HPV DNA may be a great aid to screening procedures in the near future. The value of HPV testing in both primary cervical screening and in the management of abnormal cervical cytology has been stated in recommendations from the IARC and/or in US/European guidelines (Cox and Cuzick, 2006). The Hybrid Capture 2 (hc2) high-risk HPV DNA test (Digene) is a diagnostic test that has been approved by the FDA. In this test, RNA probes are used to detect the genomic DNA of 13 high-risk HPV types. Specific RNA–DNA hybrids are formed in solution and captured by specific antibodies coated at the bottom of a microtiter plate. Additional antibodies that generate a luminescent product in the presence of hybrids are used to detect the captured hybrids, and a specialized instrument called a luminometer analyzes the signal. Note that the majority of HPV infections will be transient (clearance time 6–18 months) and conclusions from these tests need to take this fact into account.

LEADERS IN THE FIELD . . . of cancer vaccines: Douglas Lowy and John Schiller

The work of Douglas Lowy and John Schiller laid the foundation for the development of a preventative vaccine against cervical cancer. Their work investigated the role of papillomavirus in cervical cancer and showed that the capsid proteins of the virus could elicit an immune response. They also supervised the Phase I clinical trials of the vaccine, leading to FDA approval of the first HPV vaccine in 2006. Their work exemplifies the translation of basic research to applications in public health. They were presented with the Landon Award at the 100th year anniversary of the American Association for Cancer Research in 2007.

Dr Lowy received his MD from New York University School of Medicine. Dr Schiller received a PhD from the University of Washington in Seattle. Both are currently working at the Center for Cancer Research at the National Cancer Institute.

10.6 Inhibition of inflammation

Non-steroidal anti-inflammatory drugs (NSAIDs), such as aspirin, have been shown to decrease cancer risk and may be used for the treatment of cancer. One mechanism of action of NSAIDs in inhibiting inflammation is by inhibiting cyclo-oxygenase (COX) activity. There are two COX isoforms: COX1 is constitutively active and COX2 is inducible. These enzymes catalyze the synthesis of prostaglandins from arachidonic acid. Thus inhibition of COX results in the decrease of prostaglandin synthesis. Prostaglandin synthesis produces mutagenic metabolites, and prostaglandins induce the production of cytokines and stimulate cell proliferation. NSAIDs may also act via inhibition of NF-κB.

These drugs are not without side-effects; they can cause severe stomach irritation and ulcers. Since COX1 was found to have protective effects on the stomach lining, selective COX2 inhibitors were developed to eradicate these side-effects. However, this avenue of drug discovery is not without problems. Vioxx (Merck; http://www.merck.com/), a COX-2 inhibitor, had to be withdrawn from the market in 2004 due to an increased risk of heart attacks and stroke.

Another COX2 inhibitor, Celecoxib (Celebrex; Pfizer; http://www.pfizer.com/), has been approved for the disease called familial adenomatous polyposis (Chapter 8). As you may remember from Chapter 8, patients with this disease carry a germline mutation in the *APC* gene and have almost a 100% risk of colon cancer. One study has demonstrated a 30% reduction in the number of polyps in these patients after treatment with Celecoxib (Steinbach *et al.*, 2000). Additional trials of Celecoxib for cancer prevention (see Kismet *et al.*, 2004) and treatment are ongoing, although under high doses, side-effects similar to those induced by Vioxx have been reported.

Antagonists of TNF-α are being evaluated in clinical trials. Etanercept, a recombinant soluble fusion protein consisting of the ligand-binding domain of the human TNF-α receptor and the constant region of immunoglobulin G, binds to free TNF-α and antagonizes its binding with endogenous receptors. This drug is currently in PhaseI/II trials for the treatment of ovarian cancer.

Inhibiting the NF-κB pathway

Many research groups are focusing on strategies that selectively inhibit IKK activity as the most promising and effective approach to inhibit NF-κB activation. Numerous compounds have been identified by large-scale screening and combinatorial chemistry, most acting as IKK inhibitors (see Karin *et al.*, 2004). One of these compounds, PS-1145, was developed from a β-carboline natural product and was shown to prevent NF-κB activation and inhibit the growth of multiple myeloma cells. Further along, pyridyl cyanoguanidine compounds have been reported to act as anti-tumor agents in clinical trials and a patent for their use in the treatment of cancer is held by Leo Pharma.

PAUSE AND THINK

What other strategies can be used to inhibit the NF-κB pathway? Think about the molecular mechanisms involved and how NF-κB exerts its effects.

You may have thought of compounds that: interfere with NF-κB binding to DNA; block nuclear translocation; block degradation of IκB, or inhibit gene expression of IKK by antisense oligonucleotides or siRNA.

■ CHAPTER HIGHLIGHTS—REFRESH YOUR MEMORY

- Infectious agents and chronic inflammation account for 15–20% of all cancers.

- Certain criteria are used to classify an infectious agent as a carcinogen.

- Specific DNA and RNA viruses and bacteria have been classified as carcinogens.

- One hundred per cent of cervical cancers are associated with human papillomavirus.

- Common mechanisms of infectious agents and chronic inflammation in carcinogenesis include:

  induction of growth factors/signaling programs (autocrine or paracrine)
  inactivation of tumor suppressor genes
  activation of nuclear transcription factor NF-κB.

- The CagA protein is implicated in the mechanism of the induction of gastric cancer by the bacterium *H. pylori*.

- CagA is a phosphoprotein that interferes with kinase signaling and regulation in the cell.

- Considerable evidence suggests that chronic inflammation, even in the absence of infection, contributes to carcinogenesis.

- The site of chronic inflammation is characterized by cytokines, chemokines, and reactive oxygen/nitrogen species that can act as a carcinogen.

- The transcription factor NF-κB is an important mediator between inflammation and cancer.

- Bone marrow stem cells migrate to sites of inflammation and injury and may contribute to gastric carcinogenesis.

- Gardasil® (Merck), the first preventative cervical cancer vaccine, was approved in 2006.

- Current HPV vaccines are not able to protect against all HPV infection. Therefore, screening procedures must be maintained.

- Vaccination programs have been and will continue to be important preventative measures for some cancers.

■ ACTIVITY

1. Look at the paper by Watanabe *et al.* (*Gastroenterology* **115**: 642–648, 1998). Describe the model system, experimental procedure and the methods of analysis that provided *in vivo* evidence that *H. pylori* infection leads to gastric cancer.

■ FURTHER READING

Aggarwal, B.B. (2004) Nuclear factor-κB: the enemy within. *Cancer Cell* **6**: 203–208.

Aggarwal, B.B., Shishodia, S., Sandur, S.K., Pandey, M.K., and Sethi, G. (2006) Inflammation and cancer: how hot is the link? *Biochem. Pharmacol.* **72**: 1605–1621.

Balkwill, F., Charles, K.A., and Mantovani, A. (2005) Smoldering and polarized inflammation in the initiation and promotion of malignant disease. *Cancer Cell* **7**: 211–217.

Coussens, L.M. and Werb, Z. (2002) Inflammation and cancer. *Nature* **420**: 860–867.

Escarcega, R.O., Fuentes-Alexandro, S., Garcia-Carrasco, M., Gatica, A., and Zamora, A. (2007) The transcription factor Nuclear Factor-kappa B and cancer. *Clin. Oncol.* **19**: 154–161.

Farazi, P.A. and DePinho, R.A. (2006) Hepatocellular carcinoma pathogenesis: from genes to environment. *Nature Rev. Cancer* **6**: 674–687.

Hatakeyama, M. (2004) Oncogenic mechanisms of the *Helicobacter pylori* CagA protein. *Nature Rev. Cancer* **4**: 688–694.

Huang, K.-Y. and Lin, S.-R. (2000) Nationwide vaccination: a success story in Taiwan. *Vaccine* **18**: S35–S38.

Karin, M. (2006) Nuclear factor-κB in cancer development and progression. *Nature* **441**: 431–436.

Karin, M., Yamamoto, Y., and Wang, Q.M. (2004) The IKK NF-κB system: a treasure trove for drug development. *Nature Rev. Drug Discov.* **3**: 17–26.

Kelley, J.R. and Duggan, J.M. (2003) Gastric cancer epidemiology and risk factors. *J. Clin. Epidemiol.* **56**: 1–9.

Li, Q., Withoff, S., and Verma, I.M. (2005) Inflammation-associated cancer: NF-κB is the lynchpin. *Trends Immunol.* **26**: 318–325.

Lowy, D.R. and Schiller, J.T. (2006) Prophylactic human papillomavirus vaccines. *J. Clin. Invest.* **116**: 1167–1173.

Matysiak-Budnik, T. and Megraud, F. (2006) *Helicobacter pylori* infection and gastric cancer. *Eur. J. Cancer* **42**: 708–716.

Munoz, N., Bosch, F.X., de Sanjose, S., Herrero, R., Castellsague, X., Shah, K.V., Snijders, P.J.F., and Meijer, C.J.L.M. (2003) Epidemiologic classification of human papillomavirus types associated with cervical cancer. *New Engl. J. Med.* **348**: 518–527.

Pagano, J.S., Blaser, M., Buendia, M.-A., Damania, B., Khalili, K., Raab-Traub, N., and Roizman, B. (2004) Infectious agents and cancer: criteria for a causal relation. *Semin. Cancer Biol.* **14**: 453–471.

Radkov, S.A., Kellam, P., and Boshoff, C. (2000) The latent nuclear antigen of Kaposi sarcoma-associated herpesvirus targets the retinoblastoma-E2F pathway and with the oncogene Hras transforms primary rat cells. *Nature Med.* **6**: 1121–1127.

Tan, T.-T. and Coussens, L.M. (2007) Humoral immunity, inflammation and cancer. *Curr. Opin. Immunol.* **19**: 209–216.

Vogelmann, R. and Amieva, M.R. (2007) The role of bacterial pathogens in cancer. *Curr. Opin. Microbiol.* **10**: 76–81.

Zhang, X., Zhang, H., and Ye, L. (2006) Effects of hepatitis B virus X protein on the development of liver cancer. *J. Lab. Clin. Med.* **147**: 58–66.

zur Hausen, H. (2002) Papillomaviruses and cancer: from basic studies to clinical application. *Nature Rev. Cancer* **2**: 342–350.

■ **WEB SITES**

Gardasil, Merck www.merck.com/newsroom/press_releases/product/2007_0509.html

UK Cervical Cancer Statistics
http://info.cancerresearchuk.org/cancerstats/types/cervix/mortality/

■ **SELECTED SPECIAL TOPICS**

Cox, T. and Cuzick, J. (2006) HPV DNA testing in cervical cancer screening: from evidence to policies. *Gynecol. Oncol.* **103**: 8–11.

Greten, F.R., Eckmann, L., Greten, T.F., Park, J.M., Egan, L.J., Kagnoff, M.F., and Karin, M. (2004) IKKb links inflammation and tumorigenesis in a mouse model of colitis-associated cancer. *Cell.* **118**: 285–296.

Harper, D., Franco, E., Wheeler, C., Ferris, D., Jenkins, D., Schuind, A., Zahaf, T., Innis, B., Naud, P., and De Carvalho, N. (2004) Efficacy of a bivalent L1 virus-like particle vaccine in prevention of infection with human papillomavirus types 16 and 18 in young women, a randomized controlled trial. *Lancet* **364**: 1757–1765.

Houghton, J., Stoicov, C., Nomura, S., Rogers, A.B., Carlson, J., Li, H., Cai, X., Fox, J.G., Goldenring, J.R., and Wang, T.C. (2004) Gastric cancer originating from bone marrow-derived cells. *Science* **306**: 1568–1571.

Kismet, K, Akay, M.T., Abbasoglu, O., and Ercan, A. (2004) Celocoxib: a potent cyclooxygenase-2 inhibitor in cancer prevention. *Cancer Detect. Prev.* **28**: 127–142.

Naugler, W.E., Sakurai, T., Kim, S., Maeda, S., Kim, K.H., Elsharkawy, A.M., and Karin, M. (2007) Gender disparity in liver cancer due to sex differences in MyD88-dependent IL-6 production. *Science* **317**: 121–124.

Pikarsky, E., Porat, R.M., Stein, I., Abramovitch, R., Amit, S., Kasem, S., Gutkovich-Pyest, E., Urieli-Shoval, S., Galun, E., and Ben-Neriah, Y. (2004) NF-κB functions as a tumour promoter in inflammation-associated cancer. *Nature* **431**: 461–466.

Steinbach, G., Lynch, P.M., Phillips, R.K.S., Wallace, M.H., Hawk, E., Gordon, G.B., Wakabayashi, N., Saunders, B., Shen, Y., Fujimura, T., Su, L.-K., Levin, B., Godio, L., Patterson, S., Rodriguez-Bigas, M.A., Jester, S.L., King, K.L., Schumacher, M., Abbruzzese, J., DuBois, R.N., Hittelman, W.N., Zimmerman, S., Sherman, J.W., and Kelloff, G. (2000) The effect of Celecoxib, a cyclooxygenease-2 inhibitor, in familial adenomatous polyposis. *New Engl J. Med.* **342**: 1946–1952.

Villa, L.L., Costa, R.L., Petta, C.A., Andrade, R.P., Ault, K.A., Giuliano, A.R., Wheeler, C.M., Koutsky, L.A., Malm, C., Lehtinen, M., Skjeldestad, F.E., Olsson, S.E., Steinwall, M., Brown, D.R., Kurman, R.J., Ronnett, B.M., Stoler, M.H., Ferenczy, A., Harper, D.M., Tamms, G.M., Yu, J., Lupinacci, L., Railkar, R., Taddeo, F.J., Jansen, K.U., Esser, M.T., Sings, H.L., Saah, A.J., and Barr, E. (2005) Prophylactic quadrivalent human papillomavirus (types 6, 11, 16, and 18) L1 virus-like particle vaccine in young women: a randomized double-blind placebo-controlled multicentre phase II efficacy trial. *Lancet Oncol.* **6**: 271–278.

Wong, B.C.-Y., Lam, S.K., Wong, W.M., Chen, J.S., Zheng, T.T., Feng, R.E., Lai, K.C., Hu, W.H.C., Yuen, S.T., Fong, D.Y.K., Ho, J., Ching, C.K., and Chen, J.S. (2004) *Helicobacter pylori* eradication to prevent gastric cancer in a high-risk region of China: a randomized controlled trial. *J. Am. Med. Assoc.* **291**: 187–194.

Chapter 11

Nutrients, hormones, and gene interactions

Introduction

Does our diet influence whether we are the one out of three people who get cancer? Diet plays a significant role in cancer incidence. Many epidemiological studies provide evidence to support the role of diet in both causation and prevention of cancer. Approximately one-third of the variations in cancer incidence between different populations are due to differences in diet. For example, the Japanese diet has changed radically between the 1950s and 1990s, including a seven-fold increase in meat consumption (Key *et al.*, 2002). This coincides with a five-fold increase in colorectal cancer over the same period. The knowledge gained from investigations into the role of diet in cancer and cancer prevention should be integrated into lifestyle modifications in order to reduce the occurrence of the disease.

In this chapter we will see that some diets act as cancer-causative factors and others act as cancer-preventative factors. Diet and exercise also affect cell metabolism. Metabolic changes associated with tumor cells will be described. Upon examination of the mechanisms of action of nutrients it will become clear that some of these mechanisms parallel the mechanism of action of growth factors and others parallel the mechanism of action of hormones. The chapter will conclude with a discussion of the role of hormones in carcinogenesis.

Let us examine why we eat food (Figure 11.1). The basic food groups of carbohydrates, fats, and proteins provide us with glucose, fatty acids, and amino acids, respectively, that can be metabolized to produce energy. Food also provides precursors for biosynthetic reactions. For example, proteins provide a source of nitrogen needed for the synthesis of the nitrogenous bases of DNA. Vitamins and minerals provide co-factors that are essential for the function of many enzymes. Additional biologically active microconstituents have been identified in the foods we eat (Table 11.1). Many biologically active microconstituents act as **antioxidants**, compounds that significantly inhibit or delay the damaging action of ROS (see Chapter 2), often by being oxidized themselves. Plants require many phytochemicals as a defense against excess energy and oxidative damage as they absorb solar energy for photosynthesis. Many of these phytochemicals provided in the diet are important for the protection of human cells. Although humans can synthesize some required

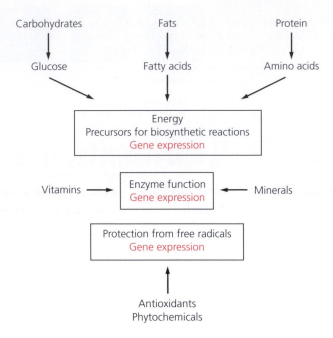

Figure 11.1 Provisions of food.

antioxidants others must be obtained by eating fruit and vegetables. The four major groups of dietary antioxidants–phytochemicals are vitamin C, isoprenoids (e.g. vitamin E), phenolic compounds (flavonoids), and organosulfur compounds. These will be discussed below. Lastly, specific nutrients and microconstituents have been shown to affect gene expression (Figure 11.1).

Information gained about the role of microconstituents in cancer prevention could be applied to the development of chemopreventative **supplements**, extra sources of dietary components taken in addition to food. However, unraveling the individual contributions of microconstituents as preventative agents against cancer is a challenge for the future. Epidemiological studies strongly suggested that diets rich in β-carotene-containing fruits and vegetables reduced lung cancer risk. Animal studies also generated supportive evidence. This led to the β-Carotene and Retinol Efficacy Trial (CARET) and the Alpha-Tocopherol Beta-Carotene Cancer Prevention Study (ATBC) which tested the effect of β-carotene supplements on smokers and those exposed to asbestos. Surprisingly, β-carotene supplementation increased lung cancer in these high-risk individuals and had no effect on healthy individuals. The results of these trials do not support the initial hypothesis formulated on pre-clinical findings (see Pause and Think, page 223).

Only recently have molecular approaches been used to investigate the molecular mechanisms of dietary constituents involved in the causation or prevention of cancer. One of the most significant insights gained is that *nutrients regulate gene expression*. The power of food has begun to be revealed. This chapter will include a sample of these findings.

Table 11.1 Microconstituents. Reprinted from Manson, M.M. (2003) Cancer prevention—the potential for diet to modulate molecular signaling. *Trends Mol. Med.* 9: 11–18, Copyright (2003), with permission from Elsevier

Food source	Class of compound	Chemical
Cruciferous vegetables	Isothiocyanate	Benzyl isothiocyanate, phenethyl isothiocyanate, sulforaphane
Cruciferous vegetables	Dithiolthione	Ohipraz
Cruciferous vegetables	Glycosinolate	Indole-3-carbinol, 3,3'-diindoylmethane, indole-3-acetonitrile
Onions, garlic, scallions, chives	Allium compound	Diallyl sulfide, allylmethyl trisulfide
Citrus fruit (peel)	Terpenoid	D-Limonene, penllyl alcohol, geraniol, menthol, carvone
Citrus fruit	Flavonoid	Tangeretin, nobiletin, ratin
Berries, tomatoes, potatoes, broad beans, broccoli, squash, onions	Flavonoid	Quercetin
Radish, horseradish, kale, endive	Flavonoid	Kaempferol
Tea, chocolate	Polyphenol	Epigallocatechin gallate, epigallocatechin, epicatechin, catechin
Grapes	Polyphenol	Resveratrol
Turmeric	Polyphenol	Curcumin
Strawberries, raspberries, blackberries, walnuts, pecans	Polyphenol	Caffeic acid, ferulic acid, ellagic acid
Cereals, pulses (millet, sorghum, soya beans)	Isoflavone	Genistein
Orange vegetables and fruit	Carotenoid	α- and β-carotene
Tomatoes	Carotenoid	Lycopene
Tea, coffee, cola, cacao (cocoa and chocolate)	Methylxanthines	Caffeine, theophylline, theobromine

PAUSE AND THINK

Propose a hypothesis to explain these seemingly conflicting results. The most likely explanation is that alternative micro-constituents in β-carotene-rich vegetables and fruits may be the active ingredient in reducing lung cancer risk, or perhaps β-carotene works in a synergistic manner with other microconstituents not present in the supplements. Interactions between different dietary constituents must be considered for a complete picture.

11.1 Causative factors

Three main aspects of our diet can be considered as causative factors of cancer. First, any given food is a very complex substance that can carry harmful factors in addition to nutritional value. The consumption of food provides a route for chemical carcinogens to be delivered to the body.

Genotoxic agents present as microconstituents in food act as dietary carcinogens. Secondly, lack of a particular essential nutrient may enhance the risk of cancer. In addition, conditions such as obesity aid in tumor promotion. In this section we will examine carcinogenic contaminants, nutritional deficiencies, and obesity, as dietary cancer-causative factors.

Carcinogenic contaminants

The carcinogenic effect of one particular food can be variable. Salmon, rich in omega-3 polyunsaturated fatty acids, and known to be an important component of a healthy diet, is one example. Salmon, being fatty carnivorous fish, accumulate pollutants and can pass genotoxic contaminants through the food chain to humans. A study of farmed and wild salmon from around the world found that in some geographical regions (e.g. Scotland), polychlorinated biphenols (PCBs) and other pesticides are present in quantities that suggested that eating farmed salmon more than once a month could increase cancer risk (Hites *et al.*, 2004). Risk was calculated based on the assumption that the risks of individual carcinogens are additive. This study raises many issues. First, it underscores that differences in the source of food can have varying consequences; farmed salmon has more contaminants than wild salmon and farmed salmon from Scotland contains significantly more contaminants than farmed salmon available in North American cities. Perhaps the results have a broader implication and point to the suggestion that the source of all food should be properly labeled to allow for consumer choice and to create competition for the production of good products. Data from this study suggested that fish feed (fish meal and fish oils) may be a distinguishing factor for the carcinogenicity of salmon, suggesting that improvements in feed composition are needed. Evaluating cancer risk associated with more than one contaminant at a time, in addition to the benefits of other microconstituents of a particular food, is an area that requires further study. Overall, the study described above underlines the complications that occur when analyzing the relationship between diet and cancer.

Food preparation can contribute to the cancer-causing properties of our diet. Heterocyclic amines produced by cooking meat at high temperatures were discussed as carcinogens in Chapter 2. After metabolic activation, their mechanism of action involves the formation of DNA adducts, resulting in base substitutions and thus mutations. Similarly, toxins produced by molds that contaminate food form DNA adducts and thus are genotoxic. **Aflatoxin** B, a fungal product of *Aspergillus flavus*, is a well-known contaminant found on peanuts, and fumonisin B is found on corn. Aflatoxin induces GC→TA transversions and is thought to be involved in hepatocellular carcinoma. Food preservatives, such as sodium

PAUSE AND THINK

Suggest an experiment to examine whether the nutritional benefit of a particular food outweighs its risk as a carcinogen.

nitrite, are regulated by government agencies because they, too, are a risk factor producing carcinogenic N-nitroso compounds.

Dietary deficiencies

Evidence is accumulating that supports the concept that micronutrient deficiencies also contribute to cancer risk. The most compelling findings suggest that a deficiency in folate increases the risk of colorectal cancer. Folate, one of the B vitamins, can accept or donate one-carbon units in metabolic reactions. Folate is a critical co-enzyme for nucleotide synthesis and DNA methylation, and these processes can affect carcinogenesis. The enzyme methylenetetrahydrofolate reductase (MTHFR) regulates the balance between nucleotide synthesis and DNA methylation by affecting the relative quantities of 5,10-methylenetetrahydrofolate (5,10-methylene THF) and methyl-tetrahydrofolate (5-methyl THF), the respective precursors of these distinct processes (Figure 11.2a). MTHFR irreversibly converts 5,10-methylene THF to 5-methyl THF. 5,10-Methylene THF and deoxyuridylate (dUMP) are reactants for the enzyme thymidylate synthase used for the production of deoxythymidylate (dTMP). 5-Methyl THF and homocysteine are reactants used to produce methionine, which regenerates S-adenosylmethionine (SAM), the methyl donor for DNA methylation.

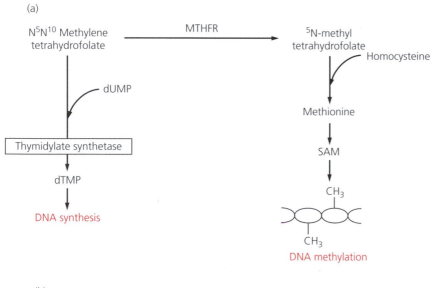

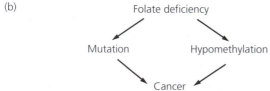

Figure 11.2 (a) Role of folate derivatives in DNA synthesis and DNA methylation. (b) Role of folate deficiency in cancer.

The depletion of folate may contribute to tumor development by interfering with both nucleotide synthesis and DNA methylation. A disruption in DNA synthesis leads to DNA instability and fuels mutation, while disruption in DNA methylation may cause genomic hypomethylation (Figure 11.2b). Deoxythymidylate synthesis is inhibited in conditions of low folate and the imbalance of the nucleotides results in the incorporation of uracil into DNA. DNA strand breaks occur as a result of attempts to repair this DNA and these breaks increase cancer risk. Both uracil misincorporation and DNA strand breaks are observed in folate-deficient humans, and both defects are reversed by folate administration. Remember that genomic hypomethylation and specific tumor suppressor gene promoter hypermethylation is characteristic of the epigenetic changes observed in cancer cells (Chapter 3). Since the methyl groups used for DNA methylation are supplied by folate, a lack of folate causes a decrease in the synthesis of methionine, and subsequently genomic hypomethylation of DNA. Genomic hypomethylation is observed in folate-deficient humans and is reversed upon folate repletion. Hypermethylation at specific 5′ gene loci have also been observed during studies of folate depletion.

Obesity

Obesity, classified as a risk factor for several cancers by the International Agency for Research on Cancer (IARC), is the excessive accumulation of fat that leads to a body weight that is greater than skeletal and physical requirements. Those with a body mass index [weight (in kg)/height (in m) squared] greater than 30 (kg/m^2) are considered obese. It has become a significant problem in the USA, affecting 25% of the population, and it has been suggested that 15–20% of all cancer deaths in the USA can be attributed to being overweight and obese. Based on epidemiological evidence, obesity increases the risk of cancer of the colon, breast, endometrium, kidney, and esophagus. Adipose tissue is an endocrine organ that can affect other tissues: it can release free fatty acids, peptide hormones, and steroid hormones. Several mechanisms of action of obesity as a cancer risk factor have been suggested. Indirectly, obesity is associated with acid reflux, which damages the esophageal epithelium and leads to adenocarcinoma of the esophagus. Secondly, obesity results in high fat deposits in adipose cells. The deposits may be used for the synthesis of estrogen from androgen by aromatase and may contribute to the risk of breast cancer (see below). Thirdly, food metabolism is linked with oxidation and an increase in ROS production can cause an increase in mutations. Lastly, obesity leads to chronically increased levels of plasma insulin due to the release of large amounts of free fatty acids from adipose tissue. Subsequent tumorigenic effects (e.g. promotion of cellular proliferation and inhibition of apoptosis) are mediated through insulin receptors and additional growth factors (e.g. insulin-like growth factor).

11.2 Preventative factors: microconstituents of fruits and vegetables

The intake of fruits and vegetables as a means of reducing cancer risk is strongly supported by epidemiological studies. Ongoing studies, such as the European Prospective Investigation into Cancer and Nutrition (EPIC), include the collection of blood samples for analysis and this will provide a valuable source of chemical and molecular data for future studies. The ability to block DNA damage caused by ROS and/or carcinogens is the most direct strategy for preventing the initiation of cancer and for slowing down the progression of disease. It is here that microconstituents found in fruits and vegetables play an important role. This is accomplished either directly by free radical scavengers (below) or indirectly by regulating the expression of Phase I (oxidative) and Phase II (conjugative) metabolizing enzymes in the body.

HOW DO WE KNOW THAT?

Analysis of DNA damage by the Comet assay (see Bub *et al.*, 2003)

The molecular effects of fruit polyphenols in humans were investigated by analyzing DNA damage in blood samples taken before, during, and after treatment. A precise schedule of fruit juice consumption (330 ml/day; over two, 2-week periods) in healthy men was executed. Two juices were tested; both contained apple, mango, and orange juice but one was enhanced with berries rich in anthocyanin and the other with green tea, apricot, and lime rich in flavanols. The single-cell microgel electrophoresis, or Comet, assay was used to detect oxidized DNA bases. Blood cells were embedded onto agarose-coated slides, lysed, treated with alkali (for unwinding) and a specific endonuclease (III) to detect oxidized pyrimidine bases and subjected to electrophoresis. Comet-like images indicating single-strand breaks and resulting from the extension of DNA into the agarose were computer-analyzed after neutralization and ethidium bromide staining. The data showed significantly lower levels of DNA base oxidation for both juices over the last treatment period (see Figure 1 in Bub *et al.*, 2003). That is, the effect was observed after the second 2-week period of consumption but not the first. The effect was not permanent since levels returned to baseline when tested 11 weeks after the experiment was terminated. The time delay indicated by this experiment suggests that ROS scavenging is not the prime mechanism and that protective detoxifying enzymes (described below) are induced.

The modulation of Phase I and Phase II metabolizing enzymes is a major defense mechanism against **xenobiotics** (foreign substances). The cytochrome P450 family of Phase I drug-metabolizing enzymes catalyzes the hydroxylation/oxidation of many drugs which often has a harmful effect by converting pro-carcinogenic molecules into ultimate carcinogens. Phase I products are often highly electrophilic (e.g. epoxides) and can

PAUSE AND THINK

In general, how would you modify Phase I and II enzyme activity to reduce tumor formation? Inhibit Phase I and induce Phase II.

damage DNA but at the same time induce enzymes required for Phase II. Phase II enzymes, such as UDP-glucuronosyltransferases or glutathione *S*-transferases, catalyze conjugation of Phase I products to hydrophilic moieties, thus making them more water soluble and aiding in their innocuous removal from the cell.

Figure 11.3 illustrates the modifications of the carcinogen aflatoxin B1 (AFB1) made by the Phase I and II metabolizing enzymes. First, aflatoxin

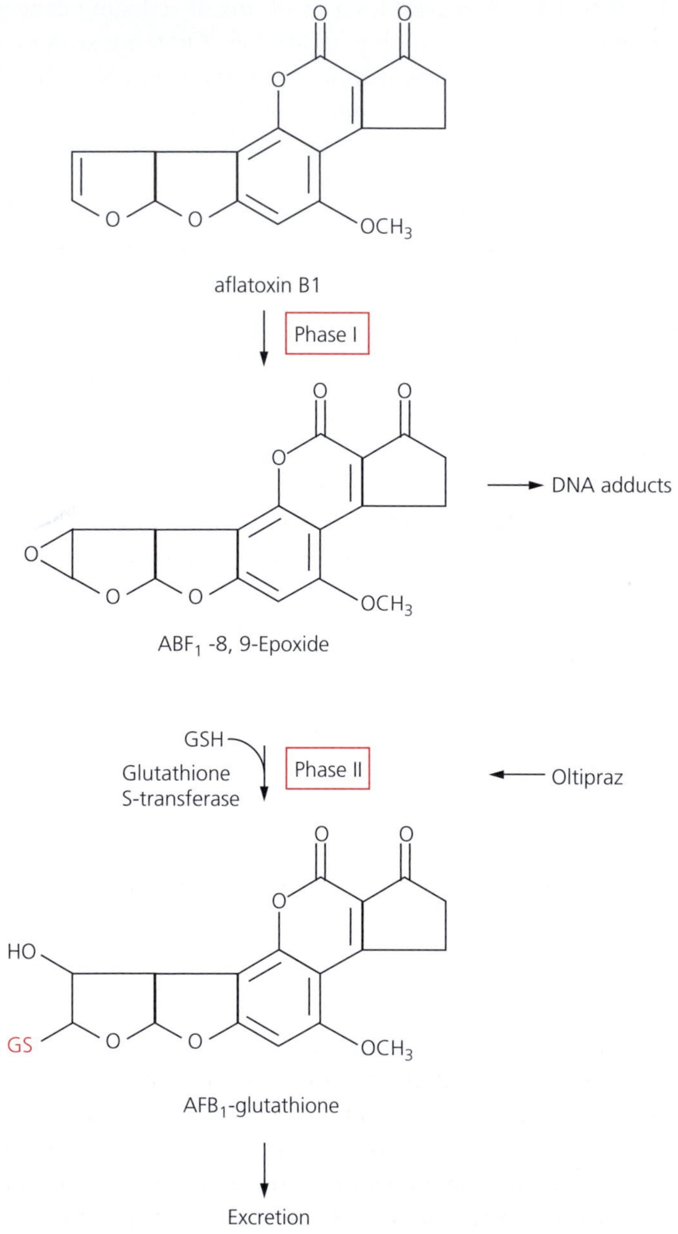

Figure 11.3 Effects of Phase I and II enzymes on aflatoxin B1. GS, glutathione. Oltipraz is a synthetic agent that can induce Phase II enzymes and is discussed in Therapeutic strategies below.

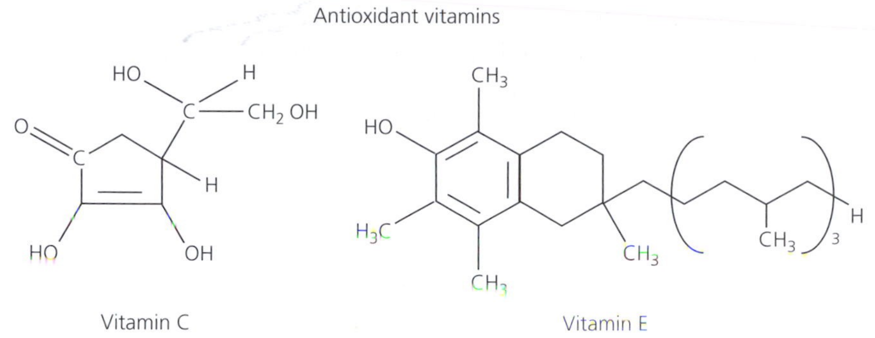

Figure 11.4 The structure of the antioxidant vitamins, vitamin C and vitamin E.

B1undergoes oxidation by Phase I cytochrome P450 to form the potent genotoxic metabolite AFB_1-8,9-epoxide. AFB_1-8,9-epoxide is conjugated to glutathione by the Phase II enzyme, glutathione *S*-transferase to produce AFB1-glutathione. This leads to detoxification and facilitates easy excretion.

Free radical scavenging

Several microconstituents in fruits and vegetables act as antioxidants that scavenge ROS. Water-soluble vitamin C (see Figure 11.4a) can donate an electron to a free radical directly, thus inhibiting its reactivity and blocking free radical chain reactions. Oxidized vitamin C forms an ascorbyl radical that is fairly stable and unreactive due to electron delocalization or resonance. An enzyme called vitamin C reductase can regenerate vitamin C from the ascorbyl radical for reuse, or the ascorbyl radical may lose another electron and become degraded. Consequently, vitamin C reserves need to replenished daily. Lipid-soluble vitamin E (Figure 11.4b) acts as a free radical scavenger in a similar manner. A resonance-stabilized structure called the α-tocopheryl radical is produced after vitamin E donates an electron to a free radical (e.g. singlet oxygen) and helps to terminate chain reactions of free radical in membranes.

Regulation of genes that code for drug-metabolizing and antioxidant enzymes

'You are what you eat' is a common expression. It has been given greater significance recently by its translation into molecular terms: some dietary constituents can affect the expression of our genes. The molecular mechanisms employed are common to those discussed in previous chapters. For example, epigallocatechin-3-gallate (EGCG), the major polyphenol found in green tea, activates MAPK signal transduction pathways (Figure 11.5a). As with the induction of this pathway by growth factors (Chapter 4), intracellular kinases modulate the activity of transcription

PAUSE AND THINK

Is the hydroxyl radical described in Chapter 2 likely to be scavenged by these microconstituents? No, in fact the menacing reactive hydroxyl radical is unlikely to be scavenged by these microconstituents because of its extremely rapid reaction time. It would take exceptionally high concentrations to prevent such interactions with molecules immediately surrounding it.

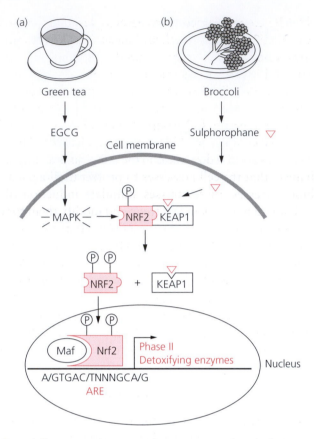

Figure 11.5 Several dietary constituents regulate gene expression via the transcription factor NRF2. (a) Green tea contains the microconstituent EGCG. EGCG can activate MAPKs. Serine/threonine phosphorylation of NRF2 by MAPK is thought to disrupt the cytoplasmic NRF2–KEAP1 complex allowing NRF2 to translocate into the nucleus. NRF2 forms a heterodimer with co-activator MAF, binds to the ARE, and stimulates the transcription of detoxifying enzymes. (b) Broccoli is a rich source of sulforophane. Sulforophane binds directly with KEAP1 causing a conformational change, and results in the release of NRF2. As in (a) above, NRF2 can then translocate into the nucleus, heterodimerize with MAF, and stimulate transcription of detoxifying enzymes.

factors by phosphorylation and the end result is the regulation of gene expression. The crucial link between nutrients and their role in preventing DNA damage was made by the identification of an antioxidant response element (ARE) (5′-A/G TGA C/T NNNGC A/G-3′) in the promoter region of the genes for several drug metabolizing and antioxidant enzymes (e.g. glutathione *S*-transferase). The ARE conferred antioxidant-dependent regulation of target genes. That is, genes containing an ARE in their promoter regions are transcriptionally activated in response to antioxidants. The transcription factor NRF2 and co-activator Maf, members of the basic leucine zipper family, bind the ARE and mediate the effects of the EGCG–MAPK signal transduction pathway. MAPK phosphorylates NRF2 and this causes NRF2 to be released from its cytoplasmic repressor, KEAP1. Upon release, NRF2 enters the nucleus, binds to its co-activator Maf, and stimulates transcription of its target genes through the ARE.

In addition, other microconstituents such as sulforophane found in broccoli also activate NRF2-regulated transcription (Figure 11.5b; see also Surh, 2003). Sulforophane (a hydrolysis product of sulfur-containing glucosinolates) contain sulfydryl groups that are able to react with cysteine residues within the cytoplasmic NRF2 repressor, KEAP1. These cysteines normally act as sensors of redox status in the cell. This is an important molecular mechanism that the cell possesses to protect itself against oxidative and xenobiotic stresses: these stresses stimulate induction of enzymes, via Keap 1, that will make them less toxic and modify them for excretion. Dietary antioxidants mimic carcinogenic ROS or electrophiles that activate stress-response genes via the NRF2–KEAP1 complex. The direct interaction of sulforophane with the cysteine residues of KEAP1 causes a conformational change in KEAP1 that releases NRF2. NRF2 is then able to translocate into the nucleus and, as a heterodimer with Maf, stimulates Phase II detoxifying enzymes. Therefore, some dietary microconstituents can aid in protecting the cell from DNA damage caused by oxidants by regulating the expression of genes that code for detoxifying enzymes.

Additional mechanisms of dietary microconstituents

Current evidence suggests several mechanisms for the cancer-preventative role of fruits and vegetables. As we have seen above, one mechanism is the ability to decrease oxidative DNA damage by free radical scavenging or inducing protective enzymes. Two other mechanisms for the role of particular vegetables in cancer prevention are modulation of apoptosis and/or cell proliferation. The microconstituents of garlic utilize all three mechanisms. The antioxidant properties of organosulfur compounds in garlic include the induction of Phase II enzymes and scavenging. Ajoene, a major compound in garlic, has been shown to induce apoptosis of leukemic cells in patients with leukemia. Particular caspases (3 and 8) and transcriptional regulators (IκB) are activated and peroxide is produced. Allicin, another major compound in garlic, has been shown to inhibit the proliferation of human mammary, endometrial, and colon cancer cells. It is suggested that some of these effects are mediated via inhibition of the NFκB signaling pathway (Chapter 10).

Another protective mechanism of dietary microconstituents that has been suggested is regulation of telomerase activity. Upon ingestion, EGCG undergoes rapid degradation and by an unknown mechanism blocks telomerase activity (Naasani et al., 2003). The inhibition of telomerase limits the replicative capacity of cells (see Chapter 3) and in this study correlates with a decrease in tumor size in mouse models.

LIFESTYLE TIP

We should use the knowledge that we have gained about the preventative role of particular foods and beverages to make better choices about what we ingest. Green tea is the second most popular beverage in the world, after water. A high intake of green tea is associated with a low incidence of several cancers (e.g. gastric and colorectal cancer). Green tea is a better choice than soda.

Although fiber is usually included in discussions of preventative agents of cancer, I have chosen to omit this topic here due to the inconsistencies of recent large studies (see references within Key *et al.*, 2002). On the other hand, the first key publication of EPIC shows a strong protective effect of dietary fiber against colorectal cancer (Bingham *et al.*, 2003). The data suggest that preventative effects were not seen in some previous studies because the range of fiber intake was much lower than those in the EPIC study (see Activity 2 at the end of this chapter).

In conclusion, a brief examination of several different foods demonstrates that the molecular mechanisms by which nutrients affect carcinogenesis are beginning to be revealed.

11.3 Metabolic changes in tumor cells

The digestion of food provides many of the compounds required for metabolism, the sum of the biochemical reactions in the body. Thus diet (and exercise) affect cellular metabolism. Some tumors cells seem to be addicted to increased glucose uptake and glycolysis. The observation that cancer cells carry out aerobic glycolysis, converting glucose to lactate in the presence of oxygen, was made in the 1920s and is called the **Warburg effect**. This metabolic alteration is thought to differ from both anaerobic (without oxygen) glycolysis and aerobic metabolism that proceeds through the Krebs cycle and electron-transport chain (see box 'A quick review about glucose metabolism'). This area of study has recently been revived, and differing viewpoints have not yet settled. Some suggest that 60–90% of tumors shift to glycolysis, others propose that the shift is time-dependent, and others suggest it may be cell-type-dependent (stem cells versus differentiated cells). Regardless of these different views, it is of interest that the Warburg effect is the basis for an important imaging technique used to detect tumors in the clinic. Positron emission tomography (PET) scans work on the basis that tumor cells exhibit a greater uptake of glucose than most normal cells. A glucose analog, [18F]fluoro-2-deoxyglucose (FDG), is injected into the bloodstream and is converted by the glycolytic enzyme hexokinase to FDG-phosphate, which can be visualized.

Data suggest that both genetic alterations (oncogenes and tumor suppressor genes) and a response to hypoxia via HIF-1α contribute to the altered metabolism observed in cancer cells. Let's examine evidence for both mechanisms.

Understanding of the pathway of a key metabolic enzyme, AMP-activated protein kinase (AMPK), is uncovering links between energy metabolism and cancer. AMPK senses the energy state of a cell and is activated under conditions of increased AMP and decreased ATP in

PAUSE AND THINK

You may remember from Chapter 9 that hypoxia-inducible factor (HIF), is composed of two subunits; the α-subunit is regulated at the protein level via regulated degradation and the β-subunit is constitutive.

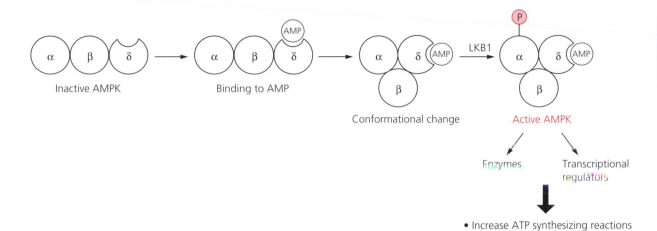

Inactive AMPK   Binding to AMP   Conformational change   Active AMPK

Enzymes   Transcriptional regulators

- Increase ATP synthesizing reactions
- Decrease ATP consuming processes

response to starvation, hypoxia, and exercise. It is composed of an α catalytic subunit and β and γ regulatory subunits. In the current model of AMPK activation (Figure 11.6), AMP binds to the γ subunit of AMPK and causes a conformational change exposing a potential phosphorylation site within the α subunit of AMPK. The serine/threonine kinase LKB1 phosphorylates (Thr172) and activates AMPK. AMPK exerts its effects through the regulation of target enzymes and transcription factors. In general, ATP-generating pathways are stimulated (e.g. fatty acid oxidation, glycolysis) and ATP-consuming pathways are inhibited (e.g. fatty acid synthesis). A link between AMPK and cancer comes from the finding that LKB1 and a downstream effector called TSC2 are tumor suppressor genes (Figure 11.7). Both have been identified as germline mutations in syndromes that predispose patients to cancer (Peutz–Jeghers syndrome and tuberous sclerosis, respectively). Although more studies are required, inhibition of growth has been reported for tumor cells in culture upon activation of AMPK. In addition, AMPK activates the 'star' tumor suppressor, p53. In this capacity, p53 acts as a metabolic checkpoint and induces cell cycle arrest in response to low cellular energy. Two new target genes of tumor suppressor p53 include an inhibitor of glycolysis and a stimulator of oxidative phosphorylation (Matoba *et al.*, 2006). Thus the mutations that drive cancer also regulate an altered metabolism. (Note: In contrast to the effect of p53 in inhibiting of glycolysis, one report suggests that AMPK stimulates glycolysis in some cell types, and thus the role of AMPK in the regulation of glycolysis is requires further study.)

Both hypoxia and oncogenic mutations in the absence of hypoxia can activate HIF-1α (Figure 11.7). The inactivation of the tumor suppressor VHL stabilizes HIF-1α in the presence of oxygen. Also, HIF-1α is increased in cells transformed with oncogenes such as Src and Ras. In addition

Figure 11.6 Activation of AMP-activated protein kinase, AMPK. When the energy of a cell decreases, AMP increases. AMP binds to inactive AMPK and causes a conformational change that allows phosphorylation of the α catalytic subunit by LKB1. The activating phosphate is shown in red.

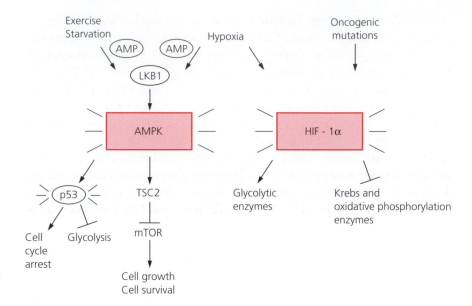

Figure 11.7 Pathways of metabolic regulators AMPK and HIF-1α (shown in red).

to regulating VEGF transcription, HIF-1α upregulates the expression of nearly all of the core enzymes of glycolysis and inhibits the expression of some enzymes involved in the Krebs cycle and oxidative phosphorylation. Thus, the increased glycolysis observed in some tumors is regulated by a specific transcriptional program, rather than only a lack of oxygen.

Further investigations regarding the mechanism of this long-observed phenomenon are needed and may have additional therapeutic implications.

A quick review about glucose metabolism

In normal cells, the glycolysis pathway involves the breakdown of glucose in the absence of oxygen (anaerobic metabolism) and the production of pyruvate. Pyruvate is converted into lactate by the enzyme lactate dehydrogenase. In the presence of oxygen, pyruvate from glycolysis is shuttled through the Krebs cycle, and NADH and FADH$_2$ are generated. These electron carriers shuttle their electrons through the electron transport chain located in the inner mitochondrial membrane. Oxygen is the terminal electron acceptor. The resulting proton motor force generates ATP.

11.4 Genetic polymorphisms and diet

It seems that some people can do all the 'wrong things' such as drink excessive amounts of alcohol and smoke heavily and still live long healthy lives. We often hear that this is due to an individual's metabolism. Cancer risk associated with diet is influenced by an individual's metabolism. Metabolic reactions are catalyzed by enzymes. Enzyme activities may vary among individuals due to small variations, often single nucleotide changes, in the genes that code for them. These genetic polymorphisms may alter the response to a particular dietary constituent. Here are two examples. A polymorphism (C→T transition at nucleotide 677) in the *MTHFR* gene reduces its enzyme activity and homozygotes for this polymorphism have a 50% decreased risk of colorectal cancer compared with those with wild-type alleles (Ueland *et al.*, 2001). These individuals have an increased availability of 5,10-methylene THF and a lower chance of disrupting nucleotide and subsequently DNA synthesis; these conditions deter mutation and carcinogenesis (see Figure 11.2). However, the polymorphism increases the risk of cancer if these individuals become deficient in folate. Under these conditions, methyl-THF becomes depleted and DNA methylation is altered in a manner that is characteristic of carcinogenesis.

Polymorphisms in the gene that codes for *N*-acetyltransferase modify the risk of specific cancers in response to the consumption of red meat. This enzyme is involved in the metabolic activation of carcinogenic heterocyclic amines produced by cooking meat at high temperatures. Individuals with the 'rapid variant' of the enzyme (a fast acetylator) who consume large amounts of red meat have an increased risk of colon cancer compared with those who have this variant and do not consume much red meat, or those who possess the 'slow variant' polymorphism who do. Therefore, the response to red meat intake with respect to an increased risk of cancer depends on a person's genotype in combination with exposure to carcinogens that result from cooking.

Inherited metabolic diseases can illustrate a more obvious role of metabolism in carcinogenesis. Here are two examples resulting from blocks in tyrosine metabolism pathways. Albinos have an inherited deficiency of the enzyme tyrosinase and are unable to produce melanin, causing the characteristic lack of pigment in their skin. The lack of pigment causes albinos to be more sensitive to the sun and results in an increased risk of skin carcinoma. Tyrosinemia type I, another disorder of tyrosine metabolism, results from a deficiency of fumarylacetoacetate hydrolase. As a result of this metabolic block, the metabolites fumarylacetoacetate and maleylacetate accumulate. Both are alkylating agents and cause DNA mutations and tumorigenesis. In brief, tyrosinemia type I is characterized by the synthesis and accumulation of carcinogens.

11.5 Vitamin D: a link between nutrients and hormone action

A precursor, or pre-vitamin, to biologically active vitamin D can be obtained through the diet (fortified dairy products and seafood) or produced in the skin from 7-dehydrocholesterol upon exposure to sunlight. The pre-vitamin, regardless of its source (skin or diet), must be metabolized first in the liver to form 25-hydroxyvitamin D (biologically inert) and then in the kidney to form the biologically active form, 1,25-dihydroxyvitamin D. Synthesis of the pre-vitamin in the skin upon UV exposure accounts for 90–95% of an individual's requirement for vitamin D; very few foods (except oily fish) naturally contain vitamin D. This is one reason why some countries fortify milk and other foods.

Epidemiological evidence has demonstrated that there is an increased risk of several cancers (particularly prostate, colon, and breast; note that prostate, colon, and breast cells contain the enzyme needed to produce 1,25-dihydroxyvitamin D) in people living at higher latitudes (van der Rhee *et al.*, 2006; see also Holick, 2006). It has been proposed that vitamin D deficiency underlies this effect, although additional effects of sun exposure may also play a role. One study evaluated the growth of colon cancer cells in **xenografts** (human cells implanted in the backs of the immunodeficient mice) in vitamin D-deficient versus vitamin D-sufficient mice (Tangpricha *et al.*, 2005). Tumors were 80% larger on average in mice that were deficient in vitamin D compared with vitamin D-sufficient mice. Collectively, epidemiological and *in vivo* evidence establish a link between vitamin D deficiency and increased cancer risk.

> **LIFESTYLE TIP**
>
> Vitamin D deficiency is now a worldwide problem. Most experts recommend 1000 IU of vitamin D is needed daily in the absence of sun exposure to maintain healthy blood levels of the pre-vitamin. Exposure to a 'sensible' amount of sunlight (depending on skin type) is also encouraged.

A little lesson about the history of vitamin D fortification of milk

Rickets, a debilitating bone-deforming disease, affected more than 80% of children living in industrialized cities in the northeastern United States and northern Europe at the beginning of the 20th century. Vitamin D fortification was introduced to try to reduce the incidence of rickets. In the United States, milk, orange juice, and some cereals are fortified with vitamin D. In Europe, fortification of foods was carried out until the late 1940s. Over-fortification of milk caused an outbreak of vitamin D intoxication in Great Britain and led to regulations that ablated vitamin D fortification throughout Europe. These remain active today. Over-fortification most likely resulted from human error or inaccurate food analysis. Since food analysis has become more reliable over the last 50 years, should vitamin D fortification be reconsidered in northern Europe and elsewhere?

The link between nutrients and molecular signaling became apparent upon the discovery that the receptors for vitamin A and D are members of the steroid hormone receptor superfamily.

Let us examine the molecular mechanisms of vitamin D action. The active form of vitamin D, 1,25-hydroxyvitamin D, acts as a ligand for the cytoplasmic vitamin D receptor, a member of the steroid hormone receptor superfamily. This receptor recognizes the vitamin D response element in gene promoter regions and regulates transcription of its target genes.

> **PAUSE AND THINK**
>
> How do steroid hormone receptors function? Remember from Chapter 3 that they are ligand-dependent transcription factors.

Current data suggest that vitamin D is a chemopreventative agent that inhibits growth and induces differentiation and apoptosis through several molecular targets. Here are a few examples: vitamin D can act as a dominant negative ligand for EGFR (epidermal growth factor receptor, Chapter 4). That is, vitamin D can bind to the ligand-binding domain of EGFR instead of EGF and prevent the binding of EGF to EGFR. As a result, vitamin D can inhibit growth. Secondly, upon binding to the vitamin D receptor, the active form of vitamin D can directly activate specific tumor suppressor genes such as *BRCA1* and *p21* through a vitamin D response element in their promoter regions. You may recall that the p21 protein is an inhibitor of cyclin-dependent kinase and that it can induce cell cycle arrest. Vitamin D promotes apoptosis through mitochondrial signaling independent of caspase activation. It induces the redistribution of two pro-apoptotic proteins BAK and BAX from the cytosol to the mitochondria. These two proteins form channels in the mitochondrial membrane and facilitate the release of cytochrome *c* and apoptosome assembly (see Chapter 7). Simultaneously, Bcl-2 and IAPs, inhibitors of apoptosis, are downregulated.

11.6 Hormones and cancer

There is group of cancers linked by a common mechanism of carcino-genesis that involves endogenous hormones as initiators rather than chemicals, viruses, or radiation. The hormone-related cancers include breast, endometrium, ovary, prostate, testis, and thyroid cancer. We will examine breast cancer as a paradigm for hormonal carcinogenesis. (Note: Links between hormones and some other hormone-related cancers are not as straightforward.)

Breast cancer is the most common type of cancer in women. **Estrogens** ◎ (estradiol and estrone) appear to play a central role in the initiation and progression of breast cancer. The principal site of estrogen synthesis in the body changes with increased age: the ovaries are the main source in pre-menopausal women and adipose tissue (fat) is the main source in post-menopausal women. Life events, such as pregnancy, affect the exposure time to estrogens and those events that prolong exposure are considered risk factors for breast cancer (Figure 11.8). Early menarche (the start of the menstrual cycle) and late menopause indicate an extended length of time when the ovaries are producing estrogen. Obesity in post-menopausal women is a risk factor because adipose cells are the primary source of estrogen at this stage in life. Obese women have an increased number of fat cells and therefore produce increased amounts of estrogen. Adipose cells use the enzyme aromatase to produce estrogen from androgens. Thus,

Breast cancer risk factors

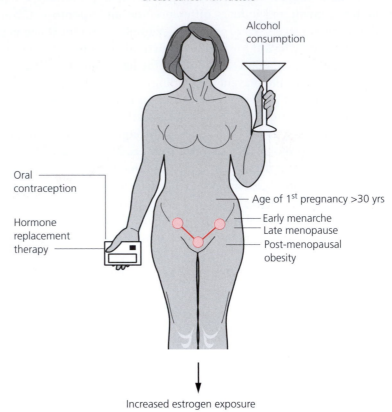

Figure 11.8 Risk factors for breast cancer.

obesity increases the risk of breast cancer through increased estrogen production. It is thought that alcohol consumption increases the risk of breast cancer through a similar mechanism of increased estrogen production. Some data suggest that one alcoholic drink per day causes a 7% increase in the risk of breast cancer. The use of exogenous hormones in oral contraceptives and in hormone replacement therapy has also been linked to increased risk of breast cancer. Conversely, factors that interrupt the menstrual cycle, such as pregnancy, lactation, and physical activity, are considered protective factors. Although a rare event, breast cancer can occur in men. Men also produce some amounts of estrogen and those with high levels appear to be more at risk.

Two predominant models for the mechanisms by which estrogens exert their effects have been proposed (Figure 11.9). It is likely that both mechanisms contribute to breast cancer.

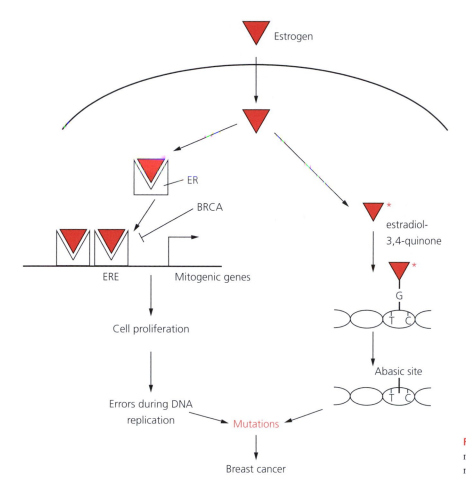

Figure 11.9 Carcinogenic mechanisms of estrogens: mitogenic and/or genotoxic.

One model is that estrogens promote cell proliferation of the breast and the high division rate allows less time for DNA repair, thus creating an opportunity for errors to occur during DNA replication. The increase in error rate translates into an increase in somatic mutations that lead to carcinogenesis. This model contrasts chemical- and radiation-induced carcinogenesis, since no specific initiator other than errors in replication is required. Estrogen does indeed act as a mitogen for cells in the breast that contain estrogen receptors. During pregnancy, estrogen levels increase and cause the mammary ducts to grow and the breasts to nearly double in size. Effects of estrogen are mediated through estrogen receptors (ERs), ◎ estrogen receptor-α and estrogen receptor-β, members of the steroid hormone receptor superfamily (see Chapter 3). The receptors bind as dimers to the estrogen response element (ERE) and regulate estrogen-responsive genes. In addition to this genomic pathway, non-genomic signaling pathways outside the nucleus have also been documented (Revankar *et al.*, 2005). The expression of the estrogen receptor isoforms changes during carcinogenesis of the breast. Estrogen receptor-α is significantly upregulated and estrogen receptor-β is downregulated in the majority of breast cancers. The reasons for these alterations are unknown at present. However, as we shall see below, blocking ER function has proved to be a successful strategy for the treatment of breast cancer.

The involvement of estrogen signaling in increasing susceptibility to breast cancer is supported by studies of the breast cancer susceptibility genes (*BRCAs*). About 5–10% of all cases of breast cancer are due to an inherited predisposition, 85% of which result from germline mutations in either the *BRCA1* or *BRCA2* gene. The *BRCA* gene products are nuclear tumor suppressor proteins that play a role in transcriptional regulation, DNA repair, and regulation of the cell cycle. BRCA1 inhibits the transcriptional activation activity of estrogen receptors and this suggests that it suppresses the proliferating effects of estrogen signaling. It has been suggested that the lost of modulation of estrogen signaling contributes to the increased risk to breast cancer in patients with an inherited mutation of *BRCA1*.

Another model suggests that estrogen and its metabolites are genotoxic. This model is consistent with the mechanism by which chemicals, viruses, and radiation initiate carcinogenesis. Estradiol is metabolized to form estradiol-3,4-quinone in cells. This metabolite covalently binds to adenine or guanine bases. The resulting adducts destabilize the bonds linking the base to the DNA backbone and result in an abasic site and, ultimately, mutations. (Note: Since adenine and guanine are purines, abasic sites that involve the loss of adenine or guanine are referred to as apurinic sites.) Estradiol quinones are present in human breast tissue. Estrogen receptor knock-out mice were used as an animal model to test the effect of estrogen in the absence of estrogen receptors. Results demonstrated that genotoxic effects occurred in the absence of estrogen receptors (Yue *et al.*, 2003). Data obtained from human breast epithelial cells *in vitro* indicated that metabolites of estrogen induce transformation *in vitro* and also induce loss of heterozygosity at chromosomal regions that have been reported to be affected in primary breast tumors (Russo *et al.*, 2003). These genotypic changes were not blocked by inhibitors of the estrogen receptor, showing that this effect was not receptor-mediated. Together, these results support the concept that estrogen metabolites contribute to breast carcinogenesis.

For this second model, predispositions to breast cancer may involve germline mutations in genes involved in estrogen biosynthesis and metabolism. Loss of the BRCA tumor suppressor proteins may leave breast cells more susceptible to the genotoxic effects of estrogen metabolites due to the normal role of BRCA tumor suppressor proteins in DNA repair.

⊚ **Therapeutic strategies**

11.7 'Enhanced' foods and dietary supplements for chemoprevention

Chemoprevention is the use of naturally occurring or synthetic agents to prevent, inhibit, or reverse the process of carcinogenesis in pre-malignant cells. Foods are not yet considered as preventative agents against cancer. However, as we learn more about the important role of nutrients in cancer and as our skills for manipulating food composition increase, this concept is set to change. The development of enhanced food products (foods that have altered levels of particular microconstituents), derived in some cases from genetically modified crops, will begin to flood the market. Foods have already been produced to have increased levels of antioxidants and may be used in future chemopreventative diets. Tomatoes have been classically bred to be bright red for consumer appeal and as a result contain more lycopene. Tomatoes have also been engineered to contain increased levels of zeaxanthin by over-expressing enzymes utilized in its synthesis. Recently, broccoli, containing high levels of glucosinolates (which are hydrolyzed to isothiocyanates including sulforophane; discussed in Section 11.2), has been developed by a traditional plant-breeding program and licensed to Seminis Inc., the world's largest developer and grower of vegetable and fruit seeds. A balance of potential advantage from enhanced foods must be tempered by the likelihood that we may have adverse reactions to food constituents at abnormally high concentrations.

Although we discussed the disappointing results of β-carotene supplementation with respect to lung cancer, an interesting observation resulting from the ATBC trial prompted further study into the effects vitamin E supplementation on the risk of prostate cancer. A significantly decreased rate of prostate cancer was observed in patients taking vitamin E (11.7 versus 17.8%) in the ATBC trial. A similar observation was observed for selenium in a separate study. The Selenium and Vitamin E Cancer Prevention Trial (SELECT), a Phase III randomized placebo-controlled trial, has recruited over 35,000 male participants to test the effects of selenium and vitamin E supplements after a minimum of 7 years (see website references at the end of the chapter for details).

The synthetic agent Oltipraz holds promise as a chemopreventative agent. Similar to sulforophane, it induces Phase II enzymes via transcription factor NRF2 and brings about the detoxification of aflatoxin (Figure 11.2). The effects of Oltipraz as a chemopreventative agent were tested in Phase I and IIa trials in Qidong, China, an area where aflatoxin contributes to a high incidence of hepatocellular carcinoma. Results demonstrated an increase in aflatoxin detoxification products, suggesting that there was a change in the metabolic phenotype of patients due to the induction of Phase II enzymes. Although this agent provides evidence for proof of concept, food-based approaches (e.g. using broccoli sprout teas) may be better alternatives, and these are also being investigated.

As we learn more about the role of nutrients in cancer prevention, it is certain that the list of trials for testing the effects of diet and supplements as chemopreventative agents will expand.

11.8 Drugs that target energy pathways

Although a fairly new strategy, the potential of targeting energy pathways may be worth exploring (Gatenby and Gillies, 2007). Since some tumor cells exhibit increased aerobic glycolysis (the Warburg effect), one obvious approach is to target hexokinase, the enzyme that catalyzes the first and rate-limiting step in glycolysis. Pre-clinical experiments testing the effects of a hexokinase inhibitor, 3-bromopyruvate (3-BrPA), have demonstrated anti-tumor effects. Numerous approaches that inhibit HIF are being developed. The small-molecule inhibitor PX-478 is one example that is due to be tested in clinical trials. Metformin is widely used for the treatment of type 2 diabetes. It activates AMPK via LKB1. Results from a pilot study have suggested that cancer risk is reduced in type 2 diabetics taking metformin (Evans *et al.*, 2005). Additional studies are ongoing.

11.9 Drugs that target estrogen

There are two strategies for the design of drugs that target estrogen action (Figure 11.10). The first is to design drugs that antagonize the actions of estrogens by interacting with estrogen receptors in order to block growth in 'estrogen-positive' tumors. These compounds are called anti-estrogens. Tamoxifen, used in the clinic for over 30 years, is the most widely used anti-estrogen to treat estrogen-receptor-positive, post-menopausal breast cancer. Tamoxifen is a competitive inhibitor that alters the folding of the ligand-binding domain of the estrogen receptor and blocks its ability to transactivate and initiate transcription of its target genes. Recently, the principle of a potentially new strategy for interfering with estrogen receptor function has been tested. Several electrophilic agents have been shown to target the estrogen receptor zinc finger domain and selectively block the receptor's DNA-binding activity. Furthermore, the progression of breast

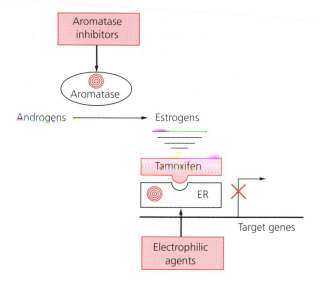

Figure 11.10 Drugs that target estrogen action (shown in red). Molecular targets are indicated by a (◉) symbol.

carcinoma was inhibited in mouse models by these drugs (Wang *et al.*, 2004). These drugs may act as lead compounds for the development of new breast cancer therapies.

The second strategy for blocking the function of estrogen in breast cancer is to design drugs that interfere with estrogen synthesis. These drugs target aromatase, the enzyme that converts androgens into estrogens. Targeting this enzyme does not interfere with the synthesis of other steroids but is rate-limiting for estrogen production. Aromatase is the main source of estrogen production in post-menopausal women because the ovaries no longer produce it. Aromatase inhibitors can be prescribed to reduce the level of estrogen in the body of post-menopausal breast cancer patients, making it appropriate for over 50% (estrogen-positive and post-menopausal) of all breast cancers. These drugs are not an option for pre-menopausal patients since aromatase is not the major estrogen producer (see Pause and Think).

Three aromatase inhibitors have gone through clinical trials and have been approved in the USA: exemestane, anastrozole, and letrozole (Brodie, 2002). The aromatase inhibitor anastrozole (Arimidex) has been used as both a first-line therapy and an adjuvant (treatment given after surgery to prevent recurrence). Results from a large-scale trial called the ATAC (Arimidex, Tamoxifen Alone or in Combination) adjuvant breast cancer trial has yielded encouraging results for the aromatase inhibitor, showing a 50% greater reduction of contralateral breast cancer at 3 years compared with tamoxifen. Further observation and evaluation for long-term side-effects including osteoporosis and bone fractures will be needed. The result from the ATAC trial is to be expected when considering the two proposed mechanisms of action of estrogen. Tamoxifen

PAUSE AND THINK

How would you design an aromatase inhibitor? One way is to model your compound after androstenedione, the endogenous substrate for the enzyme. These drugs should interact and inactivate the steroid-binding domain of aromatase.

blocks estrogen-receptor-mediated effects only. Aromatase inhibitors reduce total estrogen concentrations and therefore block both estrogen receptor mechanisms and non-receptor-mediated genotoxic events. Molecular knowledge advances drug design.

Tamoxifen has potent chemopreventative activity that may be greater than its therapeutic activity. Several studies have demonstrated that the incidence of invasive breast cancer is reduced by 49%. As a result, the US FDA has approved tamoxifen for breast cancer risk reduction. However, the perceived risk of taking tamoxifen for the recommended 5 years (increased risk for endometrial cancer and stroke) and its associated side-effects has not made it a popular option. The estrogen receptor modulator raloxifene has shown equivalent efficacy to tamoxifen and has fewer side-effects, and thus may become a better alternative. Future chemopreventative strategies need to consider the risk–benefit ratio and also improved means for the identification of high-risk individuals.

■ CHAPTER HIGHLIGHTS—REFRESH YOUR MEMORY

- Diet plays a role in both the causation and the prevention of cancer.

- In contrast to the association of a β-carotene-rich diet with reduced lung cancer incidence, β-carotene supplementation increases lung cancer in smokers.

- Diet contributes to carcinogenesis by the delivery of carcinogenic contaminants.

- Folate deficiency affects nucleotide synthesis and DNA methylation.

- Obesity and lack of specific nutrients are also causative factors in cancer.

- Nutrients may work as chemopreventative agents by blocking DNA damage via scavenging or the induction of metabolizing enzymes, inducing apoptosis, or inhibiting cell proliferation.

- The antioxidant response element (ARE) is found in the gene promoters of detoxifying and antioxidant enzymes.

- Some dietary constituents regulate gene expression of detoxifying enzymes via the transcription factor NRF2 and AREs.

- The major polyphenol of green tea, epigallocatechin gallate, inhibits telomerase.

- The Warburg effect describes the increase in aerobic glycolysis that occurs in some tumor cells.

- Genetic polymorphisms can interact with nutrient status and affect cancer risk.

- Vitamin D is a nutrient that acts through a member of the steroid hormone receptor family.

- Breast cancer is a paradigm for hormonal carcinogenesis.

- Estrogen acts as a mitogen for cells in the breast.

- Estrogen and its metabolites may damage DNA directly to initiate carcinogenesis.

- Dietary factors such as obesity and alcohol intake increase breast cancer risk by increasing estrogen production.

- Germline mutations in the *BRCA1* and *BRCA2* genes predispose patients to breast cancer.

- Enhanced food and dietary supplements are being investigated as chemopreventative agents.

- Tamoxifen is a breast cancer drug that acts as an 'anti-estrogen' and blocks estrogen binding to its receptor.

- Aromatase inhibitors, such as anastrozole, act by inhibiting the enzyme aromatase that converts androgens to estrogen.

■ ACTIVITY

1. Record what you ate and drank for dinner last night. Give a critical account of how the meal contributed either to reducing or enhancing your cancer risk. Bon appetit!

2. By reviewing the literature and using experimental evidence critically discuss the role of fiber as a cancer-preventative factor in our diet.

■ FURTHER READING

Aggarwal, B.B. and Shishodia, S. (2006) Molecular targets of dietary agents for prevention and therapy of cancer. *Biochem. Pharmacol.* **71**: 1397–1421.

Calle, E.E. and Kaaks, R. (2004) Overweight, obesity and cancer: epidemiological evidence and proposed mechanisms. *Nature Rev. Cancer* **4**: 579–589.

Choi, S.-W. and Mason, J.B. (2002) Folate status: effects on pathways of colorectal carcinogenesis. *J. Nutr.* **132**: 2413S–2418S.

Greenwald, P., Clifford, C.K., and Milner, J.A. (2001) Diet and cancer prevention. *Eur. J. Cancer* **37**: 948–965.

Henderson, B.E. and Feigelson, H.S. (2000) Hormonal carcinogenesis. *Carcinogenesis* **21**: 427–433.

Holick, M.F. (2006) Vitamin D: its role in cancer prevention and treatment. *Prog. Biophys. Mol. Biol.* **92**: 49–59.

Kensler, T.W., Egner, P.A., Wang, J.-B., Zhu, Y.-R., Zhang, B.-C., Lu, P-X., Chen, J.-G., Qian, G.-S., Kuang, S.-Y., Jackson, P.E., Gange, S.J., Jacobson, L.P., Munroz, A., and Groopman, J.D. (2004) Chemoprevention of hepatocellular carcinoma in aflatoxin endemic areas. *Gastroenterology* **127**: S310–S318.

Key, T.J., Allen, N.E., Spencer, E.A., and Travis, R.C. (2002) The effect of diet on risk of cancer. *Lancet* **360**: 861–868.

Kim, J., Gardner, L.B., and Dang, C.V. (2005) Oncogenic alterations of metabolism and the Warburg effect. *Drug Discov. Today: Dis. Mech.* **2**: 233–238.

Lamprecht, S.A. and Lipkin, M. (2003) Chemoprevention of colon cancer by calcium, vitamin D and folate: molecular mechanisms. *Nature Rev. Cancer* **3**: 601–614.

Mathers, J.C. (2003) Nutrition and cancer prevention: diet–gene interactions. *Proc. Nutr. Soc.* **62**: 605–610.

Motohashi, H. and Yamamoto, M. (2004) Nrf2-Keap1 defines a physiologically important stress response mechanism. *Trends Mol. Med.* **10**: 549–557.

Nicholls, H. (2002) Aromatase inhibitors continue their ATAC on tamoxifen. *Trends Mol. Med.* **8**: S12–S13.

Pool-Zobel, B., Veeriah, S., and Bohmer, F.-D. (2005) Modulation of xenobiotic metabolizing enzymes by anticarcinogens – focus on glutathione S-transferases and their role as targets of dietary chemoprevention in colorectal carcinogenesis. *Mut. Res.* **591**: 74–92.

Qi, R. and Wang, Z. (2003) Pharmacological effects of garlic extract. *Trends Pharmacol. Sci.* **24**: 62–63.

Shaw, R.J. (2006) Glucose metabolism and cancer. *Curr. Opin. Cell Biol.* **18**: 1–11.

Surh, Y.-J. (2003) Cancer chemoprevention with dietary phytochemicals. *Nature Rev. Cancer* **3**: 768–780.

Venkitaraman, A.R. (2002) Cancer susceptibility and the functions of BRCA1 and BRCA2. *Cell* **108**: 171–182.

Yager, J.D. and Davidson, N.E. (2006) Estrogen carcinogenesis in breast cancer. *New Engl. J. Med.* **354**: 270–282.

■ WEB SITES

World Cancer Research Fund http://www.wcrf.org/

Selenium and Vitamin E Cancer Prevention Trial (SELECT)
http://www.cancer.gov/clinicaltrials/digestpage/SELECT/allpages

■ SELECTED SPECIAL TOPICS

Bingham, S.A., Day, N.E., Luben, R., and Ferrari, P. (2003) Dietary fibre in food and protection against colorectal cancer in the European Prospective Investigation into Cancer and Nutrition (EPIC): an observational study. *Lancet* **361**: 1496–1501.

Brodie, A. (2002) Aromatase inhibitors in breast cancer. *Trends Endocrin. Metabol.* **13**: 61–65.

Bub, A., Watzl, B., Blockhaus, M., Briviba, K.L., Liegibel, U., Muller, H., Pool-Zobel, B.L., and Rechkemmer, G. (2003) Fruit juice consumption modulates antioxidative status, immune status, and DNA damage. *J. Nutr. Biochem.* **14**: 90–98.

Evans, J.M., Donnelly, L.A., Emslie-Smith, A.M., Alessi, D.R., and Morris, A.D. (2005) Metformin and reduced risk of cancer in diabetic patients. *Br. Med. J.* **330**: 1304–1305.

Gatenby, R.A. and Gillies, R.J. (2007) Glycolysis in cancer: a potential target for therapy. *Int. J. Biochem. Cell Biol.* **39**: 1358–1366.

Hites, R.A., Foran, J.A., Carpenter, D.O., Hamilton, M.C., Knuth, B.A., and Schwager, S.J. (2004) Global assessment of organic contaminants in farmed salmon. *Science* **303**: 226–229.

Matoba, S., Kang, J.-G., Patino, W.D., Wragg, A., Boehm, M., Gavrilova, O., Hurley, P.J., Bunz, F., and Hwang, P.M. (2006) P53 regulates mitochondrial respiration. *Science* **312**: 1650–1653.

Naasani, I., Oh-hashi, F., Oh-hara, T., Feng, W.Y., Johnston, J., Chan, K., and Tsuruo, T. (2003) Blocking telomerase by dietary polyphenols is a major mechanism for limiting the growth of human cancer cells *in vitro* and *in vivo*. *Cancer Res.* **63**: 824–830.

Revankar, C.M., Cimino, D.F., Sklar, L.A., Arterburn, J.B., and Prossnitz, E.R. (2005) A transmembrane intracellular estrogen receptor mediates rapid cell signaling. *Science* **307**: 1625–1630.

van der Rhee, H.J., de Vries, E., and Coebergh, J.W.W. (2006) Does sunlight prevent cancer? A systematic review. *Eur. J. Cancer* **42**: 2222–2232.

Russo, J., Lareef, M.H., Balogh, G., Guo, S., and Russo, I.H. (2003) Estrogen and its metabolites are carcinogenic agents in human breast epithelial cells. *J. Steroid Biochem. Mol. Biol.* **87**: 1–25.

Tangpricha, V., Spina, C., Yao, M., Chen, T.C., Wolfe, M.M., and Holick, M.F. (2005) Vitamin D deficiency enhances the growth of MC-26 colon cancer xenografts in Balb/c mice. *J. Nutr.* **135**: 2350–2354.

Ueland, P.M., Hustad, S., Schneede, J., Refsum, H., and Vollset, S.E. (2001) Biological and clinical implications of the MTHFR C677T polymorphism. *Trends Pharmacol. Sci.* **22**: 195–201.

Wang, L.H., Yang, X.Y., Zhang, X., Mihalic, K., Fan, Y.-X., Xiao, W., Howard, O.M.E., Appella, E., Maynard, A.T., and Farrar, W.L. (2004) Suppression of breast cancer by chemical modulation of vulnerable zinc fingers in estrogen receptor. *Nature Med.* **10**: 40–47.

Yue, W., Santen, R.J. Wang, J.-P., Li, Y., Verderame, M.F., Bocchinfuso, W.P., Korach, K.S., Devanesan, P., Todorovic, R., Rogan, E.G., and Cavalieri, E.L. (2003) Genotoxic metabolites of estradiol in breast: potential mechanism of estradiol induced carcinogenesis. *J. Steroid Biochem. Mol. Biol.* **86**: 477–486.

Chapter 12

The cancer industry: drug development and clinical trial design

Introduction

The goal of cancer research is to develop new effective and non-toxic cancer therapies. In this chapter, the process of drug development is reviewed. The development of the drug Gleevec, one of the most successful cancer therapies of recent years, is used to illustrate the process. The understanding of both the mechanism of action of this drug and the development of drug resistance is being used to produce 'second-generation' therapeutics. Investigations of the variable responses of individuals to another new drug, Iressa, will also be described. The chapter ends with a description of how to initiate a career in cancer research—just in case I have caught your interest.

12.1 Strategies of drug development

Drug development follows a series of stages (see Figure 12.1) and people with different expertise (e.g. biochemists, cell biologists, chemists, clinicians) may carry out the different stages at different facilities. In the preceding chapters we have seen many examples of important molecular targets and strategies to manipulate them (e.g. kinase inhibitors). Once a potential drug has been identified and prepared as a final product for *in vivo* delivery (drug formulation), subsequent studies can be divided into pre-clinical and clinical studies. **Pre-clinical studies** test a drug in animal models and gather data on safety and efficacy for proof of concept. These studies are required before administration of the drug to humans in **clinical trials** (discussed in Section 1.5). The concept of validating a drug target is often used in drug discovery. True cancer drug target validation occurs

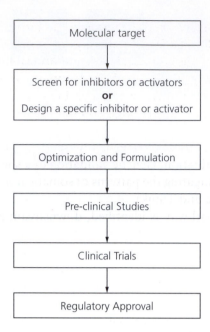

Figure 12.1 Stages of drug
development.

when a therapeutic agent is shown to act via the molecular target it was designed against and proved to be clinically effective. However, a more current use of the term 'target validation' refers only to the experimental evaluation of the role of a given gene or protein in cancer and its potential as a therapeutic target; that is, target validation may occur before clinical testing.

In order to develop a new targeted therapy, a three-step approach has been proposed for development of the drug before it goes to the clinic: identify the molecular targets/pathways that drive tumor growth; create a genetically equivalent, high-incidence animal model where tumors of interest develop in their correct anatomical locations and at a developmentally relevant time; and screen for or design inhibitors to block the molecular pathway and test their effects in the animal models (Romer and Curran, 2005).

Molecular targets and target validation

There are several different types of molecular target that may be identified and studied for drug development. The most popular are genetic lesions that have a causal role in cancer. The products of these lesions are oncogenic proteins or mutated tumor suppressor proteins. Targets include these aberrant proteins or components of the pathways they affect. Another type of molecular target may involve tissue-specific characteristics and/or differentiation pathways. For example, estrogen acts as a mitogen for the breast and inhibitors of estrogen action (e.g.

tamoxifen) are effective in the treatment of breast cancer. Similarly, knowledge of the differentiation pathways of the hematopoietic lineage has been applied for the treatment of acute promyelocytic leukemia by differentiation therapy (see Section 8.5). Another type of molecular target affects host processes rather than tumor biology. For example, molecular regulators of angiogenesis are good therapeutic targets (e.g. VEGF, VEGFR; Section 9.11).

Validating a molecular target may involve several strategies that together provide data for evaluation. Genetic validation of a specific genetic lesion is obtained by investigating the patterns of somatic mutation in a particular tumor (see Pause and Think).

Once a specific pathway is identified, downstream effectors may also prove to be important therapeutic targets. For example, EGFR has proved to be a validated drug target and its downstream effectors RAF and MEK are also validated targets. Cell-based systems are also valuable methods used for target validation. Transformation assays that rely on the introduction of putative oncogenes into normal cells are an example and have been instrumental in the field. RNA-interference techniques in cells are also important approaches to test target validation. However, perhaps the most valuable strategy is the use of transgenic animals, whereby a target may be analyzed in the context of a tumor *in situ*.

Let's look at an example. Raf, a component of the EGF signal transduction pathway (Chapter 4), is an important regulator of cell proliferation. Oncogenic mutations resulting in constitutive activation of Raf have been identified in cancers, especially melanomas and thyroid cancers. Evidence was needed to support the hypothesis that Raf is a potential therapeutic target. The results from an experiment utilizing Raf antisense oligonucleotides demonstrated growth inhibition in human tumor xenografts in mice. This provided proof-of-concept that Raf is a valid target for future drug development. (See the Activity at the end of the chapter for a discussion of an approved drug targeted against Raf.)

Animal models

There is difficulty in finding a cancer model that can reliably predict the effect of a new drug in human patients. A tumor is similar to an organ with tumor cells interacting with host cells, the immune system, blood vessels, and the extracellular matrix. The obvious difficulty in testing new drugs in cultured cells is that the system is far from replicating a true tumor environment. The next step up from cells in culture is the use of organ cultures and organotypic cultures, as these systems possess a three-dimensional aspect. Organ cultures are made of tissue slices. Organotypic cultures are made of cells grown in a specific matrix to mimic the tissue of interest. The most common model systems used in drug discovery are *in*

PAUSE AND THINK

What pattern of somatic mutation would you expect to observe? One feature to expect is that the genetic lesion is tumor-specific and occurs early in tumor development. Absence in healthy tissue would also be expected.

vivo mouse models. There are several approaches for using a mouse model system. The older approach is to use high doses of a single carcinogen, often with little relationship to the etiology and/or molecular defect of the tumor of interest. The most widely used approach is the creation of human tumor xenografts. Xenografts are generated by injecting human cancer cells under the skin of immunodeficient (nude) mice (the use of nude mice is necessary to avoid rejection of human cells by the immune system of the mouse). Disadvantages of this system are that reactions of the immune system cannot be monitored and that the environment, although *in vivo*, is foreign to the tumor. An improvement to this model is to inject human cells into the organ of the mouse from which they were derived (orthotopic). Injecting tumor cells of mice into mice (syngeneic tumor) is another alternative. The approach that offers a better alternative are genetically altered mice, created by transgenic, knock-out, or RNAi technologies. For example, the multiple intestinal neoplasia (min) mouse carries a germline truncation of the adenomatous polyposis coli gene. The min mouse develops multiple adenomas and is used to study colon carcinogenesis. Tissue-specific and inducible promoters can be used in these models to better mimic the etiology/molecular defect of the disease and the anatomical and temporal characteristics of human cancer. Also, 'instability models' creating mice with defective DNA repair, telomere dysfunction, impaired DNA damage checkpoints, etc. generates 'instability models' of cancer. The resultant genome instability gives rise to tumors with a level of complexity comparable to human tumors and thus is an important tool for further studies of carcinogenesis (see Maser *et al.*, 2007 and references within). It must be remembered that species differences exist and results from any of these models may give very different results in the clinic.

Screening

High-throughput screening is a common approach to selecting lead compounds for development (Figure 12.2). It permits the testing of millions of compounds in a short period of time. Plates containing hundreds of wells of biological material (e.g. cells) are used to test various chemical compounds for a desired biological effect (e.g. apoptosis). Robotics can be deployed to prepare plates and to analyze up to 100,000 compounds per day. Many screening protocols use synthetic molecules synthesized via **combinatorial chemistry**, methodologies that rapidly and systematically assemble molecular entities to synthesize a large number of different but structurally related compounds. Note that many successful drugs are based on natural compounds that have also been used in screening procedures. Another approach for selecting lead compounds for development is virtual screening. In this approach, computer

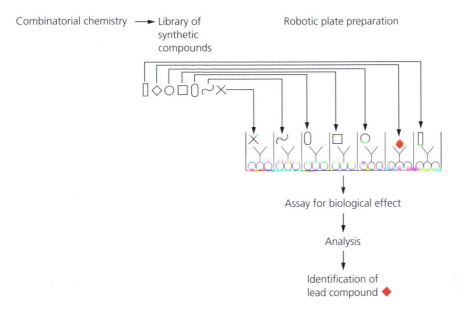

Figure 12.2 High-throughput screening. See text for details.

analysis is used to select compounds that will bind to a molecular target based on the previously known three-dimensional structural information about the target (e.g. crystal structure). Since this is an *in silico* approach, consumables are not required and the compounds examined may not necessarily exist. Studies suggest that high-throughput screening and virtual screening are complementary approaches, each yielding potentially promising results.

12.2 Development of imatinib

Let us look at the development of imatinib (Gleevec, USA; Glivec, UK, Europe) in relation to the stages of drug development (Capdeville *et al.*, 2002). It began with the understanding of a genetic lesion: the chromosomal translocation that is characteristic of chronic myelogenous leukemia. The identification of the molecular consequence of this translocation pointed to the resulting fusion protein, BCR–ABL, as a *molecular target*. Since the translocation results in elevated tyrosine kinase activity that is crucial for transformation, the obvious strategy was to develop a specific tyrosine kinase inhibitor. A lead compound (a compound that shows a desired activity, e.g. kinase inhibition) was elucidated from a chemical screen. In this case, kinase inhibition was demonstrated by the inhibition of protein kinase C. Optimization of the lead compound by the addition of small chemical groups (Figure 12.3) produced a drug that inhibited

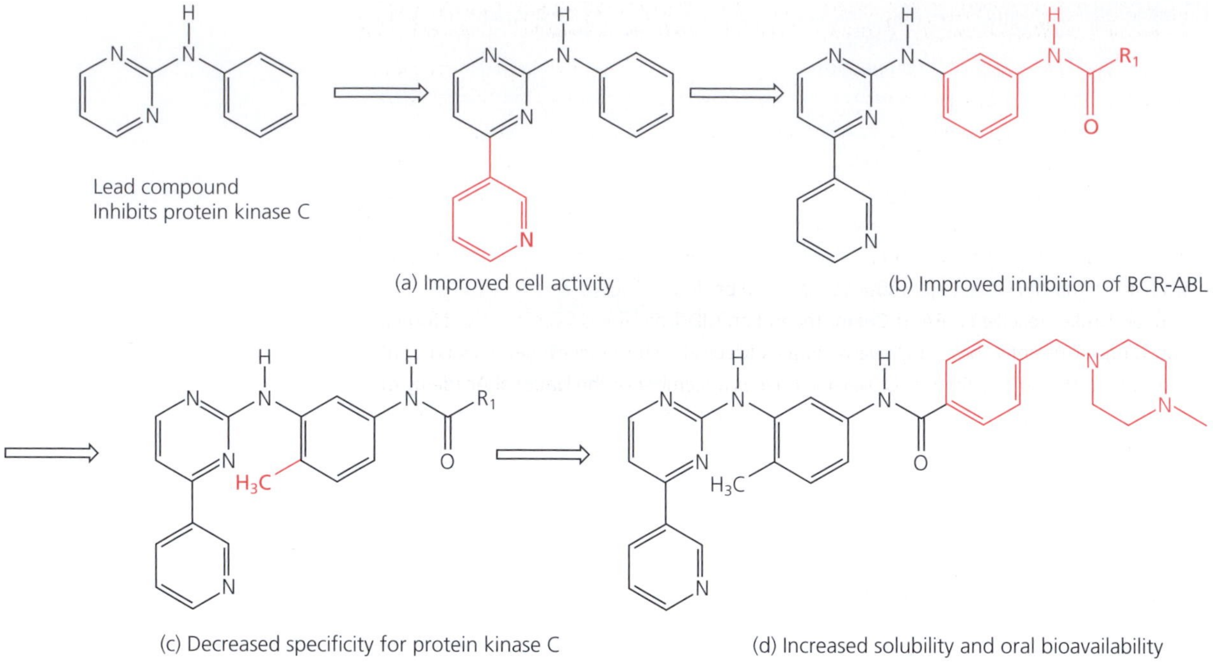

(a) Improved cell activity   (b) Improved inhibition of BCR-ABL

(c) Decreased specificity for protein kinase C   (d) Increased solubility and oral bioavailability

Figure 12.3 Optimization of a lead compound leading to production of Gleevec. Small chemical modifications are shown in red. (a) The addition of a 3'-pyridyl group enhances cellular activity. (b) An amide group conferred BCR-ABL tyrosine kinase inhibition. (c) A methyl group abolished unwanted protein kinase C activity. (d) A *N*-methyl piperazine moiety enhanced oral bioavailability and solubility.

PAUSE AND THINK

CML involves a block in differentiation that leads to an increase in white blood cells. A complete hematological response is defined as a reduction in white blood cell count to less than 10,000 per cubic millimeter (the upper limit of a normal white blood cell count) and platelet count to less than 450,000 per cubic millimeter maintained for at least 4 weeks.

BCR–ABL tyrosine kinase activity (instead of protein kinase C) and showed good bioavailability. Bioavailability relates to the ability of the drug to reach its site of action after administration. Pre-clinical testing demonstrated fairly selective inhibition of BCR–ABL kinase activity and induction of apoptosis in cell culture experiments and in leukemic cells from patients. Inhibition of tumor growth was also observed in animal models. **Clinical trials** (see Table 1.1 for phases of clinical trials) documented safety and efficacy. Results from a Phase I dose-escalation study were extremely positive: 53 out of 54 patients (98%) achieved a complete hematological response with minimal side-effects, usually within the first 3 weeks of treatment (Druker *et al.*, 2001).

Positive results continued to be demonstrated for Phase II and Phase III trials. Approval by the US Food and Drug Administration (FDA) was given on May 2001, and subsequent approval for use in Europe and Japan followed shortly afterwards. The European Medicines Evaluation Agency (EMEA) and the Japanese Ministry of Health and Welfare, together with the FDA, are working towards an internationally harmonized system for drug approval that will facilitate the delivery of drugs to more patients, more quickly.

A LEADER IN THE FIELD . . . of drug discovery: Brian Druker

Brian Druker was a major contributor to the development of Gleevec and thus has helped revolutionize drug discovery and ultimately the treatment of leukemia. In addition to being involved in pre-clinical studies, he also conducted the first clinical studies of Gleevec.

During early studies of Gleevec, several of Brian's collaborators at Novartis observed that the side-effects were minimal and were disappointed as they thought this indicated that the drug would not be effective. To everyone's delight, the drug was effective *and* showed minimal side-effects. Brian has emphasized that the connection to cancer patients through his work in the clinic is a major motivational force behind his work.

Brian Druker received a BA in Chemistry and an MD from the University of California, San Diego. Currently, he is a Howard Hughes Medical Institute Investigator working at the Oregon Health and Science University. Brian is a member of the National Academy of Sciences and, among other honors, has received the Medal of Honor from the American Cancer Society.

12.3 Second-generation therapeutics

Initial drug treatment can select for cancer cells that are resistant to the treatment, and consequently new drugs are required when the initial treatment is no longer effective. Although imatinib is a highly successful treatment for the treatment of CML in early phase disease, patients with later-phase (accelerated and blast stage) disease often develop resistance to imatinib. New drugs called *second-generation inhibitors* have been developed to block the progression of CML in those who are resistant to imatinib. Strategies in the development of these new second-generation inhibitors often rely on structural biology data that analyze drug binding (see the first panel on the cover of this book; it shows the binding of Gleevec to Abl).

 Point mutations in the *Bcr–Abl* gene that interfere with the binding of imatinib but maintain a functional tyrosine kinase domain are the most common mechanism involved in imatinib resistance. Mutations may affect physical bonding/contact points or cause changes in shape that sterically obstruct binding. Alternatively, mutations may destabilize the inactive conformation, the conformation to which imatinib binds.

 Although more than 50 different mutations associated with imatinib resistance have been identified, only six account for 60–70% of all mutations. One of these six, a mutation at Thr315 (T315I; a substitution by isoleucine; Gorre *et al.*, 2001), is noteworthy because many of the second-generation inhibitors cannot override the imatinib resistance due to this mutation. However, MK-0457 (VX-680, Merck; Figure 12.4a) is one second-generation inhibitor in clinical trials that has demonstrated an effect on this mutation.

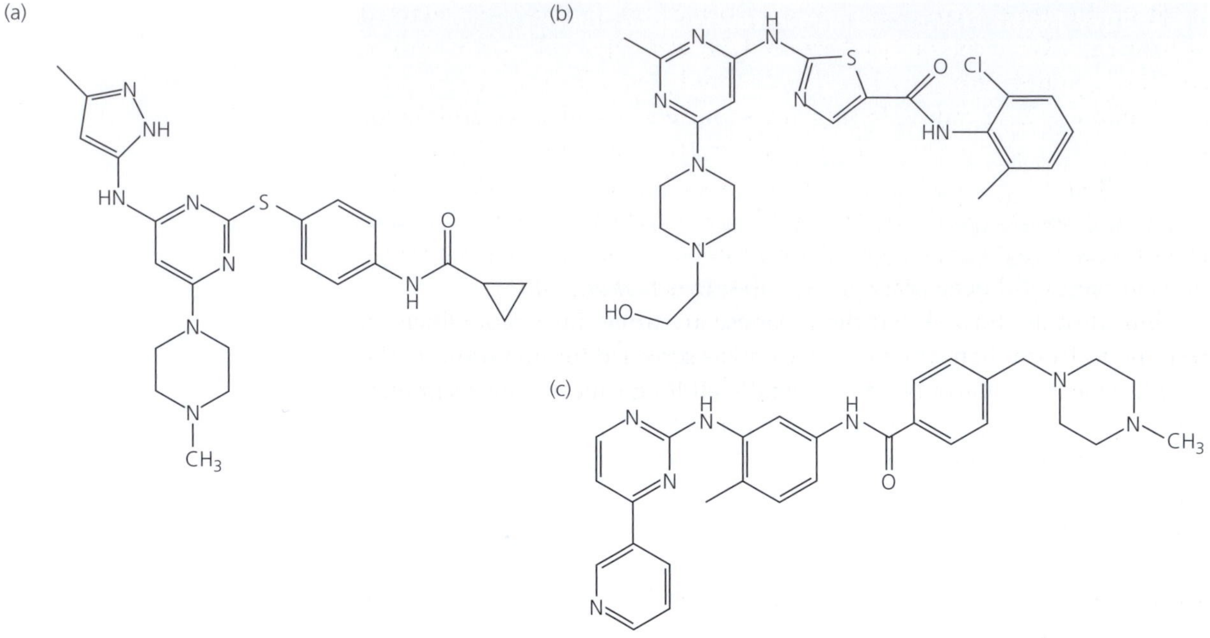

Figure 12.4 Two examples of second-generation inhibitors of BCR–ABL: (a) MK-0457 (VX-680), (b) dasatinib. Compare with (c) imatinib.

Dasatinib (Figure 12.4b) is a second-generation inhibitor that, unlike imatinib, binds to the active conformation of the ABL kinase and therefore inhibits many mutant forms of BCR–ABL. The FDA and the European Medicines Agency approved dasatinib for the treatment of imatinib-resistant CML. However, the T315I mutation noted above confers dasatinib resistance.

The origin of resistance is still not completely understood. Some data suggest that all mutant *Bcr–Abl* clones may exist *before* imatinib treatment and that clones carrying these may grow in response to selective pressure of imatinib. When a patient initially responds to a second-generation inhibitor but subsequently develops resistance with a second mutation, the new mutation responsible for the resistance is not found in addition to the first mutation but instead is identified on the original *Bcr–Abl* background. Thus, the clone carrying the new mutation may grow due to selective pressure of the second-generation inhibitor. Combinations of inhibitors may be effective in preventing the expansion of drug-resistant clones and thus such strategies are being examined.

12.4 Pharmacogenomics

Pharmacogenomics is the study of the influence of the genome on an individual's response to a drug. Gene variability in the both the individual and in the tumor may lead to differences in drug response among individuals.

Iressa (gefitinib; AstraZeneca), a tyrosine kinase inhibitor targeted against the EGF receptor (see Section 4.3), was reported to have mixed clinical responses. Approved in the USA and Japan for the treatment of non-small-cell lung cancer, Iressa causes impressive and successful tumor regression but, curiously, in only a select 10% of patients. Since non-small-cell lung cancer accounts for 80% of all lung cancers, the number of patients that respond to Iressa (10%) is significant. It has now been demonstrated that the patients who respond to Iressa carry specific mutations in the *EGFR* gene (Paez *et al.*, 2004; Lynch *et al.*, 2004).

Clinical trials showed that the Japanese are three times more likely to respond to Iressa than Americans. Scientists screened for mutations in the *EGFR* gene in two groups of non-small-cell lung cancer tumor samples: one set from a Japanese hospital and another set from an American hospital. Somatic mutations in the *EGFR* gene were found more often in Japanese patients. The mutations were either missense mutations or small deletions that were located in the coding region for the receptor tyrosine kinase active site, a region near the binding site for Iressa. Scientists then asked whether the mutations correlated with treatment response. The analysis of a small set of patients showed that those who responded to Iressa also carried the identified mutations.

The mutations produce an altered protein that increases the amount and duration of EGF-induced signal transduction compared with wild-type receptors. In other words, the receptors are hyperactive but not constitutive. These mutations that underlie aberrant tyrosine kinase signaling and drive carcinogenesis also make the tumor more susceptible to Iressa because they cluster in the sequences that code for the region where Iressa binds. This suggests that knowing the particular molecular characteristics of a tumor (e.g. mutations of the *EGFR* gene) is important for selecting the best treatment for an individual.

As mentioned in Section 4.3, Gleevec inhibits c-kit (in addition to Abl) and has been approved for the treatment of gastrointestinal stromal tumor (GIST). Similarly, mutations in the *KIT* gene affect the sensitivity of GIST to Gleevec. These and similar observations support the emergence of pharmacogenomics, the study of correlating specific gene DNA sequence information to drug response.

> **PAUSE AND THINK**
>
> Why are these particular mutations in the *EGFR* gene more common in Japanese than Americans? It may be due to a lifestyle factor such as exposure to a specific carcinogen or a genetic predisposition, or a mixture of both.

12.5 Improved clinical trial design

There are some flaws in the design of clinical trials performed today that result in an inflated number of unsuccessful drug results. A problem that is difficult to overcome is that many new drugs are tested on older patients who have advanced cancer and who have not responded to a range of conventional therapies. Drugs that may be effective in early stage cancer may fail to have an effect on late-stage cancer in clinical trials. The development of such drugs would be wrongly discontinued. Ethically acceptable suggestions are needed on how we can move forward. The inclusion of controls is strongly recommended, but surprisingly they have not been included in a majority of Phase II oncology trials in the past. Modifications are being made to the classical Phase I, II, and III trials. The FDA has approved Phase 0 Trials. Phase 0 trials allow the testing of small doses of experimental drugs in people for 7 days or less. They aim to gather data on drug targeting, action, and metabolism in the body. Initially, only small batches of a drug are required to be produced for these studies. In addition, Phase IV trials may be carried out after a drug has been approved and licensed. The purpose of Phase IV trials is to further investigate side-effects, safety, and/or long-term risks and benefits. They are also useful to help develop new applications for a given drug. Phase IV trials for the HPV vaccine Gardasil (discussed in Section 10.5), are planned to test different vaccination policies in Nordic countries and to monitor effectiveness and the occurrence of rare adverse events.

It is expected that sample size calculations for a clinical trial should be carried out properly and reported in associated publications. This is important for trial evaluation and the production of statistically meaningful results. Many researchers use computer software programs for this task. However, it may be informative to describe a basic formula (Schulz and Grimes, 2005). For trials with two outcomes (e.g. patient remains ill or patient becomes well), four components are required for calculating sample sizes. They are: type I error (α), power, event rate in the control group and event rate in the treatment group (treatment effect). Type I error is the probability of concluding that two treatments (e.g. treatment versus placebo) differ, when in fact they do not; i.e. the chance of a false-positive result. Power is derived from type II (β) error: $P = 1 - \beta$. Type II error is the opposite of type I: it is the probability of not detecting a statistically significant difference when a difference actually exists. It is the chance of a false-negative result: the treatment is different from the control but the difference is not detectable. Therefore power is the probability of detecting a statistically significant difference when a difference really exists. Investigators would usually like less than a 5% chance of making a false-positive error, and thus by convention α is usually set to 0.05. Similarly, if investigators want less that a 10% chance of making a false-negative error they will set β to 0.10. In this case, power will be $1 - 0.10 = 0.90$.

The equation below illustrates a simple formula for calculating sample size for a case with two possible outcomes, assuming $\alpha = 0.05$, power = 0.90 and an equal sample size in the two groups

$$n = \frac{10.51[(R + 1) - p_2(R^2 + 1)]}{p_2(1 - R)^2}$$

where n is sample size, p_1 is the event rate in the treatment group, p_2 is the event rate in the control group, and R is the risk ratio (p_1/p_2).

Defining the target population and clinical endpoints requires special attention in clinical trial design. Important lessons have been gained recently about defining the target population for clinical trials. The results discussed above that illustrated variable response rates among two different populations to the drug Iressa argue for the benefit of including geographically and genetically diverse populations in clinical trials. Molecular profiling of the tumor prior to and/or during clinical trials is also important in order to gain a true measure of drug efficacy. However, obtaining tumor tissue for analysis may be difficult, as in the case of the lung.

Patient selection (i.e. choosing patients who have the molecular defect that a drug is designed to target) is important so that drugs are shown to be efficient when tested on the 'right' patients. Otherwise a variable response will be observed and the observed efficacy will not be accurate. For example, as we saw above with Iressa, if a drug acts on tumor cells that contain a mutated receptor, the efficacy of the drug should be tested on patients whose tumor contains these mutations. For other drugs, patients may be selected on the basis of gene copy number rather than mutation. Digital karyotyping is a method that allows determination of DNA copy number on a genomic scale.

When designing drug trials it is important to define parameters that will indicate the effectiveness of the drug. How will we know if the drug is working? Before the initiation of the trial, clinical endpoints must be defined. Tumor shrinkage is commonly used to indicate a response, but it may not necessarily correlate with survival. In particular, cytostatic drugs inhibit tumor growth and/or metastasis and thus progression-free survival time is a more suitable endpoint, rather than tumor regression. The classical endpoints used are survival, improved time to progression, plus improvement in symptoms or quality of life.

A novel trial design is the randomized discontinuation trial design. In this design patients receive one or two cycles of a cytostatic drug and, upon completion, those who have stable disease are then randomized to placebo or to continue the same treatment. The aim of this design is to enrich the patient population with those with slowly progressive cancer and eliminate those with rapidly progressive cancer.

In addition to clinical endpoints, clinical trials that evaluate new molecular therapeutics warrant defined molecular endpoints. Molecular endpoints involve the evaluation of molecular target inhibition and are important to ensure that the drug is eliciting its effects in the expected manner. For example, testing whether Gleevec inhibits BCR–ABL tyrosine kinase activity was an important molecular endpont (data shown in Druker *et al.*, 2001). A phosphorylated substrate of Abl tyrosine kinase was used as a biomarker. A biomarker is a biochemical or genetic feature that can

HOW DO WE KNOW THAT?

Clinical trials terms and clinical endpoints

Let's examine some of the characteristics of the Phase II trial of Gardasil® reported by Villa *et al.* (2005). As the title of the article states, it is a randomized, double-blinded, placebo-controlled, multicenter, phase II study. Each term will be explained:

Randomized: treatment parameters (dose and type: treatment or placebo) were assigned to participants using computer-randomized schedules.

Double-blinded: neither participants, nor hospital staff, nor investigators knew which participants received treatment versus placebo.

Placebo-controlled: the placebo consisted of the same adjuvant used for the vaccine, so that participants in the control group received exact the same treatment as the participants in the treatment group *except* they did not receive the vaccine.

Multicenter: participants were recruited from Brazil, Europe, and the USA. Several criteria were set including age (16–23 years old) and aspects of previous medical history.

Phase II: a dose escalation study involving several hundred participants was used to access safety, immunogenicity, and efficacy. Methods used to monitor efficacy included gynecological examination, Pap test, PCR analysis to detect HPV, serum samples, and biopsies of any lesions.

The primary endpoint assessed was persistent infection by HPV6, -11, -16, or -18 or disease of the cervix or external genitals. Cervical cancer was not used as an endpoint because cervical cancer can be prevented by the treatment of pre-cancerous lesions identified by screening. Identifying pre-cancerous lesions and allowing them to progress without treating them would be unethical. Furthermore, long-term studies would be required because of the lag time between infection and cancer.

be used to measure disease progression or the effect of treatment. They may include the measurement of specific molecules (prostate-specific antigen, PSA), genetic alterations, gene expression profiles, cell-based markers (circulating cells), and **single-nucleotide polymorphisms** (SNPs).

The measurement of a biomarker has important implications for the administered dose, as maximal tolerated dose, often prescribed for conventional chemotherapies, may not be necessary. In the example above, the dose of imatinib required to inhibit substrate phosphorylation would be appropriate to test in clinical trials. Also, some studies have shown that expression levels of drug targets can change during progression of the disease, and therefore drug response may be expected to change during the course of the disease.

12.6 A career in cancer research

People are the most important asset in cancer research and drug discovery. There are several avenues to pursue for a career in cancer research. The road most often traveled is to obtain a PhD in an area that interests you. Interest is important for several reasons: first, you will be spending many hours reading and thinking about your subject; secondly, you will spend many hours in the laboratory conducting experiments which focus around your topic; thirdly, one can never predict in which area a big breakthrough will occur, so there is no sense in trying to guess. Research can be frustrating at times because you are trying to figure out something that no one knows or has really done before and progress tends to be in small steps. However, many small steps made by many individuals drives the field. It can be most rewarding to know that you have made contributions to relieving suffering and saving lives. PhD studentships are posted in the back of the leading scientific journals such as *Nature* and *Science* and on internet sites such as http://www.findaphd.com/, but a personal approach by letter to the head of a laboratory in which you are interested in working can also be successful. Alternatively, cancer research can be pursued in a pharmaceutical company with entry levels at different stages of education. In fact, working in a research laboratory after obtaining a BSc degree is another valid path for a career in cancer research.

Cancer research is expensive and requires appropriate facilities equipped with high-tech equipment. These facilities are available in universities, research institutes, hospitals, and in biotechnology and pharmaceutical companies (see Appendix 2). The relationship between these types of research providers has recently grown to be symbiotic; a close association leads to mutual benefit. Several organizations and funding agencies create opportunities that help foster collaborations between universities and industry. Such organizations also provide commercial business training for academics. A career in cancer research promises to be interesting and rewarding. You are guaranteed to meet and work with interesting, intelligent, and talented people!

■ CHAPTER HIGHLIGHTS—REFRESH YOUR MEMORY

- Drug development follows a series of stages from defining a molecular target through to approval.
- Target validation refers to the experimental evaluation of the role of a given gene or protein in cancer and its potential as a therapeutic target.
- Combinatorial chemistry in conjunction with high-throughput screening are common methodologies used in drug discovery.
- The development of Gleevec (imatinib) is a paradigm for drug development of new molecular cancer therapeutics.
- Many patients with late-phase CML often develop resistance to Gleevec.
- Only six mutations in the *Bcr–Abl* gene account for 60–70% of mutations that lead to imatinib resistance.
- Second-generation therapeutics are being developed to overcome resistance to Gleevec.
- The study of the influence of the genome on a patient's response to a drug is called pharmacogenomics.
- Iressa has shown favorable responses in patients who carry specific mutations in the *EGFR* gene.
- Phase 0 and Phase IV clinical trials have been added to the three conventional phases of clinical trials, Phases I, II, and III.
- Defining the target population and clinical endpoints are two important aspects requiring careful consideration during the design of clinical trials.
- A biomarker is a biochemical or genetic feature that can be used to measure disease progress or the effect of treatment.
- Please consider a career in cancer research.

■ **ACTIVITY**

1. Read the case history of the discovery and development of sorafenib (*Nature Rev Drug Discov.* **5**: 835–844). Compare the process with that of imatinib. Pay particular attention to the target population used in the early clinical trials. Note the timescale from discovery to approval.

■ **FURTHER READING**

Arteaga, C.L. and Baselga, J. (2003) Clinical trial design and end point for epidermal growth factor receptor-targeted therapies: implications for drug development and practice. *Clin. Cancer Res.* **9**: 1579–1589.

Benson, J.D., Chen, Y.-N.P., Vornell-Kennon, S.A., Dorsch, M., Kim, S., Leszczyniecka, M., Sellers, W.R., and Lengauer, C. (2006) Validating cancer drug targets. *Nature* **441**: 451–456.

Druker, B.J. (2002) STI571 (Gleevec™) as a paradigm for cancer therapy. *Trends Mol. Med.* **8**: S14–S18.

Klebe, G. (2006) Virtual ligand screening: strategies, perspectives, and limitations. *Drug Discov. Today* **11**: 580–594.

Romer, J. and Curran, T. (2005) Targeting medulloblastoma: small-molecule inhibitors of the sonic hedgehog pathway as potential cancer therapeutics. *Cancer Res.* **65**: 4975–4978.

Schiller, J.H. (2004) Clinical trial design issues in the era of targeted therapies. *Clin. Cancer Res.* **10**: 4281S–4282S.

Schulz, K.F. and Grimes, D.A. (2005) Sample size calculations in randomized trials: mandatory and mystical. *Lancet* **365**: 1348–1353.

Strausberg, R.L., Simpson, A.J.G., Old, L.J., and Riggins, G.J. (2004) Oncogenomics and the development of new cancer therapies. *Nature* **429**: 469–474.

Weisberg, E., Manley, P.W., Cowan-Jacob, S.W., Hochhaus, A., and Griffin, J.D. (2007) Second generation inhibitors of BCR-ABL for the treatment of imatinib-resistant chronic myeloid leukemia. *Nature Rev. Cancer* **7**: 345–356.

■ **SELECTED SPECIAL TOPICS**

Capdeville, R., Buchdunger, E., Zimmermann, J., and Matter, A. (2002) Glivec (STI571, Imatinib), a rationally developed, targeted anticancer drug. *Nature Rev. Drug Discov.* **1**: 493–502.

Druker, B.J., Talpaz, M., Resta, D.J., Peng, B., Buchdunger, E., Ford, J.M., Lydon, N.B., Kantarjian, H., Capedeville, R., Ohno-Jones, S., and Sawyers, C.L. (2001) Efficiency and safety of a specific inhibitor of the BCR-ABL tyrosine kinase in chronic myeloid leukemia. *New Engl. J. Med.* **344**: 1031–1037.

Gorre, M.E., Mohammed, M., Ellwood, K., Hsu, N., Paquette, R., Rao, P.N., and Sawyers, C.L. (2001) Clinical resistance to STI-571 cancer therapy caused by Bcr-Abl gene mutation or amplification. *Science* **293**: 876–880.

Lynch, T.J., Bell, D.W., Sordella, R., Gurubhagavatula, S., Okimoto, R.A., Brannigan, B.W., Harris, P.L., Haserlat, S.M., Supko, J.G., Huluska, F.G., Louis, D.N., Christiani, D.C., Settleman, J., and Haber, D.A. (2004) Activating mutations in the epidermal growth factor receptor underlying responsiveness of non-small cell lung cancer to gefitinib. *New Engl. J. Med.* **350**: 2129–2139.

Maser, R.S., Choudhury, B., Campbell, P.J., Feng, B., Wong, K.-K., Protopopov, A., O'Neil, J., Gutierrez, A., Ivanova, E., Perna, I., Lin, E., Mani, V., Jiang, S., McNamara, K., Zaghlul, S., Edkins, S., Stevens, C., Brennan, C., Martin, E.S., Wiedemeyer, R., Kabbarah, O., Nogueira, C., Histen, G., Aster, J., Mansour, M., Duke, V., Foroni, L., Fielding, A.K., Goldstone, A.H., Rowe, J.M., Wang, Y.A., Look, A.T., Stratton, M.R., Chin, L., Futreal, P.A., and DePinho, R.A. (2007) Chromosomally unstable mouse tumours have genomic alterations similar to diverse human cancers. *Nature* **447**: 966–971.

Paez, J.G., Janne, P.A., Lee, J.C., Tracy, S., Greulich, H., Gabriel, S., Herman, P., Kaye, F.J., Lindeman, N., Boggon, T.J., Naoki, K., Sasaki, H., Fujii, Y., Eck, M.J., Sellers, W.R., Johnson, B.E., and Meyerson, M. (2004) EGFR mutations in lung cancer: correlation with clinical response to Gefitinib therapy. *Science* **304**: 1497–1500.

Villa, L.L., Costa, R.L., Petta, C.A., Andrade, R.P., Ault, K.A., Giuliano, A.R., Wheeler, C.M., Koutsky, L.A., Malm, C., Lehtinen, M., Skjeldestad, F.E., Olsson, S.E., Steinwall, M., Brown, D.R., Kurman, R.J., Ronnett, B.M., Stoler, M.H., Ferenczy, A., Harper, D.M., Tamms, G.M., Yu, J., Lupinacci, L., Railkar, R., Taddeo, F.J., Jansen, K.U., Esser, M.T., Sings, H.L., Saah, A.J., and Barr, E. (2005) Prophylactic quadrivalent human papillomavirus (types 6, 11, 16, and 18) L1 virus-like particle vaccine in young women: a randomized double-blind placebo-controlled multicentre phase II efficacy trial. *Lancet Oncol.* **6**: 271–278.

Chapter 13

Cancer in the future: focus on diagnostics and immunotherapy

Introduction

This concluding chapter will address two issues: first is the question of whether cancer will exist in the future and, secondly, if the answer is 'yes', what changes in cancer treatment and management are likely to be implemented? As discussed in Chapter 11, chemoprevention of cancer, based on strategies that use dietary microconstituents or target hormonal signaling pathways, hold potential for reducing the incidence of some cancers in the future. Overall, however, evidence suggests that cancer will 'always be around' because mutation underlies carcinogenesis and we cannot escape from mutations. Although we may be able to avoid certain carcinogenic agents (e.g. tobacco) and processes (e.g. sunbathing), we certainly cannot avoid all of them. Furthermore, cancer is associated with aging and life expectancies are increasing. As a consequence of people living longer, the incidence of cancer is increasing.

PAUSE AND THINK

What are examples of cellular processes that can induce mutations? One example is DNA replication, which is associated with errors caused by the incorporation of incorrect nucleotides. Two other examples are normal cellular respiration and inflammation, both of which are associated with oxygen by-products that damage DNA. All three examples are cellular processes that can give rise to mutations.

On the other hand, maybe there is a lesson to be learnt from the history of medicine. In the past, there were dreaded infectious diseases such as smallpox, which are now preventable through vaccination. Could vaccination be used to eradicate cancer? The observation that the immune system could recognize and respond to tumors following bacterial infection was made over 100 years ago. More recent studies have shown that effector cells of the immune system can recognize tumor-associated **antigens** and kill tumor cells. This endogenous mechanism of protection against tumor cells by the immune system is called 'immunosurveillance' and suggests that boosting the immune system by vaccination against tumor cells may be possible.

Alternatively, if we are not able to eradicate cancer, what will it be like having cancer in future decades? It is envisaged that cancer, a disease of the genome at the cellular level, will be detected much earlier than is possible today because of the rise of genomics and its associated technologies. Instead of a positive diagnosis being linked imminently with death, cancer may become a long-term, chronic disease, like arthritis. Although a cure is preferred, the complexity of cancer may foster the development of treatments that allow people to live more comfortably with the disease rather than cure it.

In this chapter, we will examine current, far-reaching advancements in the fields of immunology and technology in order to form an educated prediction of the future of cancer. The potential for the prevention of cancer through vaccination will be examined. We will also investigate the application of improved tools, techniques, and therapeutics that are essential in order to transform cancer into a chronic, rather than a terminal, disease. These include molecular diagnostics, expression profiling for cancer classification, **bioinformatics**, and new treatment strategies including cancer vaccines as therapeutic agents.

13.1 Cancer vaccines

Our ability to harness the immune system to prevent and/or kill tumor cells is becoming evident. Vaccination is called active immunization because it tries to stimulate the individual's own immune effector cells. A vaccine is composed of antigen(s) and **adjuvant**(s). Adjuvants are vaccine additives that enhance the immune response to an antigen. This contrasts passive immunization, which involves the transfer of effectors of the immune system, such as T cells or secreted products of lymphoid cells, into the patient.

A little review of immunology basics

There are two main classes of lymphocytes (immune cells): Bone-marrow-derived (B) lymphocytes and thymus-derived (T) lymphocytes. The main function of B lymphocytes is to synthesize and secrete antibodies. The aspect of immunity mediated by antibodies produced by B cells is called humoral immunity. Antibodies contain an antigen-binding domain, and overall specific antibodies can recognize almost any antigen encountered. An antigen can be defined as any molecule that is able to generate an immune response. Since many B cells respond to an antigen, a mixture of antibodies is produced by many clones (polyclonal). Experimentally, we can grow a single clone of a specific B lymphocyte by creating a hybridoma in order to produce quantities of a specific, monoclonal, antibody. Antibodies can activate cell-mediated cell lysis. T cells are responsible for cell-mediated immunity. It is thought that the cytotoxic T-cell response is the principal anti-tumor defense of the body. Cytokines are polypeptides involved in cell signaling in the immune system.

Passive immunization

Many early attempts at cancer immunotherapy utilized passive immunization strategies. Interferon-γ, a cytokine with promising ability to modulate the immune response, was studied extensively in Phase I, II, and III trials. In general, however, poor clinical responses were observed. Tumor necrosis factor also gave disappointing results in clinical trials. Recently, however, Rosenberg (see Box 'Leaders in the field') and his group have demonstrated promising results after the transfer of selected tumor-reactive T cells into cancer patients who underwent lympho-depleting chemotherapy (destruction of endogenous lymphocytes by cytotoxic drugs) (Dudley *et al.*, 2002). Tumor-infiltrating lymphocytes were expanded *in vitro* and transferred to patients along with the cytokine adjuvant, interleukin-2, for immunization. Cancer regression was observed in patients with metastatic melanoma.

Here, we focus on vaccinations. Cancer vaccines can either be designed to prepare the immune system prior to getting cancer for cancer prevention, so-called *prophylactic vaccines*, or they can act to stimulate the immune system in order to cause tumor regression in a patient with cancer, a *therapeutic vaccine*. Most cancer vaccines are designed to be therapeutic vaccines, though we will consider both types below.

Therapeutic vaccines

The production of a vaccine involves the selection of an appropriate antigen that will stimulate an effective anti-tumor response. Tumor-associated antigens may be derived from either degradation and processing of unfolded intracellular proteins that are shuttled to the surface of the tumor cell or from damaged or dying tumor cells. These may include oncoproteins arising from oncogenic mutations or chromosomal translocations. Since T cells are the main effectors of an anti-tumor response, antigens from the vaccine must be displayed eventually on the surface of other cells, called antigen-presenting cells. A series of cellular events characterize an immune response upon administration of a cancer vaccination (Figure 13.1). Antigen-presenting cells, such as dendritic cells that reside in the tissue, are at the heart of signaling for the mission of eliciting T-cell-mediated immunity. It is the dendritic cells that (1) *acquire* and (2) *process* the antigens, and, upon maturation, migrate to the lymphoid organs to (3) *present* the antigens to the main effector T cells. The uptake of antigens by the dendritic cells is primarily by endocytosis. Antigen processing involves cleavage of the antigen into small peptides by proteases (depicted by scissors in Figure 13.1). The adjuvant in a cancer vaccine induces the maturation of the antigen-presenting cells and their migration to the lymphoid organs. Processed antigen is translocated to the cell surface for presentation in association with proteins from the major

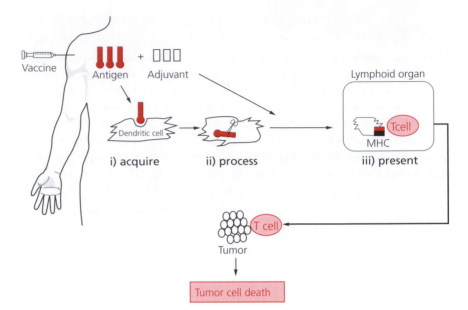

Figure 13.1 Cellular events in an immune response following vaccination.

histocompatibility complex (MHC; details of which are beyond the scope of this book). It is the CD8+ cytotoxic T cells that recognize the antigen on the tumor cell membrane and proceed to kill the tumor cells by releasing cytotoxic granules or inducing apoptosis.

Cancer vaccines are required to overcome tumor protective mechanisms. Tumor cells possess mechanisms, such as the secretion of particular growth factors, which allow them to evade and suppress the immune system. For example, transforming growth factor β obstructs dendritic cell maturation and interferes with antigen presentation to T cells. Let us examine several strategies used for producing cancer vaccines.

Whole-cell vaccines

Vaccines against infectious diseases are composed of bacteria or viruses whose ability to produce disease has been reduced or **attenuated** by different processes such as passage through an unnatural host, chemical treatment, or irradiation. The first cancer vaccines were composed of irradiated tumor cells, being modeled after successful, attenuated pathogen vaccines.

PAUSE AND THINK

The term vaccination comes from the Latin word 'vacca' or cow because the first vaccine, reported in 1798 by Edward Jenner, used cowpox virus for immunization against smallpox. As a doctor in the English countryside during a smallpox outbreak, Jenner noticed that milk maids were less likely to contract smallpox, although these women were often exposed to cowpox infection. He hypothesized that cowpox infection was the cause of the resistance to smallpox and carried out experiments that supported his hypothesis.

All of the antigens expressed by a specific tumor are included in the whole-cell vaccine design. These first cancer vaccines demonstrated immune responses in mouse models but were disappointing in clinical trials, causing either a weak response from the immune system (a weak immunogenic response) or a response against normal cells (autoimmunity). This may be due to the under-representation of immunogenic antigens relative to the total number of antigens and stimulation against normal gene products, respectively. For example, vitiligo, an autoimmune disease that targets melanocytes, was observed in studies of a melanoma vaccine, suggesting that the induced immune response also targeted normal antigens and thus normal cells. Some modifications of whole-cell vaccines are being pursued. For example, gene-modified tumor cells that express stimulatory molecules for T cells double as antigens and adjuvants. However, regardless of their degree of success, whole-cell vaccines have been important stepping-stones towards antigen-specific vaccines.

Peptide-based vaccines

Another strategy for the development of cancer vaccines is to use tumor-associated antigens to generate an immune response. This involves the identification and characterization of specific molecules on the tumor cells that are recognized by T cells rather than using whole cells from tumors as was described above. Tumor-specific antigen molecules have qualitative or quantitative differential expression patterns in tumor cells compared with normal cells. Many of these antigens elicit an immunogenic response without autoimmunity. This has led to the production of antigen-specific peptide vaccinations. The peptides used are short sequences of amino acids that code for a part of the tumor-associated antigen and can be produced as synthetic or recombinant proteins.

PAUSE AND THINK

What is the difference in methods between making synthetic and recombinant protein? Synthetic peptides are made in the laboratory by linking amino acids together in a specific order while recombinant proteins are synthesized *in vivo* from genetically engineered molecules that include a DNA sequence encoding the specified amino acids.

A growing list of breast tumor antigens, including HER2, mucin1, and carcinoembryonic antigen (CEA), provide the basis for the production of breast cancer vaccines. Several melanoma tumor antigens have also been characterized. A peptide-based vaccine targeting the melanoma-associated antigen glycoprotein 100 (gp100) was successful in producing a therapeutic clinical response in melanoma patients as reported by Rosenberg (see Box 'A leader in the field of vaccination') and colleagues. The gp100 antigen is an antigen that is expressed in normal melanocytes, melanomas, and pigmented retinal cells. The study used a modified gp100 peptide that had an increased ability to generate reactive cytotoxic T cells, along with cytokine adjuvant, interleukin-2 (IL-2). Forty-two percent of patients (13 of 31 people) demonstrated cancer regression in metastases from different locations.

A LEADER IN THE FIELD . . . of vaccination: Steven A. Rosenberg

The Institute for Scientific Information reported in 1999 that Rosenberg was the most cited clinician in the world in the field of oncology for the 17 years between 1981 and 1998. Rosenberg is the author of over 820 scientific articles covering various aspects of cancer research and has written eight books.

Rosenberg helped to develop the first effective immunotherapies for selected patients with advanced cancer. He was also the first person successfully to insert foreign genes into humans, pioneering the development of gene therapy for the treatment of cancer. Along with his research group, he cloned the genes encoding cancer antigens and used these as the basis to develop cancer vaccines for the treatment of patients with metastatic melanoma. His recent studies, involving the transfer of anti-tumor lymphocytes and their repopulation in cancer patients, demonstrated cancer regression.

Rosenberg received his BA and MD degrees at Johns Hopkins University in Baltimore, Maryland and a PhD in Biophysics at Harvard University. After completing his residency training in surgery in 1974, Dr Rosenberg became the Chief of Surgery at the National Cancer Institute, a position he still holds at the present time. Rosenberg is also currently a Professor of Surgery at the Uniformed Services University of Health Sciences and at the George Washington University School of Medicine and Health Sciences in Washington, DC.

Dendritic cell vaccines

Vaccines may also be composed of human dendritic cells, cells that are critical antigen-presenting and stimulatory cells for the induction of a T-cell-dependent immune response. Dendritic cells originate in the bone marrow, and reside in an immature state in peripheral tissues. As described above, upon receiving inflammatory signals, they differentiate or mature and migrate to lymph nodes where antigens are presented and the T-cell response is initiated. *In vivo*, tumors secrete several factors that suppress dendritic cell differentiation and migration, and may contribute to the immunosuppression observed in cancer patients.

For the purpose of vaccination, dendritic cells must be isolated from an individual patient and cultured *in vitro* during which time they can be loaded or pulsed with specific antigens, DNA, or RNA via their high capacity for endocytosis (Figure 13.2) (or other means of transfection such as electroporation). Subsequently, they are reintroduced into the patient. Thus, dendritic vaccines are labor intensive and expensive. Initial clinical trials using loaded dendritic cells have shown positive clinical responses and no significant toxicity. An antigen-loaded dendritic cell vaccine called

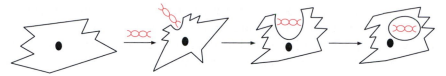

Figure 13.2 Dendritic cell loading.

Provenge (Dendreon Corporation, Seattle, WA) was produced for the treatment of prostate cancer by the following steps:

(1) a dendritic cell precursor-enriched fraction was isolated;

(2) the cells were matured *in vitro* by incubation with a recombinant fusion protein (consisting of prostatic acid phosphatase linked to granulocyte–macrophage colony-stimulating factor (GM-CSF)) that targets the GM-CSF receptor present on dendritic cells;

(3) the mature dendritic cells, now carrying the prostate cancer antigen, are administered.

Phase III trial results demonstrated an effect on time to disease progression in some patients with intermediate disease (see http://www.dendreon.com/). Dendritic cell vaccines continue to be actively investigated. CEA (mentioned above) is also over-expressed in more than 95% of colorectal cancers and has provided a target for colorectal cancer vaccination. CEA RNA pulsed dendritic cell vaccines are in clinical trials. Ongoing clinical trials for colorectal cancer can be viewed at the National Cancer Institutes web site (http://www.nci.nih.gov/). Expanding and loading dendritic cells *in vivo*, though not yet possible, is a promising idea for the future that would eliminate the dangers (e.g. contamination) associated with cell transfers and reduce labor and costs.

Overall the optimization of therapeutic vaccines needs to be pursued. The correct patient population (i.e. with respect to age, cancer stage, molecular signature of tumors) and timing of vaccine administration needs to be a focus. These vaccines may also become a tool for cancer management since many trials have shown vaccination results more often in a stable disease response rather than a complete curative response. Side effects of vaccines are usually minimal in contrast to conventional chemotherapies.

Vaccines for cancer prevention

The therapeutic vaccines discussed above are aimed at the tumor. Vaccines generated from shared tumor antigens have been successful as prophylactic vaccines in animal models but have not been tested in humans. However, there are a few select types of cancer that are caused by pathogenic carcinogens (i.e. bacteria or viruses), and in these cases conventional prophylactic vaccines that target the pathogen can be produced. As we saw in Chapter 10, human papillomavirus (HPV) is the causative factor of cervical cancer; that is, cervical cancer is 100% attributable to viral infection. The recent approval (2007) of a vaccine against several HPV strains (see Chapter 10) will prevent a large proportion of deaths due to cervical cancer in the near future.

Large strides are being made in the development of prophylactic vaccines for breast cancer. As mentioned above, several promising breast-cancer antigens have been characterized. Prophylactic breast cancer vaccines are likely to be an important alternative to prophylactic mastectomies and/ or oophorectomies or chemoprevention in women who carry germline mutations in the *BRCA1* and *BRCA2* genes (see Section 11.6). Safety and immune responses have been demonstrated for therapeutic vaccines in several Phase I and II trials in patients with breast cancer but prophylactic trials are needed. Reluctance to carry out large-scale trials comes from the fear of autoimmunity against normal breast tissue, though auto-immune attack of normal breast tissue may be tolerable and may not have more severe consequences than mastectomies.

Hurdles to jump

There are several problems that need to be overcome for the full potential of vaccine development to be reached. First, the immune system becomes less effective with aging and is suppressed by conventional chemotherapy. It is rare that pre-clinical studies are performed in old mice or mice that have been pre-treated with chemotherapy and this may help to explain the discrepancies between outcomes in mice and humans; positive immuno-logical responses in mice are often not reproducible in humans. It may be that therapeutic cancer vaccines may be more successful in pediatric cancer patients than older patients. Such comparisons need to be carried out. Secondly, many vaccines may be most effective in early stage cancer patients, although trials using such patients are unlikely to receive approval. In addition, resistance against therapeutic vaccines may arise. Antigen-negative tumor cell clones evolve due to selective pressure exerted by the vaccine. Mutations that alter antigen expression will allow tumor cells to evade the immune response and survive.

Also, vaccines need to be tested in all appropriate contexts. Vaccines against tumor-specific antigens are being tested in humans exclusively as therapeutic agents, and not as prophylactics, even though the success of these agents in pre-clinical trials has been demonstrated almost exclusively as prophylactics. Note that since human tumors can only be grown in immune-deprived mice (e.g. **nude mice**), immunotherapy studies on human tumors cannot be performed in existing pre-clinical models and results from animal models may be species-specific. We cannot assume that what is successful in mice will be successful in humans because some aspects of physiology between the two are different. Prophylactic vaccines aimed at tumor-specific antigens (not including those directed against pathogens, e.g. HPV) have not been tested in clinical trials because the test population will be healthy individuals and the consequences and/or side-effects are unknown. However, at some point, vaccines as prophylactics need to be tested in humans.

13.2 Microarrays and expression profiling

Microarrays and their associated technologies have enabled the expression of thousands of genes to be analyzed easily. This technique is a tremendous asset providing data sets that are not available by other methods. Previous methods could only examine individual genes or, at most, small sets of genes at a time. The applications of microarrays in cancer biology are far-reaching. Since cancer is a disease of the genome at the cellular level, the changes in gene expression of genes that are involved in carcinogenesis can be identified. Different gene expression signatures can be identified for specific cancers. The data generated may suggest new tumor classifications and lead to the development of more precise diagnosis. The molecular signatures may also allow for the prediction of disease outcome and prescription of the most efficient treatment available for a particular tumor type. A futuristic vision is to be able to develop tailor-made therapies for individual patients based on the genetic profile of their primary tumor.

Experimental procedure

Microarrays are grids, usually made on glass slides or silicon chips. They hold DNA representing thousands of genes that act as probes (i.e. sequences that are complementary and can hybridize to specific RNAs) for RNA. The RNAs that are in a sample indicate genes that are expressed (transcribed) in that sample. A typical protocol will be described. Thousands of gene-specific hybridization probes are applied to a glass slide or silicon chip (Figure 13.3a). The DNA is usually bound to defined locations on the grid by robotic or laser technology. RNA is isolated from a biological sample, such as a tumor, and copied to incorporate fluorescent nucleotides or a fluorescent tag (Figure 13.3b). The chip is then incubated with labeled RNA or complementary DNA (cDNA) from the tumor sample (Figure 13.3c). Unhybridized RNA is washed off and the microarray is then scanned under a laser and analyzed by computer (Figure 13.3d). A sample microarray image is shown in Figure 13.3e (see also Plate 7). By analyzing the fluorescent intensities of the RNA or cDNA hybridized to

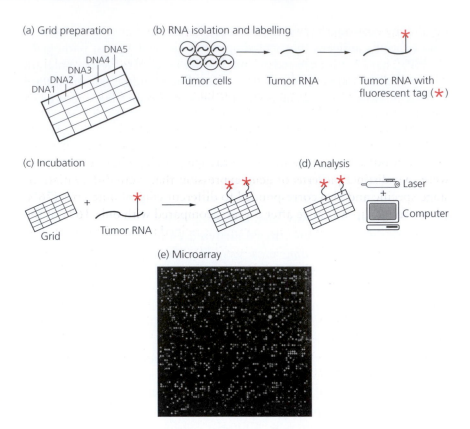

(a) Grid preparation

DNA5
DNA4
DNA3
DNA2
DNA1

(b) RNA isolation and labelling

Tumor cells   Tumor RNA   Tumor RNA with
                                    fluorescent tag (✱)

(c) Incubation

Grid   Tumor RNA

(d) Analysis

                                    Laser
                                    +
                                    Computer

(e) Microarray

Figure 13.3 (a–d) The basic protocol for microarrays. (e) Sample microarray. See color plate.

the probes using computerized scanners, gene expression can be quantified. There are two common types of microarray: cDNA microarrays and oligonucleotide microarrays. The difference between the two is due to the nature of the probes. In cDNA microarrays each probe has its own ideal hybridization temperature (based on factors such as GC content) and thus intensities of a test sample must always be compared with a control sample processed at the same time. In oligonucleotide microarrays, the synthetic probes are designed such that all the probes have identical hybridization temperatures allowing absolute values of expression to be measured within one sample. Results from microarrays can be visualized in different formats. One type of data display format is a heat map that uses color to represent levels of gene expression (see Plate 8). Genes may be arranged in rows and time points may be arranged in columns. A red box may be used to indicate an increase in expression relative to a control; a green box may be used to indicate a decrease in expression relative to a control; and a black box to represent no change. Similarities in the patterns of gene expression can then be depicted in clusters in a cluster analysis diagram. Modifications of the technique, including protein microarrays and antibody microarrays, demonstrate that the microarray design has far-reaching potential.

Application of microarrays to cancer classification

Let us examine one example of how a microarray was applied to characterize subclasses of a specific cancer. The application of a lymphochip, a microarray that screens for genes important to cancer, immunology, and lymphoid cells, helped to define two molecularly distinct forms of a particular lymphoma (Alizadeh *et al.*, 2000). Diffuse large B-cell lymphoma is clinically heterogeneous, whereby 40% of patients respond to treatment and 60% do not. Results from the lymphochip showed that there were two distinct patterns of gene expression that were differentiation-stage specific and also corresponded to different clinical outcomes (76% of one subgroup was alive after 5 years, compared with only 16% of the other). The classification of one cancer was refined to two distinct cancers. These findings have important implications for cancer management and have stimulated the rethinking of the current treatment strategy. Currently all patients of diffuse large B-cell lymphoma undergo chemotherapy first. Those who have a poor response are then named candidates for bone marrow transplantation. Perhaps some patients, as defined by their molecular signature, should be directed for bone marrow transplantation immediately. DNA arrays are being used to refine molecular classifications of other cancers, including breast cancer.

13.3 Diagnostics and prognostics

It is well established that early diagnosis of cancer is crucial for a good prognosis. The power of biomarkers is being applied to the field of diagnostics and prognostics. The measurement of a biomarker indicates whether it falls within either a 'normal' or 'abnormal' range and this helps to suggest a diagnosis or prognosis. Biomarkers exist in different forms and include mammograms, circulating antigens, and expression profiles. The future promises new and improved biomarkers.

Let us examine some progress that has been made in the detection of prostate cancer, the second leading cause of cancer-related deaths in men. Prostate-specific antigen (PSA) has been the conventional prostate tumor marker, whereby elevated levels can be detected in blood. However, improvements are needed to prevent subsequent negative biopsy rates (70–80%). Negative biopsy rates are due to the fact that PSA is not specific for prostate cancer. Elevated levels are also detected in benign prostate conditions such as prostatitis. Diagnostics based on genomics are leading to improvements in prostate cancer detection. $DD3^{PCA3}$ is a gene that has been identified as the most prostate cancer-specific gene described thus far. $DD3^{PCA3}$ is only expressed in prostate tissue and is strongly over-expressed

(10–100-fold) in more than 95% of prostate tumors. Urinalysis that detects $DD3^{PCA3}$ RNA, using a nucleotide amplification method called quantitative reverse transcriptase-PCR, has been designed for the diagnosis of prostate cancer. The test has been carried out on urine samples collected after prostate massage to help transport tumor cells into the urethra and the results (67% sensitivity) hold great promise as a non-invasive diagnostic tool that may reduce the number of unnecessary biopsies (Hessels *et al.*, 2003). Cancer blood tests that can provide comprehensive molecular information may one day become a reality with further study focused around the observation that circulating DNA from tumor cell death is released into the bloodstream. Another futuristic idea is that it may become possible to implant a gene chip under the skin to monitor changes in the expression of specific genes, thus speeding up diagnosis and facilitating early treatment.

As we saw in Chapter 3, hypermethylation of particular gene promoters is characteristic of specific tumors. The promoter regions of two genes, *p16* and O-6-methyl-guanine-DNA methyltransferase (*MGMT*), are frequently methylated in lung cancer. The p16 gene product is a tumor suppressor that plays a role in the regulation of the cell cycle while the latter is involved in the repair of DNA damage caused by alkylating agents. Methylation-specific PCR (see Chapter 3) has been used to detect the aberrant methylation of these two genes in the sputum of patients both at the time of lung cancer diagnosis and up to 3 years prior to diagnosis (Palmisano *et al.*, 2000). This suggests that aberrant DNA methylation may be an applicable non-invasive molecular diagnostic marker.

Many of the therapies described in this book will only be successful on tumors that have the appropriate molecular profile. For example, Herceptin and Erbitux will be effective for tumors that over-express HER2 and BCL2 antagonists such as Genasense will be effective for tumors that over-express BCL2. A diagnostic to identify EGFR-positive tumors (Dako, Copenhagen) received FDA approval in 2004 for use with Erbitux.

Microarrays will play a prominent role in diagnosis. Interestingly, approximately 5% of gene expression distinguishes any normal tissue from its corresponding cancerous tissue. In addition, pre-cancerous lesions can be distinguished from normal and cancerous tissue by expression profiling. These facts can be applied to diagnostics and prognostics. One study has reported that the diagnosis of multiple cancers could be achieved solely on the basis of molecular classification from data gathered by DNA microarray analysis (Ramaswamy *et al.*, 2001). This suggests that in the future DNA microarrays will play a vital role in the molecular diagnosis in the clinic.

Several groups have used microarrays to identify a number of marker genes whose expression can predict metastasis and/or prognosis (Shipp *et al.*, 2002; Van't Veer *et al.*, 2002). As a result, the first patient gene expression profiling tests were launched in 2004. Oncotype DX (Genomic

Health, Redwood City, CA) and Mammaprint (Agendia, Amsterdam) have designed tests that can predict breast cancer progression. Sixteen genes selected from a total of 250 and 70 genes from a total of 25,000, respectively, have been identified to indicate good or bad prognosis. The main purpose of analyzing these selected genes is to identify tumors that are unlikely to metastasize in order to spare patients the trauma of chemotherapy. Only a small proportion of patients whose breast cancer has not spread to the lymph nodes develop metastases (20%) and really require chemotherapy. Most node-negative breast cancer patients are cured by surgery and radiotherapy. Until a gene expression profiling test is generally in place, and its ability to vigorously distinguish between the two groups in the clinic confirmed, many patients will be receiving unnecessary chemotherapy in order to prevent metastasis in the unidentified few, for whom it is essential.

13.4 Imaging

In the past, imaging has been restricted mainly to anatomical features. The future of imaging will reside in molecular and functional imaging (MFI), using several techniques (modalities) to investigate molecular pathways and tissue function during routine use in the clinic (Glunde *et al.*, 2007). A brief description of each of the main imaging modalities is shown in Table 13.1. Molecular features that may be examined by MFI include over-expression of receptors, gene expression, or cellular location. Functional aspects may include aspects of angiogenesis (e.g. vascular volume, vascular permeability, hypoxia) and metabolism (e.g. glycolytic activity).

Molecular and functional imaging promises to have a major impact on early diagnosis as well as on the monitoring of disease progression upon treatment. Note, in general, that the detection of early stage (stage 1)

Table 13.1 The main imaging modalities used in cancer medicine

Imaging modality	Mechanism	Comments
Computed tomography (CT)	X-rays	
Positron-emission tomography (PET)	Positrons	Requires radiotracer. Can create a cross-sectional image (see Plate 9)
Optical imaging	Fluorescent/bioluminescent probes	
Magnetic resonance imaging (MRI)	Radiofrequency pulse is applied to tissue in the presence of a static magnetic field	
Ultrasound imaging (US)	High-frequency sound waves	

cancers is associated with a 5-year survival rate of more than 90%. Refined imaging may also decrease the number of biopsies taken in the clinic. Molecular and functional imaging is another approach that will help match tumor to therapy. Such imaging will also serve as a guide to the administration of future molecular therapeutics such as siRNA and nano- and microdevices. One of the main things preventing new imaging techniques from reaching the clinic is economics.

13.5 Cancer research bioinformatics

Physicians currently make decisions about patient treatment on the basis of population-based statistics, but the future holds hope for a time when physicians will rely on individual differences instead. The time will soon come when hospitals and health services will easily be able to subject an individual tumor to genomic analysis.

PAUSE AND THINK

So how close are we to being able to sequence an individual's genome? This has already been done in 2007 for one famous person, James Watson the co-discoverer of the structure of DNA. The 2-month project was the result of a collaboration between 454 Life Sciences and the Baylor College of Medicine Human Genome Sequencing Center and cost under a million dollars (to learn how they did it, see Activity 2 at the end of this chapter). Thus, the idea is feasible but too costly to be routine at the present time.

  Such genomic analysis could take place over the course of the tumor's known history: upon detection, during, and after treatment (Figure 13.4). This type of information could be pooled from thousands of geographic locations and thousands of clinical trials, providing an extraordinary tool for future treatment and research. The molecular profile of an individual patient will be able to be compared and analyzed in order to select the best-known therapy available. Researchers will be able to identify cancer-specific molecular targets for drug design more rapidly. Several new bioinformatics initiatives have been launched in 2004. The US National Cancer Institute and the UK National Cancer Institute will collaborate in developing tumor information databases and networks (see web sites below). These initiatives will make tissue data, biological contexts or ontologies, and clinical trial information readily available to researchers. Computer capabilities and facilities will need to be expanded and enhanced to handle the enormous number of data generated. Some improvements in image compression have already been made allowing histological images to be analyzed over the internet.

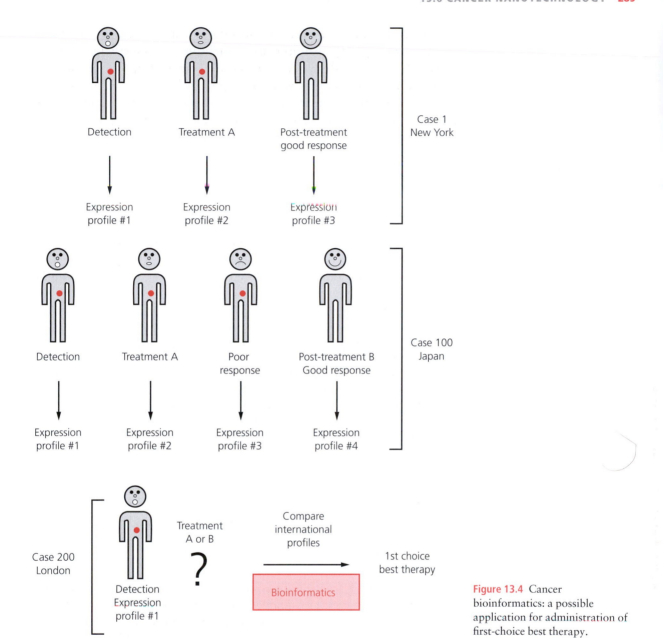

Case 1
New York

Detection   Treatment A   Post-treatment good response

Expression profile #1   Expression profile #2   Expression profile #3

Case 100
Japan

Detection   Treatment A   Poor response   Post-treatment B Good response

Expression profile #1   Expression profile #2   Expression profile #3   Expression profile #4

Case 200
London

Detection
Expression
profile #1

Treatment
A or B

?

Compare
international
profiles

Bioinformatics

1st choice
best therapy

Figure 13.4 Cancer bioinformatics: a possible application for administration of first-choice best therapy.

13.6 Cancer nanotechnology

A multidisciplinary field that promises to make a huge impact on cancer in the future is cancer nanotechnology. Nanotechnology is the study of devices (or their essential components) that are made by humans and have at least one dimension in the 1–1000 nm range. For scale, the size range is similar to the size of a few atoms to the size of subcellular structures. Nanotechnology has many potential applications in the field of cancer and a selection of these applications will be briefly described below.

The problem of targeting a cancer drug specifically to a tumor must be better addressed in the future. We are all aware of the harsh side-effects observed with conventional therapies which are due to the exposure of healthy tissue to these agents. Nanostructures that can be filled with anti-cancer drugs and which also contain targeting moieties on their surface are called nanovectors. Nanovectors hold promise in accomplishing efficient tumor-specific drug delivery. Lipid-based nanovectors, called liposomes, were mentioned in Section 9.10 (Figure 9.12) and some are used in the clinic for treatment of Kaposi's sarcoma and breast cancer. In addition, nanovectors will be used as imaging contrast agents that greatly amplify signals detected by various imaging techniques. It is easy to envision that nanotechnology will refine microarrays to greater-capacity 'nanoarrays'.

Lastly, and perhaps most uniquely, nanotechnology will lead to bio-molecular sensors that are able to detect many biomarkers simultaneously and will be used for refined diagnosis, prognosis, and treatment monitoring. Two specific designs, the nanocantilever and nanowires, currently show promise. Both can be coated with molecules that bind to biomarkers. Nanocantilevers are deflected upon binding to a biomarker (in a manner similar to piano keys when they are tapped). Lasers are used to detect the deflections. Nanowires undergo a change in conductance upon binding and this change is detected electronically. Both may change the way and speed at which cancer is monitored.

In summary, nanotechnology may enable specific cancer drug targeting, leading to better therapeutic results and fewer toxic side-effects. It promises to enhance imaging and biomarker detection for improved diagnosis. Used as biomolecular sensors, this technology may replace the need for biopsies.

LEADERS IN THE FIELD . . . of nanotechnology: Robert Curl, Harry Kroto, and Richard E. Smalley

Robert Curl, Harry Kroto, and Richard E. Smalley shared the Nobel Prize for Chemistry in 1996 for the discovery of buckyballs (fullerenes). Full autobiographies of all three can be found at http://nobelprize.org/.

What I find interesting in reading autobiographies is learning about the varied backgrounds and life events that inspire people to enter a career in science. For example, Richard Smalley claims that his principal impetus for choosing a science career was the success of the Sputnik launch in 1957. This event convinced him that science and technology was going to be where the action was in the future. Indeed the field of nanotechnology, in which he made enormous contributions, still promises to be where the action will be in the future, especially in applications to cancer management. Ironically, Smalley died of cancer at the age of 62. ➜

→ Smalley received his PhD in Chemistry from Princeton University. He became chair of the chemistry department and a professor in the physics department at Rice University in Texas. Smalley was also the founding director of the Center for Nanoscale Science and Technology at Rice University.

13.7 Treating cancer symptoms

In order for cancer to become a chronic disease, symptoms that are associated with it and that contribute to the high mortality rates and poor physiological function must be addressed. The alleviation of cancer pain is one area towards which many pharmaceutical companies are directing their research. Successful drugs will greatly increase the quality of life of cancer patients. Cachexia, a metabolic defect that is characterized by progressive weight loss due to the deletion of adipose tissue and skeletal muscle, is another common symptom of cancer. It is the early loss of skeletal muscle that makes cachexia dissimilar to starvation. In starvation, fat is lost prior to muscle in order to preserve lean body mass. The mechanism for cachexia involves the upregulation of catabolism or a defect in anabolism. Nutritional supplements and inducers of appetite are unable to relieve the process. Since patient survival is directly related to the total weight loss, therapeutic strategies based on anabolic and anticatabolic pathways must be designed. Eicosapentaenoic acid (EPA) or fish oil combined with an energy-dense supplement have been shown to be clinically effective for increasing lean body mass. Fish oils repress the transcription of genes whose products play a role in protein catabolic pathways, such as the ubiquitin-proteasome pathway (Tisdale, 2002). Further work in this area is needed.

13.8 Are we making progress?

Do you think we are making progress? Despite several media articles that raise doubts, the real answer to this question is almost certainly 'Yes'! The statistics are available. For example, the overall survival for all stages of prostate cancer combined has increased from 67% to 89% over the past 20 years. The increased survival is attributable to both earlier and better detection and advances in therapeutics. Furthermore, the total number of cancer deaths has finally shown a decrease in the last two consecutive years in the United States (Jemal *et al.*, 2007; see Chapter 1). Although our knowledge about cancer has grown enormously, there is still so much more to learn. Perhaps there are some secrets held in the heart—literally. Primary cardiac tumors, of which only one-quarter are malignant, are rare

(0.02%). Investigations into why cancer is rare in this particular tissue may lead to knowledge of protective mechanisms that can be applied to other tissues.

You will notice that most of the newly approved therapies, shown in Table 13.2, are directed against molecules that are tyrosine kinases (e.g. EGFR, VEGFR, ABL). There are several tyrosine kinases that are known to play important roles in carcinogenesis (e.g. fibroblast growth factor receptor, FGFR) but have yet to become targets for new drugs in clinical trials. However, although we can design new cancer therapies against molecular targets, tumor cells may undergo additional mutations that can result in drug-resistant clones. This suggests that combinations of drugs and drug strategies are important for future treatment regimens. As we saw in previous chapters, there are many potential molecular therapies, such as angiogenesis inhibitors, anti-endocrine drugs, apoptotic inducers, cell cycle inhibitors, HDAC inhibitors, and inhibitors of cell renewal signaling pathways, in development. (I regret that some strategies have not been discussed, e.g. proteasome inhibitors.) For many of these drugs, the therapeutic index is enhanced compared with conventional chemotherapies. We await the elongation of the list of newly approved molecular cancer therapeutics shown below.

Table 13.2 Targeted cancer therapeutics approved in 2007

Trademark	Drug	Description	Target	Cancer	Company
Avastin	Bevacizumab	Humanized mAb	VEGF	Colorectal	Genentech
Erbitux	Cetuximab	Humanized mAb	EGFR	Colorectal	Imclone
Gleevec (USA), Glivec (UK, Europe)	Imatinib	Small-molecule inhibitor	BCR–ABL, KIT, PDGFR	CML, GIST	Novartis
Herceptin	Trastuzumab	Humanized mAb	HER2	Breast	Genentech
Iressa	Gefitinib	Small-molecule inhibitor	EGFR	NSCLC	AstraZeneca
Nexavar	Sorafenib	Multi-kinase inhibitor	Raf, VEGFR, PDGFR, KIT, RET	Renal cell carcinoma	Bayer Pharm
Sprycel	Dasatinib	Small-molecule inhibitor	BCR-ABL, Src family	Imatinib-resistant leukemias	Bristol-Myers Squibb
Sutent	Sunitinib (SU11248)	Small-molecule inhibitor	PDGFR, VEGFR, KIT	Renal cell carcinoma, GIST	Pfizer
Tarceva	Erlotinib	Small-molecule inhibitor	EGFR	NSCLC, pancreatic	Genetech, OSI Pharm
Tykerb	Lapatinib	Small-molecule inhibitor	EGFR, HER2	Breast	GlaxoSmithKline
Velcade	Bortezomib	Proteasome inhibitor		Myeloma	Millennium Pharm
Zactima	Vandetanib (ZD6474)	Small-molecule inhibitor	VEGFR, EGFR, RET	Orphan drug for rare types of thyroid cancer	AstraZeneca
Zolinza (Vorinostat)	SAHA (suberoylanilide hydroxamic acid)	Small molecule inhibitor	HDAC	Non-Hodgkin's lymphoma	Merck & Co.

Abbreviations: mAB, monoclonal antibodies; CML, chronic myelogenous leukemia; GIST, gastrointestinal stromal tumor; NSCLC, non-small-cell lung cancer.

■ CHAPTER HIGHLIGHTS—REFRESH YOUR MEMORY

- Cancer vaccines can be designed to be prophylactic or therapeutic.

- Therapeutic vaccines use whole-cell, peptide, or dendritic cell strategies.

- Conventional prophylactic vaccines can be aimed at cancer caused by pathogens, e.g. the human papillomavirus.

- Microarrays analyze the expression of thousands of genes at once.

- Microarrays have several applications, including identifying new oncogenes, helping to refine cancer classifications, and predicting cancer prognosis.

- Molecular profiling of individual tumors may allow for tailor-made therapies.

- Molecular and functional imaging investigates molecular pathways and tissue function.

- The sequencing of an individual's genome (that of James Watson) has been accomplished.

- New bioinformatic initiatives have been launched to coordinate the organization and sharing of data from cancer studies.

- Nanovectors are/will be used for tumor-specific drug delivery.

- Biomolecular sensors using nanocantilevers and nanowires are being developed.

- Cachexia, a metabolic defect resulting in the progressive loss of fat and protein, may be a symptom associated with cancer. It is a symptom that needs future attention.

- We *are* making progress in the field of molecular cancer therapeutics.

■ ACTIVITY

1. An enzyme involved in the functional activity of phosphorylation sites, called Pin1, has been identified. Discuss the molecular mechanisms of the action of Pin1, its role in oncogenesis, and its use as a molecular diagnostic tool. (Hint: Start with Lu, K.P. (2003) *Cancer Cell* **4**: 175.)

2. If you are interested in learning how James Watson's genome was sequenced, read 'How genome sequencing is done' at http://www.454.com/watson/.

■ FURTHER READING

Antonia, S., Mule, J.J., and Weber, J.S. (2004) Current developments of immunotherapy in the clinic. *Curr. Opin. Immunol.* 16: 130–136.

Blattman, J.N. and Greenberg, P.D. (2004) Cancer immunotherapy: a treatment for the masses. *Science* 305: 200–205.

Chang, J.C., Hilsenbeck, S.G., and Fuqua, S.A.W. (2005) Utility of microarrays in the management of breast cancer patients. *Drug Discov. Today: Ther. Strategies* 2: 307–311.

Dalton, W.S. and Friend, S.H. (2006) Cancer biomarkers – an invitation to the table. *Science* 312: 1165–1168.

Ferrari, M. (2005) Cancer nanotechnology: opportunities and challenges. *Nature Rev. Cancer* 5: 161–171.

Figdor, C.G., de Vries, I.J., Lesterhuis, W.J., and Melief, C.J.M. (2004) Dendritic cell immunotherapy: mapping the way. *Nature Med.* 10: 475–480.

Finn, O.J. (2003) Cancer vaccines: between the idea and the reality. *Nature Rev. Immunol.* **3**: 630–641.

Finn, O.J. and Forni, G. (2002) Prophylactic cancer vaccines. *Curr. Opin. Immunol.* **14**: 172–177.

Frazer, I.H. (2004) Prevention of cervical cancer through papillomavirus vaccination. *Nature Rev. Immunol.* **4**: 46–54.

Jemal, A., Siegel, R., Ward, E., Murray, T., Xu, J., and Thun, M.J. (2007) Cancer Statistics, 2007. *CA Cancer J. Clin.* **57**: 43–66.

Lollini, P.-L., Cavallo, F., Nanni, P., and Forni, G. (2006) Vaccines for tumour prevention. *Nature Rev. Cancer* **6**: 204–216.

Liu, E.T. (2003) Classification of cancers by expression profiling. *Curr. Opin. Genet. Dev.* **13**: 97–103.

Schuler, G., Schuler-Thurner, B., and Steinman, R.M. (2003) The use of dendritic cells in cancer immunotherapy. *Curr. Opin. Immunol.* **15**: 138–147.

Weissleder, R. (2006) Molecular imaging in cancer. *Science* **312**: 1168–1171.

Zeh, H.J. III, Stavely-O'Carroll, K., and Choti, M.A. (2001) Vaccines for colorectal cancer. *Trends Mol. Med.* **7**: 307–313.

■ WEB SITES

Bioinformatics initiatives: Cancer Biomedical Informatics Grid https://cabig.nci.nih.gov/ and NCRI Informatics Initiative http://www.cancerinformatics.org.uk/.

Clinical trials: National Cancer Institute http://www.cancer.gov/

Drugs: US Food and Drug Administration, Listing of approved oncology drugs with approved indications http://www.fda.gov/cder/cancer/druglistframe.htm

■ SELECTED SPECIAL TOPICS

Alizadeh, A.A., Eisen, M.B., Davis, R.E., Ma, C., Lossos, I.S., Rosenwald, A., Boldrick, J.C., Sabet, H., Tran, T., Yu, X., Powell, J.I., Yang, L., Marti, G.E., Moore, T., Hudson Jr., J., Lu, L., Lewis, D.B., Tibshirani, R., Sherlock, G., Chan, W.C., Greiner, T.C., Weisenburger, D.D., Armitage, J.O., Warnke, R., Levy, R., Wilson, W., Grever, M.R., Byrd, J.C., Botstein, D., Brown, P.O., and Staudt, L.M. (2000) Distinct types of diffuse large B-cell lymphoma identified by gene expression profiling. *Nature* **403**: 503–511.

Dudley, M.E., Wunderlich, J.R., Robbins, P.F., Yang, J.C., Hwu, P., Schwartzentruber, D.J., Topalian, S.L., Sherry, R., Restifo, N.P., Hubicki, A.M., Robinson, M.R., Raffeld, M., Duray, P., Seipp, C.A., Rogers-Freezer, L., Morton, K.E., Mavroukakis, S.A., White, D.E., and Rosenberg, S.A. (2002) Cancer regression and autoimmunity in patients after clonal repopulation with anti-tumor lymphocytes. *Science* **298**: 850–854.

Glunde, K., Pathak, A.P., and Bhujwalla, Z.M. (2007) Molecular-functional imaging of cancer: to image and imagine. *Trends Mol. Med.* **13**: 287–297.

Hessels, D., Klein Gunnewiek, J.M.T., van Oort, I., Karthaus, H.F.M., van Leenders, G.J.L., van Balken, B., Kiemeney, L.A., Witjes, and J.A., and Schalken, J.A. (2003)

DD3^{PCA3}-based molecular urine analysis for the diagnosis of prostate cancer. *Eur. Urol.* **44**: 8–16.

Palmisano, W.A., Divine, K.K., Saccomanno, G., Gilliland, F.D., Baylin, S.B., Herman, J.G., and Belinsky, S.A. (2000) Predicting lung cancer by detecting aberrant promoter methylation in sputum. *Cancer Res.* **60**: 5954–5958.

Ramaswamy, S., Tamayo, P., Rifkin, R., Mukherjee, S., Yeang, C.-H., Angelo, M., Ladd, C., Reich, M., Latulippe, E., Mesirov, J.P., Poggio, T., Gerald, W., Loda, M., Lander, E.S., and Golub, T.R. (2001) Multiclass cancer diagnosis using tumor gene expression signatures. *Proc. Natl. Acad. Sci. USA* **98**: 15149–15154.

Rosenberg, S.A. (2001) Progress in human tumor immunology and immunotherapy. *Nature* **411**: 380–384.

Shipp, M.A., Ross, K.N., Tamayo, P., Weng, A.P., Kutok, J.L., Aguiar, R.C.T., Gaasenbeek, M., Angelo, M., Reich, M., Pinkus, G.S., Ray, T.S., Koval, M.A., Last, K.W., Norton, A., Lister, A., Mesirov, J., Neuberg, D.S., Lander, E.S., Aster, J.C., and Golub, T.R. (2002) Diffuse large B-cell lymphoma outcome prediction by gene-expression profiling and supervised machine learning. *Nature Med.* **8**: 68–74.

Tisdale, M.J. (2002) Cachexia in cancer patients. *Nature Rev. Cancer* **2**: 862–870.

Van't Veer, L.J., Dai, H., van de Vijver, M.J., He, Y.D., Hart, A.A.M., Mao, M., Peterse, H.L., van der Kooy, K., Marton, M.J., Witteveen, A.T., Schreiber, G.J., Kerkhoven, R.M., Roberts, C., Linsley, P.S., Bernards, R., and Friend, S.H. (2002) Gene expression profiling predicts clinical outcome of breast cancer. *Nature* **415**: 530–535.

APPENDIX 1: CELL CYCLE REGULATION

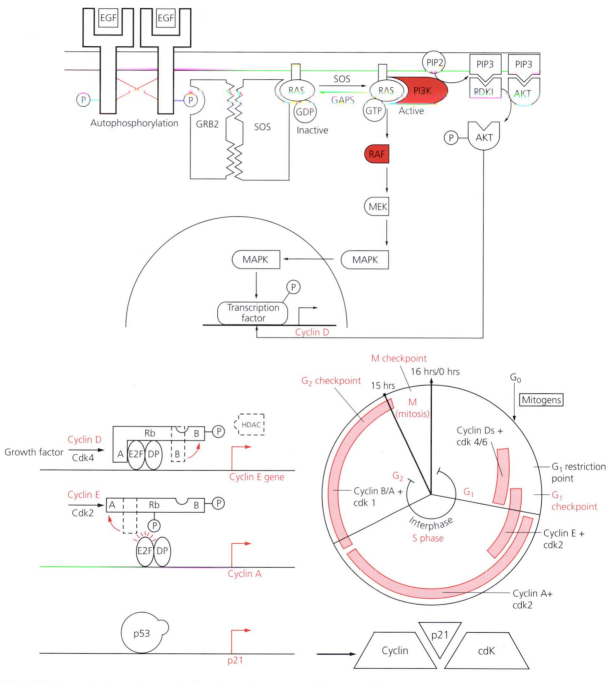

Figure A1 Key molecular pathways of cell cycle regulation. Growth factor signaling results in the expression of target genes, including cyclin genes. Cyclin proteins are key for progression of the cell cycle and are involved in the regulation of the tumor suppressor protein, RB. The protein product of the *p21* gene acts as an inhibitor of cyclin–cdk (cyclin-dependent kinase) complexes. These pathways are discussed in detail in the text.

APPENDIX 2: CENTERS FOR CANCER RESEARCH

Please note that the list below is a small sample of cancer research centers and companies in the USA and UK: many others exist.

Web sites

The National Cancer Institute designated cancer centers:
http://www.cancer.gov/cancertopics/factsheet/NCI/cancer-centers
Cancer Careers: http://www.cancercareers.org/

USA—labs/institutes

Cancer Research Laboratory
University of California, Berkeley
447 Life Sciences Addition MC2751
Berkeley
CA 94720-2751, USA
Tel.: 1510 642 4711
Fax: 1510 642 5741
Central E-mail: cslatten@uclink4.berkeley.edu
Central URL: http://biology.berkeley.edu/crl/

Cold Spring Harbor Laboratory
1 Bungtown Road
PO Box 100
Cold Spring Harbor
NY 11724 USA
Tel.: 1516 367 8455
Fax: 1516 367 8496
Central E-mail: pubaff@cshl.org
Central URL: http://www.cshl.edu/

Fels Institute for Cancer Research and
Molecular Biology
Temple University School of Medicine
3307 N. Broad Street
Philadelphia
PA 19140, USA
Tel.: 1215 707 4307
Fax: 1215 707 1454
Central E-mail: preddy@sgil.fels.temple.edu
Central URL: http://www.temple.edu/medicine/
                     departments_centers/research/fels.htm

Fred Hutchinson Cancer Research Center
1100 Fairview Avenue North
Seattle
WA 98109-1024, USA
Tel.: 1206 667 5000
Fax: 1206 667 7005
Central E-mail: commrel@fhcrc.org
Central URL: http://www.fhcrc.org

H. Lee Moffitt Cancer Center and Research Institute
12902 Magnolia Drive
Tampa
FL 33612, USA
Tel.: 1813 972 4673
Fax: 1813 972 8495
Central URL: http://www.moffitt.usf.edu

Ludwig Institute for Cancer Research—San Diego
University of California, San Diego
9500 Gilman Drive, Mail Code 0660
La Jolla
CA 92093, USA
Tel.: 1858 534 7802
Fax: 1858 534 7750
Central URL: http://sandiego.licr.org/

Memorial Sloan-Kettering Cancer Center
1275 York Avenue
New York
NY 10021, USA
Tel.: 212 639 2000
Central URL: http://www.mskcc.org

The Ohio State University Comprehensive Cancer Center
The Arthur G. James Cancer Hospital and Richard J.
Solove Research Institute
Suite 519
300 West 10th Avenue
Columbus
OH 43210, USA
Tel.: 1 800 293 5066 (The James Line)
Central E-mail: cancerinfo@jamesline.com
Central URL: http://www.jamesline.com

Salk Institute Cancer Center
10010 North Torrey Pines Road
La Jolla
CA 92037, USA
Tel.: 1858 453 4100
Fax: 1858 457 4765
Central E-mail: eckhart@salk.edu
Central URL: http://www.salk.edu/

Shands Cancer Center at the University of Florida
1600 S. W. Archer Road
Box 100286 HSC
Gainesville
FL 32610, USA
Tel.: 1352 395 05 58
Fax: 1352 395 05 72
Central E-mail: gail@surgery.ufl.edu
Central URL: http://www.ufscc.ufl.edu/

University of Pittsburgh Cancer Institute
200 Lothrop Street
Pittsburgh
PA 15261, USA
Tel.: 412 692 4670
Fax: 412 692 4665
Central E-mail: herbermanrb@msx.upmc.edu
Central URL: http://www.upci.upmc.edu

University of Texas M. D. Anderson Cancer Center
1515 Holcombe Blvd
Houston
TX 77030, USA
Tel.: 1713 792 2121
Fax: 1713 799 2210
Central URL: http://www.mdanderson.org

UK—labs/institutes

Beatson Institute for Cancer Research
Garscube Estate
Switchback Road
Bearsden
Glasgow G61 1BD
Scotland, UK
Tel.: 0141 330 3953
Fax: 0141 942 6521
E-mail: beatson@gla.ac.uk
Central URL: http://www.beatson.gla.ac.uk/

Cancer Research UK, National Office
PO Box 123
Lincoln's Inn Fields
London WC2A 3PX, UK
Tel.: 020 7242 0200
Fax: 020 7269 3100
Central URL: http://www.cancerresearchuk.org

Christie Hospital NHS Trust
Wilmslow Road,
Manchester M20 4BX, UK
Tel.: 0845 226 3000
Central URL: http://www.christie.nhs.uk

Gray Cancer Institute
PO Box 100
Mount Vernon Hospital
Northwood
Middlesex HA6 2JR, UK
Tel.: 01923 828611
Fax: 01923 835210
Central URL: http://www.gci.ac.uk/

The Institute of Cancer Research
123 Old Brompton Road
London SW7 3RP, UK
Tel.: 020 7352 8133
Fax: 020 7370 5261
Central URL: http://www.icr.ac.uk

The Institute of Cancer Research
Chester Beatty Labs
Fulham Road
London SW3 6JB, UK

The Institute of Cancer Research
Sutton
15 Cotswold Rd, Belmont
Sutton, Surrey SM2 5NG, UK

Ludwig Institute for Cancer Research
University College London Branch
91 Riding House Street
London W1W 7BS, UK
Tel.: 020 7878 4000
E-mail: webmaster@ludwig.ucl.ac.uk
Central URL: http://www.ludwig.ucl.ac.uk/

Ludwig Institute for Cancer Research
Imperial College Faculty of Medicine
St Mary's Campus
Norfolk Place
London W2 1PG, UK
Tel.: 020 7724 5522
Fax: 020 7724 8586
Central URL: http://www.med.ic.ac.uk/ludwig/home.htm

The Medical Research Council
20 Park Crescent
London W1B 1AL, UK
Tel.: 020 7636 5422
Central URL: http://www.mrc.ac.uk

University College London Cancer Institute
The Paul O'Gorman Building
University College London
Gower Street
London WC1E 6BT, UK
Tel.: 020 7679 6697
Central URL: http://www.ucl.ac.uk/cancer/

The Weatherall Institute of Molecular Medicine
University of Oxford
John Radcliffe Hospital
Headington
Oxford OX3 9DS, UK
Tel.: 01865 222443
Fax: 01865 222737
Central URL: http://www.imm.ox.ac.uk

Companies

Amgen Inc.
One Amgen Center Drive
Thousand Oaks
CA 91320, USA
Phone: 1805 447 1000
Fax: 1805 447 1010
URL: http://www.amgen.com

AstraZeneca UK Ltd
Horizon Place
600 Capability Green
Luton, Beds LU1 3LU, UK
Tel.: 01582 836 000
Fax: 01582 838 003
E-mail: medical.informationgb@astrazeneca.com
URL: http://www.astrazeneca.co.uk

Chiron UK Ltd
PathoGenesis House
Park Lane, Cranford
Hounslow TW5 9RR, UK
Tel.: 020 858 04000
Fax: 020 858 04001
URL: http://www.chiron.com

Eli Lilly and Company
Lilly Corporate Center
Indianapolis
IN 46285, USA
Tel.: 1317 276 2000
URL: http://www.lilly.com/

Genentech, Inc.
1 DNA Way
South San Francisco
CA 94080-4990, USA
Tel.: 650 225 1000
Fax: 650 225 6000
URL: http://www.gene.com/

Genzyme Ltd
Haverhill Office
37 Hollands Road
Suffolk CB9 8PU, UK
Tel.: 01440 703522
Fax: 01440 707783
URL: http://www.genzyme.co.uk/

GlaxoSmithKline UK
Stockley Park West
Uxbridge, Middx UB11 1BT, UK
Tel.: 020 8990 9000
Fax: 020 8990 4321
E-mail: customercontactuk@gsk.com
URL: http://www.gsk.com

Hoffmann-La Roche Inc.
340 Kingsland Street
Nutley, NJ 07110, USA
Tel.: 1973 235 5000
Fax: 1973 235 7605
URL: http://www.rocheusa.com/

ImClone Systems Inc.
180 Varick Street
New York, NY 10014, USA
Tel.: 212 645 1405
Fax: 212 645 2054
URL: http://www.imclone.com/

Merck & Co., Inc.
One Merck Drive
PO Box 100
Whitehouse Station,
NJ 08889-0100, USA
Tel.: 1908 423 1000
URL: http://www.merck.com

Novartis Pharmaceuticals UK Ltd
Frimley Business Park
Frimley, Camberley
Surrey GU16 5SG, UK
Tel.: 1276 698 370
Fax: 1276 698 449
URL: http://www.novartis.co.uk/

Pfizer Limited
Walton Oaks
Dorking Road
Tadworth
Surrey KT20 7NS, UK
Tel.: 01737 331 111
Fax: 01737 332 507
URL: http://www.pfizer.co.uk

Procter & Gamble Pharmaceuticals UK Ltd
Lovett House
Lovett Rd
Staines, Middx TW18 3AZ, UK
Tel.: 01784 495 000
Fax: 01784 495 253
URL: http://www.pgpharma.com

Schering-Plough Ltd
Shire Park
Welwyn Garden City
Herts AL7 1TW, UK
Tel.: 01707 363 636
Fax: 01707 363 763
URL: http://www.schering-plough.com

GLOSSARY

Adenocarcinoma a malignant tumor of a gland.

Adjuvant a vaccine additive that enhances the immune response to an antigen.

Aflatoxin a carcinogenic compound produced by the mold *Aspergillus flavus* that contaminates some food products such as peanuts.

Alkylating agent a chemical that introduces an alkyl group onto DNA; they act as carcinogens but are also used in chemotherapy.

Allele an alternative form of a gene at the same locus or relative position in a chromosomal pair. One allele may be dominant over the other.

Allograft a transplant of tissue from one individual to another (e.g. a heart transplant).

Angiogenesis the process of forming new blood vessels from pre-existing ones by the growth and migration of endothelial cells in a process called 'sprouting'. The induction of angiogenesis is a hallmark of cancer.

Anoikis apoptosis triggered in response to a lack of extracellular matrix ligand binding.

Antibody a protein produced by lymphocytes in response to an antigen, and which can specifically bind the antigen as part of an immune response.

Antigen a molecule capable of generating an immune response.

Antimetabolite an agent that resembles an endogenous metabolite and blocks a metabolic pathway.

Antioxidant a compound that significantly inhibits or delays the damaging action of reactive oxygen species, often by being oxidized themselves.

Antisense oligonucleotide synthetic nucleotide fragments that hybridize to complementary DNA or RNA in order to inhibit gene expression.

Apoptosis a process of 'neat' programmed cell death. It plays a role in tumor suppression; inhibition of apoptosis is a hallmark of cancer.

Attenuated reduced virulence (infectivity) of a pathogenic microorganism.

Autoimmunity a condition in which an individual's immune system starts reacting against their own tissues, causing disease.

Autophagy a process whereby proteins and organelle components that are no longer required are targeted to the lysosomes for degradation. Excessive autophagy leads to a specific type of non-apoptotic cell death program.

Basement membrane an acellular support of endothelial, epithelial, and some mesenchymal cells made up of a complex mix of extracellular matrix proteins, including laminins, collagens, and proteoglycans. It acts as a passive barrier that separates tissue compartments.

Benign characteristic of a tumor that does not invade surrounding tissues or metastasize.

Bioinformatics the use of computers and information technology to store and analyze nucleotide and amino acid sequences and related information.

Biomarker a biochemical or genetic feature that can be used to measure the progression of disease or the effect of treatment.

Cachexia a metabolic defect often associated with cancer that is characterized by progressive weight loss due to the depletion of adipose tissue and skeletal muscle.

Cancer stem cells cells within a tumor that have the ability to self-renew and to give rise to phenotypically diverse cancer cells.

Carcinogen a chemical or form of energy that causes cancer.

Carcinogenesis the process of inducing cancer.

Carcinoma a malignant tumor of epithelium.

Caspases specific aspartate proteases (that cleave target proteins at aspartate residues) involved in apoptosis.

cDNA the DNA sequence that is complementary (c) to a messenger (m)RNA.

Cell cycle the sequence of stages that a cell passes through between one cell division and the next. The cell cycle can be divided into four main stages: the M phase, when nuclear and cytoplasmic division occurs; the G_1 phase; the S phase in which DNA replication occurs; and the G_2 phase.

Chemoprevention is the use of naturally occurring or synthetic agents to prevent, inhibit, or reverse the process of carcinogenesis in pre-malignant cells.

Chromatin fibers made up of DNA, RNA, and protein that form chromosomes.

Chromosome a structure composed of a DNA molecule and associated RNA and protein. Humans have 46 chromosomes in the nucleus of their somatic cells.

Chronic refers to a long-lasting condition; opposite of acute.

Clinical trials involve the testing of a new drug in humans under medical supervision to test for drug safety and efficacy. Clinical trials proceed in sequential and defined phases: Phases I, II, and III.

Clonal originating from one cell.

Combinatorial chemistry methodologies that rapidly and systematically assemble molecular entities to synthesize a large number of different but structurally related compounds.

CpG islands regions of DNA that contain clusters of CG dinucleotides. They are often located in the promoter regions of genes and normally are not methylated. CpG islands of tumor suppressor genes may be found methylated in cancer cells, resulting in epigenetic gene silencing.

Cytostatic drug a drug that stops cell growth.

Cytotoxic drug a drug that kills cells.

Differentiation the functional specialization of a cell as a result of the expression of a specific set of genes.

DNA response elements short sequences of DNA that act as binding sites for transcription factors in gene promoters.

Dominant negative a mutation that produces a protein that interacts with and/or interferes with the function of a wild-type protein.

Downstream refers to DNA sequences that are nearer 3′ as a point of reference. Note that by convention a DNA sequence is read from the 5′ end to the 3′ end.

Dysplastic abnormal development or growth of cells, tissues, or organs.

Electromagnetic radiation a naturally occurring energy that moves as waves resulting from the acceleration of electric charge and the associated electric and magnetic fields. The characteristics of the radiation depend on its wavelength.

Electromagnetic spectrum the range of wavelengths over which electromagnetic radiation extends. The longest waves (wavelength 10^5–10^{-3} m) are radio waves and the shortest are gamma rays (wavelength 10^{-11}–10^{-14} m).

Electrophilic molecules that are electron-deficient and are therefore attracted to compounds with a net negative charge.

Embryonic stem cells cells derived from the inner cell mass of an early embryo. When transferred into another early embryo they combine with the inner cell mass cells of the host and contribute to embryo formation.

Epigenetic refers to inheritable information that is encoded by modifications of the genome and chromatin components and affects gene expression. It does not include changes in the base sequence of DNA.

Epithelium mesenchymal transition (EMT) involves cells leaving an epithelial layer and becoming a loose mass of mesenchymal cells which can migrate individually. EMT is crucial to gastrulation and early development.

Estrogens steroid hormones secreted by the ovary, but also produced by adipose cells, that act to maintain female characteristics and as a mitogen for breast cells.

Extravasation the process whereby a cancer cell exits a blood vessel or lymphatic vessel.

First-pass organ the first organ *en route* via the bloodstream that lies downstream from the primary tumor site.

Gene a region of DNA that occupies a specific position on a chromosome and includes the regulatory region and coding region for a protein.

Gene amplification the multiple replication of a section of DNA that results in the production of many copies of the genes involved.

Gene expression the process by which the information encoded by a gene is converted for the making of a protein. In terms of molecular biology, this usually refers to transcription.

Genomics the study of all the genes contained in a set of chromosomes.

Genotoxic the ability of a substance to damage DNA.

Genotype the genetic characteristics of a cell or organism. Also the combination of the alleles at a particular locus.

Germline mutation a mutation in either egg or sperm cell DNA (as opposed to a somatic mutation). Mutations in germ cells only can be passed on to the next generation.

Hematopoietic refers to tissue that can give rise to blood cells in the process of hemopoiesis.

Heterodimer a functional protein that is made up of two different subunits.

Heterozygous having different alleles at a given locus on homologous chromosomes.

Histones basic proteins within chromatin that bind DNA at regular intervals.

Homodimer a functional protein that is made up of two identical subunits.

Homozygous having the same two alleles at a given locus on homologous chromosomes.

Hypoxia a state of low levels of oxygen.

Incidence the number of new cases of cancer (or other disease) in a defined population over a defined period of time.

Intravasation the process whereby a cancer cell enters a blood vessel or lymphatic vessel.

Invasion spread of tumor cells into surrounding tissue.

Kinase an enzyme that transfers phosphate groups to a protein at serine, threonine, or tyrosine amino acids.

Knock-out mice mice in which both alleles of a gene have been inactivated experimentally. These mice are often used to study gene function.

Lead compound a compound identified during the development of a drug that shows a desired activity, e.g. kinase inhibition.

Leucine zipper a protein domain that mediates dimer formation and is normally adjacent to a basic DNA-binding domain. It is characterized by a pattern of five leucine residues each separated by six residues.

Leukemia a type of cancer characterized by the overproduction of white blood cells or their precursors in the blood or bone marrow.

Ligand an agent that binds to a receptor. A specific hormone is a ligand for its corresponding hormone receptor.

Linear energy transfer (LET) rate of energy loss to the surrounding medium, in a radiation track (unit: keV/μm).

Loss of heterozygosity loss of the second allele of a gene.

Lymphoma a solid tumor of T or B lymphocytes in the lymph nodes, thymus, or spleen.

M phase the phase of the cell cycle whereby the cell divides to produce two daughter cells and includes mitosis and cytokinesis.

Malignant characteristic of a tumor that is capable of invading surrounding tissue and of metastasizing to secondary locations.

MAP kinases mitogen-activated enzymes that phosphorylate serine and threonine residues on proteins. Also known as extracellular signal-related kinases (ERKs).

Metastasis the process of cancer cells spreading from a primary site to secondary sites in the body.

Microarray (DNA) is a grid of known DNA samples attached to a solid support and probed with cDNA or genomic DNA. It can be used to monitor gene expression of thousands of genes simultaneously.

Missense mutation a type of mutation that converts one codon to another, specifying a different amino acid.

Mitogen a substance that can cause cells to divide (i.e. undergo mitosis).

Mitosis the division of the nucleus that occurs in somatic cells. The process maintains a complete set of chromosomes ($2n$) for each of the two daughter cells.

Morphology the study of form and structure of organisms.

Mutagen a chemical or form of energy that can cause a mutation.

Mutation a heritable change in the bases of DNA, which may include transitions, transversions, deletions, insertions, or translocations.

Nanotechnology the study of devices (or their essential components) that are made by humans and have at least one dimension in the 1–1000 nm range. For scale, the size range is similar to the size of a few atoms to the size of subcellular structures.

Necrosis a type of cell death characterized by membrane disruption and the release of lytic enzymes. This 'sloppy' way of dying contrasts with cell death by apoptosis.

Non-genotoxic carcinogen a substance that causes cancer without damaging DNA.

Nonsense mutation a type of mutation that converts a codon that specifies an amino acid to one of the 'stop' codons, thus signaling termination of translation and the formation of an incomplete polypeptide.

Nude mice immunodeficient mice (usually hairless) that have no cell-mediated immunity due to the absence of the thymus gland. They can be used experimentally to grow human tumors.

Oncogene a gene whose product is capable of transforming a normal cell into a cancer cell. Oncogenes result from the mutation of normal genes (proto-oncogenes).

Oncogene addiction is the dependence of a cancer cell on a specific oncogene for its maintenance.

Oncomir a microRNA (miRNA) that can function as a tumor suppressor or oncogene when mutated or mis-expressed.

Ontogeny the development of an individual.

Phagocytosis the process whereby particles or cells are engulfed by cells, such as macrophages. Cells that undergo apoptosis are consumed by phagocytosis.

Pharmacogenomics the study of the influence of the genome on an individual's response to a drug. Gene variability may lead to differences in drug response among individuals.

Phenotype the observable characteristics of a cell or organism.

Phosphorylation the addition of a phosphate group (PO_4^{3-}) to a biomolecule. Phosphorylation may cause conformational changes in proteins or activate particular enzymes.

Polymorphism the occurrence of two or more alleles for a given locus in a population where at least two alleles appear with frequencies of more than 1%.

Polyp a tumor that projects from an epithelial surface (e.g. polyps of the colon).

Pre-clinical study a study to test a drug or medical treatment in animals and to gather data regarding safety and efficacy for proof of concept. Pre-clinical studies are required before clinical trials.

Pre-metastatic niche is the site of future metastasis. Signals from the primary tumor direct the migration of bone marrow cells to these sites where they are involved in altering the local micro-environment before arrival of the tumor cells.

Prognosis a forecast or future outlook for a disease.

Promoter the regulatory region of a gene that initiates transcription; usually DNA sequences located 5′ to the coding sequences but which may be located in other regions such as introns and 3′ sequences.

Protease an enzyme that degrades proteins.

Proteasome a complex of proteases in the cytoplasm that degrades proteins marked by covalent modification with ubiquitin.

Proteolysis enzymatic protein degradation involving cleavage of peptide bonds.

Proto-oncogene a normal cellular counterpart of a mutated gene that can cause tumors.

Purine the nitrogenous bases, adenine and guanine, found in DNA.

Pyrimidine the nitrogenous bases, cytosine, thymine, and uracil, found in DNA or RNA.

Radiolysis the use of ionizing radiation to produce chemical reactions.

Reactive oxygen species (ROS) in this book used to classify reactive intermediates of oxygen (e.g. hydroxyl radicals, hydrogen peroxide, and superoxide radical) although broader definitions exist.

Receptor a transmembrane, cytoplasmic, or nuclear molecule that binds to a specific factor, such as a growth factor or hormone.

Recessive an allele that is expressed only when present in the homozygous or hemizygous state (i.e. two such alleles must be present).

Relapse reappearance of a disease.

Remission reduction in the severity of cancer as a result of treatment.

Response element a short sequence of DNA within a gene promoter that is recognized by a specific protein and contributes to the regulation of the gene.

Retinoblastoma cancer of the retinal cells of the eye. A germline mutation in the retinoblastoma (*Rb*) gene is found in familial cases.

S phase the phase of the cell cycle in which DNA synthesis occurs.

Sarcoma a malignant tumor of the mesenchyme, e.g. bone cancer.

Self-renewal the process whereby a stem cell (or progenitor cell) gives rise to a daughter cell with equivalent developmental potential. For example, a stem cell divides to give rise to two daughter cells: another stem cell and perhaps another more differentiated cell.

Senescence irreversible cell cycle arrest.

Signal transduction the transfer of information along a pathway of a cell that converts a signal received from the outside of the cell to the inside, to generate a cell response.

Single nucleotide polymorphism (SNP) a single base change in DNA that differs from the usual base at that position. Some cause disease and others are normal variation in the DNA sequence.

Somatic cell all cells other than egg or sperm cells. Mutations in somatic cells cannot be passed on to the next generation.

Sporadic cancer is non-hereditary cancer. It arises in the absence of germline mutations that predispose individuals to an increased risk of developing a specific cancer.

Stem cell a cell that can self-renew and give rise to more differentiated cell types.

Supplements extra sources of dietary components taken in addition to food.

Telomerase an enzyme that extends telomere length. Elevated levels are observed in many cancer cells.

Telomere repeated DNA sequences that are located at the ends of chromosomes. The structures shorten upon each round of cell replication.

Therapeutic index the difference between the minimum effective dose and the maximum tolerated dose of a drug. The larger the value, the safer the drug.

Transcription the process of transferring the information encoded by DNA into RNA; also refers to the process that occurs when a gene is expressed.

Transfection the transfer of exogenous DNA into cells by experimental procedures such as microinjection or electroporation.

Transformation the changes that occur as a normal cell converts into a cancer cell.

Transgenic mice mice that carry foreign DNA, experimentally introduced, in every cell of their bodies.

Transition a DNA mutation whereby a purine (A or G) is exchanged for another purine (G or A) or a pyrimidine (C or T) is exchanged for another pyrimidine (T or C).

Translation the process of transferring the information encoded by RNA into protein using the genetic code.

Translocation a DNA mutation whereby the part of one chromosome is transferred to, or exchanged for, another part of a different chromosome.

Transversion a mutation whereby a purine is exchanged for pyrimidine, or vice versa.

Tumor an abnormal growth of cells that can be either benign or malignant.

Tumor suppressor gene a gene whose product performs functions that inhibit tumor formation and therefore loss or mutation of (usually both copies of) these genes leads to tumor formation; also, a gene in which a germline mutation predisposes individuals to cancer.

Ubiquitin a small polypeptide (76 amino acids) that is covalently attached to proteins at lysine residues as a marker for protein degradation (proteolysis) by proteosomes.

Upstream refers to DNA sequences that are nearer 5′ as a point of reference. Note that, by convention, a DNA sequence is read from the 5′ end to the 3′ end.

Warburg effect an observation originally made by Otto Warburg that tumor cells utilize glycolysis for glucose metabolism even in the presence of oxygen (aerobic glycolysis).

Wavelength a characteristic of a wave. It is the distance in meters between successive points of equal phase in a wave. For example: the distance between successive peaks.

Xenobiotics substances foreign to living systems.

Xenograft the transfer of tissue from one species to another. A common xenograft model used in cancer research is the transfer of human tumor cells into immunodeficient mice.

■ INDEX

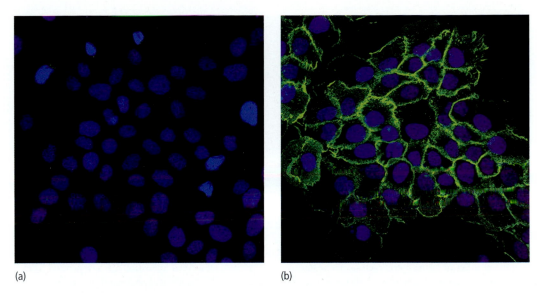

(a)   (b)

Plate 1. Phosphorylation of EGFR after EGF treatment detected by Phospho-EGF Receptor (Tyr992) Antibody (no. 2235; green). A human epithelial carcinoma cell line was analyzed by confocal immunofluorecence microscopy. (a) Untreated cells. (b) EGF-treated cells. DNA was stained with a blue fluorescent dye. Courtesy of Cell Signaling Technology, MA, USA (http://www.cellsignal.com/). See Chapter 4.

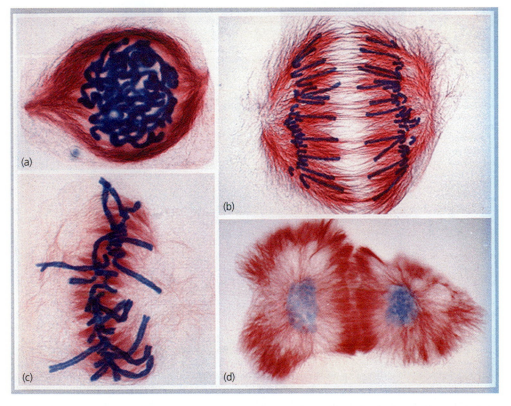

Plate 2. Cells in the four stages of mitosis: (a) prophase, (b) metaphase, (c) anaphase, (d) telophase (all magnified about 2700 times). DNA (blue); microtubules (red). Coutesy of Donald A. Levin, University of Texas. See Chapter 5.

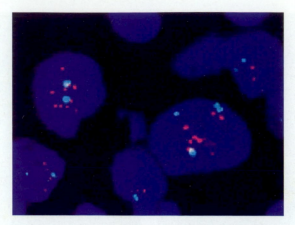

Plate 3. Fluorescent *in situ* hybridization (FISH) analysis used to detect amplification of the cyclin D_1 gene. A tissue section of non-melanoma skin cancer analyzed by FISH. Directly labeled DNA probes were used to detect copies of the cyclin D gene (red) in relation to the number of centromeric regions of chromosome 11 (green). Described in Section 5.6. (Reprinted from Figure 1A in Utikal, J., Udart, M., Leiter, U., Kaskel, P., Peter, R.U., and Krahn, G. (2005) Numerical abnormalities of the Cyclin D_1 gene locus on chromosome 11q13 in non-melanoma skin cancer. *Cancer Lett.* **219**: 197–204. Copyright (2005), with permission from Elsevier.) See Chapter 5.

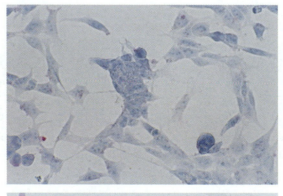

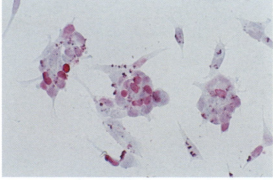

Plate 4. TUNEL staining. The induction of apoptosis in a human neuroblastoma cell line was analyzed by TUNEL staining (described above). Control (top) and induced (bottom) cells. Apoptotic cells (red) are detected using an alkaline phosphatase-conjugated anti-fluorescein antibody. (Reprinted from Lui, X.-H., Yu, E.Z., Li, Y.-Y., Rollwagen, F.M., and Kagan, E. (2006) RNA interference targeting Akt promotes apoptosis in hypoxia-exposed human neuroblastoma cells. *Brain Research* **1070**: 24–30, Figure 1. Copyright (2006), with permission from Elsevier.) See Chapter 6.

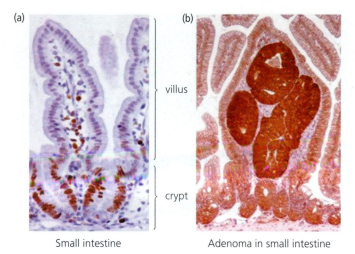

villus

crypt

Small intestine

Adenoma in small intestine

Plate 5. Comparison of normal epithelium and adenomas in the small intestine of a mouse. (a) Normal epithelial in the small intestine. Proliferative cells are stained for a cell cycle marker (brown nuclei). (b) An adenoma residing inside the villus in mouse small intestine. Tissue was stained for β-catenin (brown). An accumulation of β-catenin is seen throughout cells in the adenoma and aberrant crypt. (From Radtke, F. and Clevers, H. (2005) Self-renewal and cancer of the gut: two sides of a coin. *Science* 307: 1904–1909. Reprinted with permission from the AAAS.) See Chapter 8.

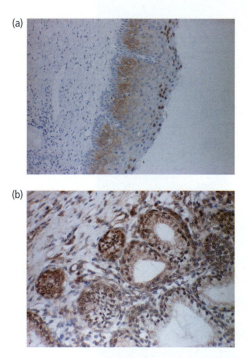

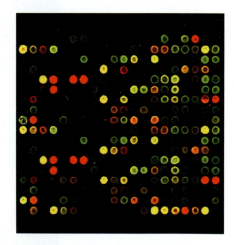

Plate 7. A sample microarray. See Chapter 13, Section 13.2.

Plate 6. Immunocytochemical analysis of HPV in cervical carcinoma. (a) Pre-malignant cervical tissue incubated with HPV16 mouse monoclonal antibody. (b) Invasive cervical carcinoma tissue incubated with HPV18 mouse monoclonal antibody. Antibodies against HPV16 and HPV18 were detected by using a horseradish peroxidase/diaminobenzidine (DAB) system. In the presence of horseradish peroxidase label and hydrogene peroxide, DAB is oxidized to a brown polymer that can be analyzed by light microscopy. Courtesy of Emma Weir. See Chapter 10.

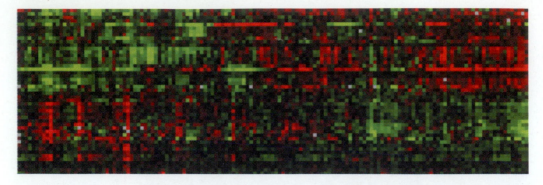

Plate 8. A representative heat map. This is a microarray data display format that uses color to represent levels of gene expression. Genes are arranged in rows and time points are arranged in columns. A red box is used to indicate an increase in expression relative to a control; a green box is used to indicate a decrease in expression relative to a control; and a black box represents no change. See Chapter 13.

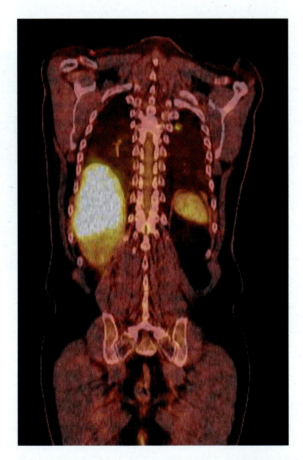

Plate 9. A positron-emission tomography (PET) image. Picture courtesy of Siemens Medical Solutions. See Chapter 13.